Communications
in Computer and Information Science 413

Editorial Board

Simone Diniz Junqueira Barbosa
Pontifical Catholic University of Rio de Janeiro (PUC-Rio),
Rio de Janeiro, Brazil

Phoebe Chen
La Trobe University, Melbourne, Austra

Alfredo Cuzzocrea
ICAR-CNR and University of Calabria, I

Xiaoyong Du
Renmin University of China, Beijing, China

Joaquim Filipe
Polytechnic Institute of Setúbal, Portugal

Orhun Kara
TÜBİTAK BİLGEM and Middle East Technical University, Turkey

Igor Kotenko
St. Petersburg Institute for Informatics and Automation
of the Russian Academy of Sciences, Russia

Krishna M. Sivalingam
Indian Institute of Technology Madras, India

Dominik Ślęzak
University of Warsaw and Infobright, Poland

Takashi Washio
Osaka University, Japan

Xiaokang Yang
Shanghai Jiao Tong University, China

Michael J. O'Grady   Hamed Vahdat-Nejad
Klaus-Hendrik Wolf   Mauro Dragone
Juan Ye   Carsten Röcker   Gregory O'Hare (Eds.)

Evolving Ambient Intelligence

AmI 2013 Workshops
Dublin, Ireland, December 3-5, 2013
Revised Selected Papers

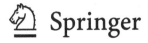 Springer

Volume Editors

Michael J. O'Grady
University College Dublin, Ireland
E-mail: michael.j.ogrady@ucd.ie

Hamed Vahdat-Nejad
University of Birjand, Iran
E-mail: vahdat.nejad@gmail.com

Klaus-Hendrik Wolf
Peter L. Reichertz Institute for Medical Informatics
Braunschweig, Germany
E-mail: klaus-hendrik.wolf@plri.de

Mauro Dragone
University College Dublin, Ireland
E-mail: mauro.dragone@ucd.ie

Juan Ye
University of St Andrews, UK
E-mail: jy31@st-andrews.ac.uk

Carsten Röcker
RWTH Aachen University, Germany
E-mail: roecker@comm.rwth-aachen.de

Gregory O'Hare
University College Dublin, Ireland
E-mail: gregory.ohare@ucd.ie

ISSN 1865-0929   e-ISSN 1865-0937
ISBN 978-3-319-04405-7   e-ISBN 978-3-319-04406-4
DOI 10.1007/978-3-319-04406-4
Springer Cham Heidelberg New York Dordrecht London

Library of Congress Control Number: 2013957188

CR Subject Classification (1998): H.4, H.5, K.4, H.3, I.2, J.4

© Springer International Publishing Switzerland 2013
This work is subject to copyright. All rights are reserved by the Publisher, whether the whole or part of the material is concerned, specifically the rights of translation, reprinting, reuse of illustrations, recitation, broadcasting, reproduction on microfilms or in any other physical way, and transmission or information storage and retrieval, electronic adaptation, computer software, or by similar or dissimilar methodology now known or hereafter developed. Exempted from this legal reservation are brief excerpts in connection with reviews or scholarly analysis or material supplied specifically for the purpose of being entered and executed on a computer system, for exclusive use by the purchaser of the work. Duplication of this publication or parts thereof is permitted only under the provisions of the Copyright Law of the Publisher's location, in ist current version, and permission for use must always be obtained from Springer. Permissions for use may be obtained through RightsLink at the Copyright Clearance Center. Violations are liable to prosecution under the respective Copyright Law.
The use of general descriptive names, registered names, trademarks, service marks, etc. in this publication does not imply, even in the absence of a specific statement, that such names are exempt from the relevant protective laws and regulations and therefore free for general use.
While the advice and information in this book are believed to be true and accurate at the date of publication, neither the authors nor the editors nor the publisher can accept any legal responsibility for any errors or omissions that may be made. The publisher makes no warranty, express or implied, with respect to the material contained herein.

Typesetting: Camera-ready by author, data conversion by Scientific Publishing Services, Chennai, India
Printed on acid-free paper

Springer is part of Springer Science+Business Media (www.springer.com)

Preface

The 4th International Joint Conference on Ambient Intelligence (AmI 2013) was held in Dublin in December 2013. As is usual with this conference series, a number of workshops were held before the main conference event. The purpose of these workshops was to explore a range of topics necessary for the fulfilment of the ambient intelligence vision. Significant research must be undertaken if the attainment of this vision is to be achieved. Five workshops explored a variety of topics pertinent to the evolution of ambient intelligence.

One of the cherished objectives of AmI is the improvement of quality of life in all its diverse facets. Thus the International Workshop on Intelligent Environments Supporting Healthcare and Well-being (WISHWell 2013) focused on one key aspect, that of the effective provision of social and healthcare to those who need it.

Middleware offers an intuitive paradigm for delivering sufficient software artifact abstractions when designing and implementing arbitrary systems. Increasingly, such systems cannot function in isolation but rather require additional contextual information to enable effective operation. The Third International Workshop on Pervasive and Context-Aware Middleware (PerCAM 2013) sought to explore issues pertinent to the design and implementation of context-aware middleware platforms.

Increasingly, there is a need for integrating robots with both new and preexisting infrastructures. This poses many challenges while giving rise to exciting possibilities. The Second International Workshop on Adaptive Robotic Ecologies (ARE 2013) sought to explore how robots may collaborate with a smart device network so as to complete arbitrary tasks in a coordinated and goal-oriented fashion.

Within the broad domain of smart environments, a critical challenge is to design for the acceptance and adoption of services. Fundamental to this objective is the issue of design, and particularly aesthetic design. Thus the International Workshop on Aesthetic Intelligence (AxI 2013) focused on the nature of the design process in smart space contexts.

Ambient intelligence straddles a multitude of dimensions; inherent in each dimension is the issue of uncertainty. To successfully deliver human-centric infrastructures, it is essential that uncertainty be managed robustly and effectively. As a step toward this objective, the First International Workshop on Uncertainty in Ambient Intelligence (UAmI 2013) strove to identify strategies for managing uncertainty at all stages of the software development process.

In conclusion, and on behalf of the chairs of AmI 2013, I would like to thank all of those involved in the organization and conduct of the workshops. Such endeavors always demand significant commitment in terms of time and effort on the part of those involved. I trust that the production of this volume will provide a useful and lasting contribution to the evolution of ambient intelligence.

December 2013   Michael O'Grady

Table of Contents

Intelligent Environments Supporting Healthcare and Well-Being

Adaptive Robotic Ecologies

Uncertainty in Ambient Intelligence

Aesthetic Intelligence

Pervasive and Context-Aware Middleware

Introduction to the 5th International Workshop on Intelligent Environments Supporting Healthcare and Well-Being (WISHWell13)

Klaus-Hendrik Wolf, Holger Storf, John O'Donoghue, and Juan Carlos Augusto

[1] Peter L. Reichertz Institute for Medical Informatics, Braunschweig, Germany
Klaus-Hendrik.Wolf@plri.de
[2] Mainz University Medical Center, Germany
holstorf@uni-mainz.de
[3] University College Cork
john.odonoghue@ucc.ie
[4] Middlesex University, London, UK
j.augusto@mdx.ac.uk

This workshop is designed to bring together researchers from both industry and academia from the various disciplines to discuss how innovation in the use of technologies to support healthier lifestyles can be moved forward. There has been a growing interest around the world and especially in Europe, on investigating the potential consequences of introducing technology to deliver social and health care to citizens (see for example [1]). This implies an important shift on how social and health care are delivered and it has positive as well as negative consequences which must be investigated carefully. On the other hand there is an urgency provided by the changes in demographics which is putting pressure on governments to provide care to specific sectors of the population, especially older adults, a group which is growing thanks to advances in medicine and greater knowledge on the relationships between lifestyles and health.

As a result companies, governments, research centres and consumer groups are developing a growing interest in a number of areas which we explore in this event. A partial list of this is: Ambient assisted living, Mobile health monitoring, Health enabling technologies, Next generation telehealth/telecare, Systems to encourage healthy lifestyles, Wearable sensor systems, Health monitoring from the home and work, Support for independent living, Support for rehabilitation, Environments supporting carers, Decision Support Systems (DSS), Data management architectures, Body area networks, Ambient Intelligence applied to health and social care, etc. We believe these topics will require a careful and long examination because although there seems to be a potential to examine how they can support independency and comfort for some citizens, the technology is not yet mature to reassure users of their efficacy and safety. Progress is steady and encouraging however some of these technologies are associated with safety critical scenarios and require extra validation.

This year the workshop joins forces with the International Workshop PervaSense Situation recognition and medical data analysis in Pervasive Health environments that is its fifth edition as well. This event will build up on the topics discussed during the previous editions of WISHWell (in Barcelona during IE09, Kuala Lumpur during IE10, Nottingham during IE11, and Guanajuato during IE12), and on the previous editions

M.J. O'Grady et al. (Eds.): AmI 2013 Workshops, CCIS 413, pp. 1–2, 2013.
© Springer International Publishing Switzerland 2013

of PervaSense (during PervasiveHealth in London 2009, Munich 2010, Dublin 2011, and San Diego 2012). Healthcare environments (within the hospital and the home) are extremely complex and challenging to manage from an IT and IS perspective, as they are required to cope with an assortment of patient conditions under various circumstances with a number of resource constraints. Pervasive healthcare technologies seek to respond to a variety of these pressures by integrating them within existing healthcare services. It is essential that intelligent pervasive healthcare solutions are developed and correctly integrated to assist health care professionals in delivering high levels of patient care. It is equally important that these pervasive solutions are used to empower patients and relatives for self-care and management of their health to provide seamless access for health care services. There are multiple synergies between WISHWell and PervaSense which we think are worth exploring and this first joint event will aim at consolidating this confluence for the future.

We would like to take this opportunity to thank everyone involved in the making of this edition, first and foremost the authors and participants as this event is theirs, the program committee which helped to select from those submitted a number of good quality papers to be presented, and the conference organizers who are providing the infrastructure for the meeting to take place.

Reference

1. Augusto, J.C., Huch, M., Kameas, A., Maitland, J., McCullagh, P., Roberts, J., Sixsmith, A., Wichert, R. (eds.): Handbook on Ambient Assisted Living - Technology for Healthcare, Rehabilitation and Wellbeing. Ambient Intelligence and Smart Environments series, Book Series, vol. 11. IOS Press (January 2012)

Measuring the Effectiveness of User Interventions in Improving the Seated Posture of Computer Users

Paul Duffy[1] and Alan F. Smeaton[1,2]

[1] School of Computing
[2] INSIGHT: Data and Analytics Research Centre
Dublin City University, Glasnevin, Dublin 9, Ireland
alan.smeaton@dcu.ie

Abstract. Extended periods of time sitting in front of a computer give rise to risks of developing musculoskeletal disorders. In the workplace, computer use contributes considerably to employee injury and results in significant costs to the employer in terms of sick leave and injury claims. Due to these risks there has been significant research into the areas of posture classification and subject intervention to improve posture in an office environment. The Kinect[TM] has been shown to be a suitable hardware platform for posture classification. This paper presents a system for posture classification and novel subject intervention that leverages each of three distinct forms of persuasive computing and explores the success of each type. Our results show significant improvement in posture results from the most effective of our intervention types.

1 Introduction

It is known that poor ergonomic posture during computer use is a risk factor in developing musculoskeletal disorders and as a result, approximately one third of lost-day cases in the US workplace have been attributed to musculoskeletal disorders [3]. A key contributor to the prevalence of such disorders in the office workplace is the use of computers for prolonged periods of time [6]. A variety of ergonomic systems have been proposed, several of them now available as commercial products. The common thread across such systems is to detect an undesired behavior that is known to increase the risk developing musculoskeletal symptoms and to provide a user intervention to attempt to change behavior.

Persuasive technologies [5] are an emergent trend in human-computer interaction and are a means to influence subjects to perform or adopt to a chosen behavior. The work reported in this paper explores the idea that an ergonomic system to monitor and correct posture will be more effective if its design is approached with the concepts of persuasive technology at its core.

M.J. O'Grady et al. (Eds.): AmI 2013 Workshops, CCIS 413, pp. 3–12, 2013.
© Springer International Publishing Switzerland 2013

2   Background

2.1   Existing Methods of Posture Classification

Evidence exists that there is a relationship between seated posture in the workplace and musculoskeletal symptoms such as neck and back pain [6]. Research has shown that the increase in daily computer usage results in a greater likelihood of symptom reporting [1]. During the study it was shown that exceeding 3 hours of continuous computer usage led to a 50% higher likelihood of reporting musculoskeletal discomfort.

Several systems for monitoring posture exist, one of which is manual posture assessment by means of observation. In this method, a trained ergonomist carries out an observation-based assessment of a participant and classifies the person's movement against set posture scales. A study [9] was carried out into the accuracy of such observational measurements where observers were required to classify a participant's elbow and shoulder posture based on a three value scale <40, [40-80], or >80. Results showed an average probability of misclassification of 30.1%. This highlights the need for better tools which can classifying posture, automatically or at least which can assist a manual classification.

Another example system provides an holistic solution for posture monitoring [8] with real time feedback and summarisation of a person's postures throughout the day. This system uses a video camera and microphone placed on top of the participant's computer monitor to ambiently log the subject's activities. Based on classifications the subject can be alerted through an on-screen dialog and can also choose to review a summary of the time spent sitting in different postures over the course of the day. Other posture classification approaches based on accelerometers have not been as successful as camera-based.

Research into the use of the Kinect™ into analysis of postural control and balance has shown that it is a device capable of making classifications of a person's joint movements with high accuracy [2]. The Kinect™ was favourably benchmarked against a more commonly-used 3D camera motion capture system made up of several video cameras and 19 markers placed on the body.

2.2   Influencing Subjects to Change Behaviour

Research has been carried out on how best to interrupt a user from their everyday office work in order to inform them of their poor posture, and to do so with the smallest impact to their workflow and productivity [7]. The three options that were proposed were graphical feedback, physical feedback and haptic feedback. *Graphical feedback* was in the form of a popup window on the subject's desktop while *physical feedback* was in the form of a toy flower placed on the subject's desk, connected to a USB interface that would mimic the subject's posture by bending its leaves and stem. The *haptic feedback* was provided using the vibrations from a game console controller. A pilot was run and the performance of each intervention method was assessed where subjects were surveyed to gather information on how disruptive each medium was. Results favoured the physical feedback approach as the haptic feedback was considered too disruptive by a considerable number of the pilot's participants. It was also found that subjects were more likely to ignore or postpone graphical, compared to physical alerts.

Using computers as a persuasive technology has been described as any inter- active technology that attempts to change a person's behaviour [5]. This can motivate behaviour change by providing experiences and sensations that cre- ate a cause and effect relationship between the person and the computer. One researcher proposes an 8-step system for successful design of persuasive technolo- gies [4] which include the selection of a simple behaviour to target, designing for a receptive audience, identifying what is currently preventing the behaviour and choosing an appropriate technology channel for communications. In the case of our study we are targeting poor posture and will attempt to use three different technology channels to trigger behavior change.

3   Experimental Methods

3.1   Units of Measurement

In designing a posture classification system we need to decide on what mea- surements yield a good approximation of seated posture, enough to differentiate between good, and bad. The Kinect^{TM} is capable of tracking torso, limb and head movements, however the nature of tracking a subject seated at a desk with the Kinect^{TM} mounted on the computer screen means that the line of sight may be blocked by objects in the environment. We know the subject's head is the least-occluded body part and we believe that measuring its angle, relative to the plane of the sensor, could provide a valid and usable approximation of overall posture.

An experiment was setup to validate what body parts can be reliably tracked using the Kinect^{TM} while a subject is seated in an office cubicle, operating a desktop computer. Software was written to log the tracking state of each of the subject's joints. In total the Kinect^{TM} sensor is able to track up to 20 joints of a subject as shown in Figure 1. Using the Kinect^{TM} SDK we can create a skeleton data stream that provides information on each of our subjects' 20 joints. This information includes joint position in 3D space, joint angle and a state variable indicating the type of tracking on the joint. The state of each joint can be *Tracked, Not Tracked* or *Inferred*, the later being a joint whose position is determined indirectly, based on its connecting joints. For this experiment we discarded inferred data from the data stream and just logged those joints in a *Tracked* state. Data was gathered at the rate of one frame per second over a period of 4 hours, and the state of each joint was logged for each frame.

The subject remained seated for 4 hours and performed their normal office working routine, moving around the chair, twisting and turning to reach things, answer the phone, etc., and generally reflecting the regular, dynamic movements which are characteristic of good seating behaviour. The logged data was analysed and the result presented in Table 1. Joints not listed had 0% detection. Skeletal tracking was most successful on the subject's head, directly in front of the sensor

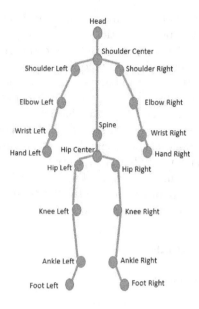

Fig. 1. Kinect^TM 20 point skeleton

Table 1. % time each joint was successfully tracked over a 4-hour period

Joint	% Time	Joint	% Time
Head	99.98%	Shoulder Centre	99.08%
Right Shoulder	87.83%	Left Shoulder	89.65%
Right Elbow	70.56%	Left Elbow	58.52%
Right Wrist	68.42%	Left Wrist	56.62%
Right Hand	68.08%	Left Hand	55.98%

and not in contact with any objects from the environment. It is possible that the raised back on the subject's chair interfered with the tracking of the shoulder joints. Tracking of the subject's right elbow, wrist and hand was more successful than tracking the subject's left side. We noted that the subject used the mouse with their right hand so their arm was resting out to the side of their body for much of the experiment. The sensor was unable to track the position of the subject's spine, hips, knees, ankles or feet as expected. Based on this, we use motion tracking of subjects' head as the basis for posture classification.

3.2 Classifying Posture

This experiment involved measuring the sensor's response to changes in the seated position of 3 subjects who were simulating various types of poor posture. Firstly a reference measurement was taken of each subject sitting in a comfortable upright position. Next they moved between four poses, sitting forward with their back hunched over, leaning back on their chair, resting heavily on their left arm rest and then on their right arm rest. During each pose a measurement was taken from the sensor.

The experiment was carried out twice for each of three subjects, once in a well-lit room and again in a poorly-lit room. This allowed us to validate the sensor's ability to measure posture on a range of people and in different lighting conditions. A camera was setup on a tripod to document each pose with photos taken at the same time as each measurement.The results t are shown in Table 2, where values are expressed in terms of the difference in the angle of the subject's head compared to the reference measurement for each pose.

Table 2. Delta in degrees from resting position

Position	Axis	Subject A	Subject B	Subject C	Lighting
Lean Fwd	Z	11	8	14	Bright
Lean Fwd	Z	8	10	13	Dim
Lean Back	Z	2	2	3	Bright
Lean Back	Z	3	5	6	Dim
Lean Left	X	13	11	14	Bright
Lean Left	X	11	11	10	Dim
Lean Right	X	16	14	14	Bright
Lean Right	X	12	15	11	Dim

Our analysis reveals that estimating posture based on head position is least sensitive to leaning backwards and that change in lighting had little effect on results. Our system now defines any posture that results in a delta of $+10$ degrees on either X or Z axis to be considered as bad posture.

3.3   Implementation of the Posture Classifier

Our posture classifier was implemented in C# .Net using the Kinect^{TM} developer toolkit and it models the subject's posture as a state machine with 4 possible states, Unknown, Good, Z Bad and X Bad. Unknown represents the subject's posture when tracking is not possible, for example when the subject is away from the desk or computer or is standing at the desk. Good posture is any posture where the subject's head stays within 10 degrees of their reference position. Z Bad is a state to represent forward leaning or slouching by the subject. A state of X Bad indicates the subject is leaning to either their left or right sides. The state machine raises events to the application layer and allows us to deliver interventions to the subject.

The software only uses the 3D depth sensor components of the Kinect^{TM}meaning it can operate with the built-in RGB camera and microphone disabled. As such, it offers a viable option for posture classification in a environment where privacy is necessary, such as an office environment. The information gathered on each subject who used our posture intervention system was limited to just the angle as measured by the sensor of their head on both the X and Z axes, captured once per second throughout each session.

3.4 Intervention Design

We used three methods of delivering interventions, the first of which controls the brightness of the monitor. Whenever the subject's posture moves into a bad state for more than a threshold period of time, the intervention triggers and the screen dims. Once the subject corrects their posture the screen returns to normal brightness. This method was intended to create a cause-effect relationship between the subjects and the computer and to train the subject into knowing that if they keep sitting up straight they will not be interrupted yet when the intervention does happen the subject can still see the screen and continue working without interruption if the subject is at a critical phase of work.

The second intervention is purely information based. It consists of a popup window that is displayed to the subject once per hour. A dialog window displays a summary showing the number of minutes spent sitting with good posture, the number of minutes sitting leaning forward and the number of minutes leaning to one side. Again, the subject can choose to ignore the intervention and the intervention was delivered once per hour, regardless of how good the subject's posture was during that time period. The final intervention was also delivered as a popup message with a set of encouraging messages which provide positive re-enforcement to the subject when they use good posture. In general, because these latter two interventions occur once per hour we expect them to be less effective than the real-time response of the monitor brightness change.

3.5 User Trials

Having defined and developed the software for our three intervention types, the next phase was to trial each method with subjects to anyalyse what effect each had on their posture. We selected 4 subjects to take part in the trial and each subject was required to use the software for four days. On each day of the three interventions was used, with the fourth day being a day with no interventions at all. Reserving one day per subject to just record posture and not intervene allows us to gather information on how much each person normally corrects their posture and gauge the impact of each intervention.

Each subject's posture throughout each day was recorded by the sensor and logged for analysis. In order to ensure there were no biasing effects from the order in which each intervention was delivered, a Latin square's approach was used to provide a different ordering of interventions for each subject.

In order to facilitate this experimental approach, each subject was given a set of daily activation keys and instructions on which day to use each key. When the application loaded up they were prompted to enter a key which in turn selected the form of intervention they would be receive for that day. After completing a short sensor calibration exercise the software began monitoring their posture and delivering interventions as appropriate. At the end of a four-hour session the subject simply exited the application and logging was stopped.

4 Results

4.1 Overall Posture

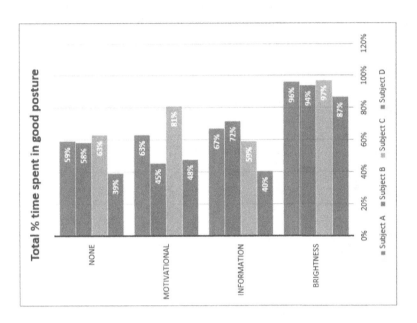

Fig. 2. Percentage time spent in good posture by subject and intervention type

The first thing we did was to extract the total amount of time spent sitting in a good posture per subject for each intervention type they received, and this information is graphed in Figure 2. For our motivational intervention we see that all four subjects showed improved posture over their day with no intervention at all. For the information-based intervention we see that two subjects showed notable improvement in their posture, however Subject C showed poorer posture compared to the day with no intervention and Subject D only showed a marginal 1% improvement. Our brightness intervention showed the most significant improvement of each intervention type with all subjects showing an increase of more that 30% of their time being spent in good posture.

4.2 Periods of Poor Posture

Next we analysed our data to find the longest period of continuously poor posture for each subject, again divided out by intervention type as shown in Figure 3. From this data we can see that two of our subjects had their longest period of poor posture on the day with no interventions. Our motivational intervention resulted in improvement for only two out of the four subjects, with subjects C and D showing longer times spend sitting in poor postures.

Our information-based intervention performed better with three of our subjects showing an improvement, however subject C spent more than three times longer sitting continuously in poor posture than they had with no intervention at all. The brightness intervention showed the most notable effect on the time spent sitting continuously with poor posture. All of our subjects showed a decrease in the number of consecutive minutes spent sitting with poor posture.

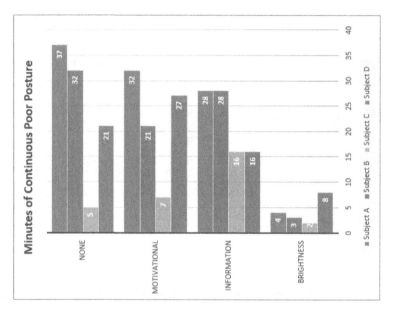

Fig. 3. Longest continuous period of poor posture by subject and intervention type

4.3   Posture Transitions

Finally we extracted the number of times our subjects posture shifted from good to poor and back again. From Figure 4 we can see that the number of transitions per subject when no intervention was delivered was quite widely dispersed, ranging from 110 to 375 transitions in a period of four hours. This may indicate the different sitting habits of each of our subjects. Data for our motivational intervention shows that the number of transitions decreased for two subjects which may indicate a heightened awareness of their posture, however the number of transitions increased for the other two subjects. Likewise, our information intervention showed improvement in two subjects and dis-improvement in the other two. Our brightness intervention is the only intervention to provide a decrease in the number of posture transitions for all four subjects.

This is interesting as it indicates that subjects maintained a more constant posture throughout the experiment when receiving the brightness intervention.

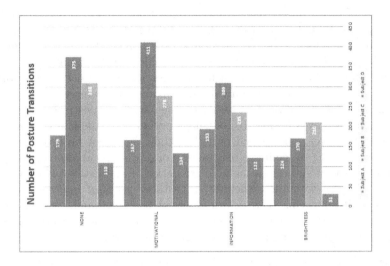

Fig. 4. Total number of posture transitions

Our brightness intervention is designed to immediately correct the subject's posture when it moves out of a good position, and as such it could have been expected that subjects would have a higher number of transitions due to the number of interventions. Instead we see that subjects have fewer transitions, meaning they are more aware of what their good posture position is and they are better able to maintain it.

We also noted some comments from the subjects in our trial, all four subjects remarked that the brightness intervention was the most intuitive and found they were more conscious of their posture during that day's session. One subject noted that simply the presence of the sensor pointed at them made them more aware of their posture during the trials. Another subject noted that they forgot about the presence of the sensor until they received interventions on days with the information and motivational interventions.

5 Conclusions

From our results we can see that the most successful intervention type was that based on monitor brightness. This proves our original hypothesis that an intervention based around an immersive subject experience will be the most effective way to correct a person's posture. While the motivational and information based interventions provided some improvements to our subject's posture the degree of improvement was significantly less than with our monitor brightness intervention. We can also conclude that the Kinect^{TM} can be used to effectively monitor a person's posture in an office environment and can do so without the need for image or video capturing of the subject. This is vital for providing a posture intervention system that protects the person's privacy.

In terms of future work, there are questions that remain to be investigated. Our study was limited to subjects using desktop PCs in an office environment and required the sensor to be mounted on a stand behind the subject's computer screen. We would like to explore sensors embedded in a monitor to provide the same intervention experience with a less intrusive presence in the working environment. Since our software only used a portion of the Kinect's[TM] capability, we could design an ever lower cost sensor for the purpose of posture classification.

Since our study was limited to four days per subject, the effects of each intervention type over a prolonged period of time could not be investigated. It would be interesting to see if the information or motivational interventions have a stronger effect on subjects after a longer period. Finally, the question of how willing people are to subject themselves to these types of interventions with the purpose of improving their posture has not been explored. Neither has the impact of these interventions of a person's productivity or concentration while carrying out work on a computer. Once again, these are for further study.

Acknowledgements. This research was supported by Science Foundation Ireland SFI/12/RC/2289.

References

1. Chang, C.-H.J., Amick, B.C., Menendez, C.C., Katz, J.N., Johnson, P.W., Robertson, M., Dennerlein, J.T.: Daily computer usage correlated with undergraduate students' musculoskeletal symptoms. American Journal of Industrial Medicine 50(6), 481–488 (2007)
2. Clark, R.A., Pua, Y.-H., Fortin, K., Ritchie, C., Webster, K.E., Denehy, L., Bryant, A.L.: Validity of the microsoft kinect for assessment of postural control. Gait & Posture 36(3), 372–377 (2012)
3. Fang, S., Dropkin, J., Herbert, R., Triola, D., Landsbergis, P.: Workers' compensation experiences of computer users with musculoskeletal disorders. American Journal of Industrial Medicine 50(7), 512–518 (2007)
4. Fogg, B.J.: Creating persuasive technologies: an eight-step design process. In: Persuasive, p. 44 (2009)
5. Fogg, B.J.: Persuasive computers: perspectives and research directions. In: Proceedings of the SIGCHI Conference on Human Factors in Computing Systems, pp. 225–232. ACM Press/Addison-Wesley Publishing Co. (1998)
6. Gerr, F., Marcus, M., Monteilh, C.: Epidemiology of musculoskeletal disorders among computer users: lesson learned from the role of posture and keyboard use. Journal of Electromyography and Kinesiology 14(1), 25–31 (2004)
7. Haller, M., Richter, C., Brandl, P., Gross, S., Schossleitner, G., Schrempf, A., Nii, H., Sugimoto, M., Inami, M.: Finding the right way for interrupting people improving their sitting posture. In: Campos, P., Graham, N., Jorge, J., Nunes, N., Palanque, P., Winckler, M. (eds.) INTERACT 2011, Part II. LNCS, vol. 6947, pp. 1–17. Springer, Heidelberg (2011)
8. Jaimes, A.: Sit straight (and tell me what i did today): a human posture alarm and activity summarization system. In: Proceedings of the 2nd ACM Workshop on Continuous Archival and Retrieval of Personal Experiences, pp. 23–34. ACM (2005)
9. Lowe, B.D.: Accuracy and validity of observational estimates of shoulder and elbow posture. Applied Ergonomics 35(2), 159–171 (2004)

Design and Field Evaluation of REMPAD:
A Recommender System Supporting Group
Reminiscence Therapy

Yang Yang[1,*], Niamh Caprani[1], Adam Bermingham[1], Julia O'Rourke[2],
Rónán Collins[2], Cathal Gurrin[1], and Alan F. Smeaton[1]

[1] INSIGHT: Data Analytics Research Centre, Dublin City University, Ireland
{yangyang,adam.bermingham,cgurrin}@computing.dcu.ie,
{niamh.caprani,alan.smeaton}@dcu.ie
[2] Department of Speech & Language Therapy, Adelaide & Meath Hospital, Tallaght, Ireland
{julia.orourke,ronan.collins2}@amnch.ie

Abstract. This paper describes a semi-automated web-based system to facilitate
digital reminiscence therapy for patients with mild-to-moderate dementia,
enacted in a group setting. The system, REMPAD, uses proactive recommendation technology to profile participants and groups, and offers interactive multimedia content from the Internet to match these profiles. In this paper, we focus
on the design of the system to deliver an innovative personalized group reminiscence experience. We take a user-centered design approach to discover and
address the design challenges and considerations. A combination of methodologies is used throughout this research study, including exploratory interviews,
prototype use case walkthroughs, and field evaluations. The results of the field
evaluation indicate high user satisfaction when using the system, and strong
tendency towards repeated use in future. These studies provide an insight into
the current practices and challenges of group reminiscence therapy, and inform
the design of a multimedia recommender system to support facilitators and
group therapy participants.

Keywords: Reminiscence therapy, dementia, recommender systems, user
interface.

1 Introduction

Reminiscence is the process of recalling personally experienced events from one's
past. Reminiscence therapy (RT) is a popular psychosocial intervention used for
people with dementia. Used either within a structured group or in a one-on-one session, it aims to stimulate senses in order to encourage memory recollection. Studies
have shown that RT intervention can lead to positive outcomes in enhancement of
self-esteem, increased life satisfaction, improved social interaction, as well as reduced
depression [1]. Reminiscence and RT involve the deliberate use of prompts or cues,

---

* Corresponding author.

M.J. O'Grady et al. (Eds.): AmI 2013 Workshops, CCIS 413, pp. 13–22, 2013.
© Springer International Publishing Switzerland 2013

for example photographs, music, and smells, to promote the recall of pleasant memories and group RT is an example of direct therapeutic intervention for individuals with dementia [2]. Advances in information technology have made it possible to bring group RT into the digital age, introducing multimedia obtained from the internet.

This paper outlines the design process for a novel computerized reminiscence system, REMPAD (Reminiscence Therapy Enhanced Material Profiling in Alzheimer's and other Dementias). The main purpose of the system is to address limitations in the way current group RT is conducted by automatically recommending content. The contribution of this paper is to investigate the current practices and challenges experienced by facilitators and use this to guide the design and evaluation of REMPAD.

1.1   Public Content for Personal Meaning

Reminiscence therapy and life review, a process of examining one's life, success and failures, have proven to be successful methods to improve the mood of older people, including those with dementia [1]. For this reason, many digital solutions have focused on personal content to support people with dementia. For example, Yashuda et al. [4] proposed a system to use personalized content with predefined themes; Sarne-Flaischmann et al. [5] concentrated on patients' life stories as reminiscent content; and Hallberg et al. [6] developed a reminiscence support system to use lifelog entities to assist a person with mild dementia.

Public or more generalised content are now being recognised as valuable reminiscence prompts, from which individuals obtain personal meaning. The benefit of this type of content is that different people have their own memories associated with a public event, which can stimulate conversation about shared experiences and interests, as well as personal reminiscence. André and colleagues [7] explored the concept of workplace reminiscence by creating personally evocative collections of content from publicly accessible media. Other studies examined the use of interactive systems, displaying generalized content to support people with dementia in clinical settings, such as hospitals or nursing homes. For example, Wallace et al. [8] designed an art piece for people with dementia and hospital staff to interact with. This consisted of a cabinet containing themed globes, which when placed in a holder initiated videos displayed on a TV screen, which were based on the associated theme, for example nature, holiday, or football. CIRCA, an interactive computer system designed to facilitate conversation between people with dementia and care staff, used a multimedia database of generic photographs, music and video clips to support reminiscence [9]. Astell et al. maintain that generic content is more beneficial than personal content as it promotes a failure-free activity for people with dementia, as there are no right or wrong memories in response to the stimuli.

However, what all these systems have in common is that their content is static and requires uploading and selection by either system developers or reminiscence facilitators. Multimedia websites potentially hold a wide range of subject matter that can be easily accessed. One question naturally arises: can we leverage the extensive range of online multimedia content, so that the reminiscence experience is maximized? We postulate that video sharing websites, such as YouTube[1], are a valuable tool in promoting interaction and social engagement during group RT [10].

2   The REMPAD System

REMPAD is a software system designed to facilitate group RT for people with Alzheimer's and other dementias. REMPAD offers a novel solution for group RT in that it uses intelligent classifiers to recommend publicly accessible videos from the Internet (e.g. YouTube) based on the group participants' profile, interests and hobbies [3]. The system also learns and adapts to group preferences with continued usage. This is obtained through a short feedback form which the facilitator fills out after each video clip and again at the end of the RT session. By automatically recommending video clips that are relevent to the group members experiences, the facilitors can focus on the group members' conversations, rather than the technology.

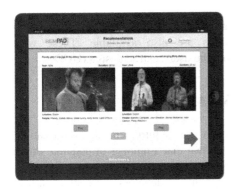 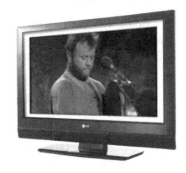

Fig. 1. The REMPAD system: facilitator view on tablet PC (left) and therapy participants view on large TV monitor (right)

The system has two hardware components: (1) a tablet computer, such as an iPad, which the RT facilitator interacts with, and (2) a TV monitor which displays video clips to the group members (see Fig. 1). Video clips are curated and annotated to ensure only high quality videos are displayed in the therapy session. This process is described in [3]. There are three main functions of REMPAD:

1. Participant profile – Personal information is recorded on a one off basis for each person who attends an RT session. This includes life history (age, locations of residence etc.) and their personal interests (music, fishing etc.) and is used to inform the system about which cues are likely to stimulate conversation.

---

[1] YouTube is a video sharing website on which users can upload, view and share video content, including movie, TV and music video clips, as well as amateur content (www.youtube.com)

2. Video recommendations – Once the RT facilitator logs onto the system they can begin an RT session. The aim is to provide cues to stimulate reminiscence and conversation. A binary choice of video clip is presented to the facilitator with video annotation. The facilitator can verbally relay this choice to the group. If one of these options act as a cue, the facilitor can select it to play on the TV screen. If the facilitator believes the group would benefit from seeing the choice, the facilitator can show a still image of both video clips side-by-side on the TV screen. If one of the options prompts reminiscence, the facilitator can select the video for the group to view. If neither are appropriate the facilitator can view the next two recommended videos. The videos are presented in a ranked order according to the group's aggregated profile.

3. Video feedback – While a video is being viewed by the group participants, the facilitator has the option to complete a short feedback form where they can rank on a 5-point scale the group satisfaction with the video, and also whether the video stimulated a positive, neutral or negative reaction for each participant. This information has potential value for both the facilitator's reports, and also to improve automatic recommendations.

Additional functions, such as providing end of session feedback, access to favourite and previously viewed video clips are also available. These were specifically requested by facilitators throughout the user-centred design (UCD).

3   Design and Evaluation of REMPAD

Healthcare systems are characterized by complex user requirements and information-intensive applications. Usability research has shown that a number of potential errors can be reduced by incorporating users' perspectives into the development life cycle [11]. Thus, employing a UCD approach throughout the development cycle, can lead to high quality intelligent healthcare systems. In order to conduct a UCD research study, we need to define user characteristics, tasks, and workflow to understand different stakeholder needs.

3.1   Participant Sample

The primary stakeholders of the REMPAD system are the facilitators who lead group RT sessions and interact directly with the system. For this study we focused on how the system supports these users to conduct the RT sessions. The participant sample consisted of 14 health professionals, including 7 speech and language therapists (SLTs) and 7 activity coordinators with nursing, counselling or social care qualifications. All participants currently run RT sessions in hospitals, day care centres or residential nursing homes. The 7 SLTs participated in Study 1 (interviews) and 2 (prototype testing), and the 7 activity coordinators participated in Study 3 (field evaluation). Throughout this paper we refer to the group RT leaders as *facilitators*.

The secondary stakeholders of the system are the *therapy participants* – people with dementia who attend the RT sessions. Although these participants do not directly interact with the tablet PC, information is displayed to the group through the TV monitor and information is also relayed through the facilitator. Current practice requires the facilitator to make subjective judgments after a session regarding the success of the material used in RT sessions to support inter-group interaction and their communication, mood and well-being. This was the method we used to gauge secondary stakeholder satisfaction in our field trials in Study 3.

3.2   User-Centred Design Process Overview

The study was designed in 3 parts: (1) exploratory interview, (2) low-fidelity prototype test, and (3) field evaluation. We implemented findings from each stage into the system design which we then re-examined. We now discuss these methods.

3.3   Study 1: Exploratory Interviews

Interviews. The purpose of the exploratory interviews was to understand current RT practices, the types of technology used in these sessions if any, and the challenges that facilitators experience during these sessions. The interviews were semi-structured in that a standard set of questions were prepared, however if the facilitator introduced a new topic, this was further explored. The types of questions that the facilitators were asked included: *what types of technology do you use during a RT session? Do you prepare material before a group session? What are the challenges you experience?* The interviews were audio recorded and later analysed by the research team for emerging trends. The findings are divided into four categories: current practices; technical skills; session challenges; and technical challenges.

Current Practices. The facilitators spoke to us about their current RT practices using physical and digital prompts. It was common for them to run RT in blocks e.g., one session per week over six weeks. Each facilitator may work with several groups, in several different locations. It was most common for them to use paper-based objects in these sessions, such as photos, newspaper clippings, and printed images. Physical objects were selected for their texture and smell to stimulate memories, for example polish or lavender. Music and video clips displayed on a TV screen or passed around via a laptop were also used. It was noted that shorter clips are preferable because these can hold the group's attention for longer.

The most common method used throughout the RT sessions was to begin with general or current themes. The reason for this was because the facilitator may not know participants' background or interests, and also to gently inform them of current issues, such as presidential elections etc. The conversation would then develop from these prepared topics. After the session, the facilitator would write up a report on what material or topics worked well to help prepare them for the following session.

Technical Skills. Through the interviews, we learned that the facilitators had different levels of technological expertise, from novice (n = 1), average (n = 5), to above average (n = 1) skills, and some (43%) had little or no exposure using tablet PCs. There were varying levels of exposure to video sharing websites, ranging in use from twice a week for RT sessions to not at all. These characteristics pose a need for clear and intuitive interfaces with easy-to-use interaction modalities. Despite this, all participants embraced the idea of using a tablet device for promoting interaction, and using online videos as stimulus to help them conduct group RT sessions.

Technical Challenges. The facilitators reported experiencing several challenges when using technology in the RT sessions. For example, internet connectivity might be very good in some sections of a hospital but poor in others, and this needs to be taken into consideration when planning a session. Some locations also have blocked access to certain websites, including YouTube, and facilitators have to acquire permission to access it. This problem was resolved in the locations where access to Internet content was considered necessary for therapy sessions.

Another challenge that facilitators experienced was technology availability. The therapy participants require a large screen with high volume to accommodate those with vision and hearing difficulties. One of the participants said that when she accesses material on a computer it is necessary to pass the computer around the group so that each of them can see it. It was also reported that there is pressure to maintain the conversation with the group, ensuring all participants are included, while also trying to prepare material for the next topic.

Session Challenges. Facilitators told us that most of their working time is spent preparing for sessions, searching for appropriate material based on previous discussions or group preferences. On one hand, this meant that the facilitators were confident that the material would stimulate conversation, but it also meant that topics were fixed and did not allow for spontaneous deviation. Five of the seven facilitators had used video websites (such as YouTube) during their sessions to support spontaneous deviation. They reported difficulties finding content about a topic before the conversation drifts onto another topic. Currently, the practice is to prepare a number of video clips prior to the RT session to ensure that they are good visual and sound quality. These are used as a fall-back strategy if new videos are not successful. The facilitators also said that they prepare paper-based prompts should technical issues arise. However these prompts are static and require the facilitator to carry around a large bag of material with them. It was also mentioned that it would be preferable to use video clips or images that had positive results in the past, but these can be difficult to re-locate, particularly when the facilitator is under pressure to maintain conversation during a session.

The facilitators commented on the challenge of preparing for a group RT session when they do not know the participants' or group's preferences. This is most likely at the beginning of a block of sessions, as each week the facilitator will learn about the group interests. However, it was noted that there can be challenges learning about an individual's interests if they are unable to suggest topics or interact with the group, and it can be unhelpful to direct attention to them by putting them on the spot.

These findings highlight how facilitators would benefit from having easy access to participants' profile information, interests, and automatically recommended material that is inclusive for all (or as many as reasonably possible) group members.

3.4   Study 2: Low-Fidelity Prototype Testing

Use Case Walkthrough. The best way to present the technology behind the proposal is through a worked example. Based on the functional requirements provided, we created initial wireframe prototypes of the REMPAD system, consisting of a series of use cases. Wireframes were designed for facilitator interaction on the tablet computer and the TV display for therapy participants. In total, 12 use cases were created. Example use cases include: *Start a new session*; *Edit an existing group*; *Browse video clips*; and *Enter feedback* (see Fig. 2). A use case walkthrough was undertaken to familiarize participants (7 SLTs from Study 1) with the proposed task flow and interaction paradigm of the prototype system. Immediately after the walkthrough, there was a discussion with the facilitators to gather feedback on the system design.

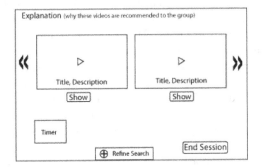 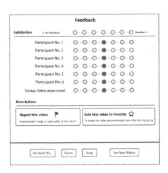

Fig. 2. Example wireframe screens used in use case walkthrough method

Findings. Participants expressed high enthusiasm and positive response towards the initial prototype design. Overall, the facilitators thought the design was simple and straightforward, and that users with low technology experience would feel comfortable interacting with it. The main areas of discussion were focused on content recommendation and session feedback.

Content Recommendation. One of the crucial elements of an intelligent reminiscence system is to offer customizable content to users. Diversity exists inside a group in areas of individual backgrounds, interests and preferences. As one of the facilitators mentioned, *"the biggest challenge is finding relevant videos"*. The facilitators were very enthusiastic about this feature and emphasised the importance of including the age of the person and place of birth into the recommender criteria. It was noted that automatic recommendation would save facilitators a significant amount of time, which is currently used planning RT sessions and would allow them to interact with the group rather than searching for appropriate material. Furthermore, as the system continues to learn about group preferences through facilitator feedback, new videos are continuously being recommended, enhancing the dynamic nature of the sessions.

The presentation of the videos was also discussed with the facilitators. It was decided that an option of two videos at a time was preferable as the facilitator could then relay this choice to the group without overloading them. Information about the video is also necessary so that the facilitator can have some knowledge about the subject being discussed. Finally, facilitators emphasised the importance of having control over topics. Maintaining the current practice of beginning a session with general topics and moving into more specific topics, facilitators said that they would use the recommended videos for the most part, but would like to have the option to search for a video based on how a conversation develops. Design alternatives were displayed to participants to search for a topic, or refine by category. We decided that the most appropriate design would be to include a search bar, which the user could refine according to a different year or decade. The ability to save successful video clips into a *favourites* section for future sessions was also requested by participants.

Session Feedback. Another challenge highlighted in building an intelligent reminiscence system is to ensure content is of high quality. In order to maximize group reminiscence experience, it was proposed that the recommendation engine should monitor patients' engagement levels, and adapt based on real-time user feedback. We designed the feedback screen layout as showed in Fig. 2. After each video, the group facilitator enters individual patient and group reactions to the presented video, so the selection of videos is improved in future sessions. However, we were unsure whether this function would add too much burden on the facilitator. During the discussion stage, participants unanimously confirmed that this level of feedback was achievable and understood and valued the benefit. The facilitators reported that they currently use pictures and icons to rate group satisfaction and topics discussed etc., in order to keep track of group progress. It was suggested that an end of session feedback report also be included in the system for the facilitator's records. This feedback was used to improve user interface design and justify design decisions, which were then implemented into a fully functional REMPAD system.

3.5   Study 3: Usability Evaluation

The REMPAD system was trialled over 54 RT sessions with 7 facilitators in 6 different locations over a period of several weeks. The facilitators used video clips recommended by the REMPAD system, sourced from YouTube, as cues to encourage reminiscence and conversation in the RT sessions. The purpose of the field trial was to investigate the use and usability of the system. We were also interested in investigating the performance of different configurations of our recommender algorithim, the results of which are discussed in [3]. The facilitators were given a post-trial usability and user experience questionnaire to complete which asked for feedback on the perceived usefulness of the system and system features, the ease of use for individual tasks, their satifaction with the system output and the overall usability of the system.

Findings. Overall, 362 recommended video clips were played during the RT sessions with an average of 6.7 per session. The facilitators reported the main benefit of REMPAD as being easy to use and requiring no preparation time. They also said that the therapy participants responded positively to the system, many being excited about seeing new technology. We asked facilitators to rate on a 5-point Likert scale the

Table 1. Participants reports for the usefulness of REMPAD features (left) and the usability of the system (right), 5-point Likert scale from negative to positive (1-5)

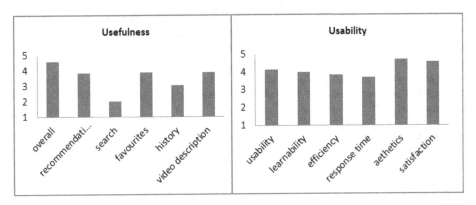

usefulness and usability of the system. The results of these can be seen in Table 1. Overall the feedback was very positive. The facilitators found that the automatically recommended videos worked well for the therapy participants and the group as a whole. Only the search feature was rated as not very useful and it could be seen from our activity logs that this feature was rarely used.

The usability, learnability, efficiency to access information, response time, aesthetics and satisfaction using the system were all rated highly. The participants also reported the system tasks to be easy, such as setting up the system before a session, logging in, setting up participant profiles and groups, choosing relevant videos and entering video feedback. It was also found that the visual quality of videos was consistently good. However, intermittent problems did arise. For example, slow Internet connection in 3 of the locations meant that in some situations the videos took time to load and the therapy participants would lose interest. Problems with the sound being inconsistent were also reported. The facilitators suggested that a wider range of therapy participants other than older adults with dementia would benefit from REMPAD use, for example older and younger adults with acute brain injury.

In summary, the field evaluation provided us with a deeper understanding of how a multimedia recommender system is used in group RT sessions. The results from our trials are positive and indicate where future developments are needed. These findings will guide the next generation of REMPAD towards the deployment of the system into clinical settings.

4   Conclusions

In this paper we described the design and evaluation of a multimedia recommender system for group RT. We applied UCD techniques to address the challenges of current RT practices and explore potential solutions to these challenges. The problems that RT facilitators reported with their current methods included: spending a large portion of their time preparing material for the sessions; not knowing enough personal information about therapy participants to prepare relevant cues; and finding appropriate digital content whilst at the same time maintaining a conversation with the group. REMPAD supports facilitators by providing content that is relevant to an individual's interests and life history, as well as the shared interests for the group as a whole. Automatically recommending appropriate video content to cue group reminiscence could significantly reduce a facilitator's workload, allowing them to focus their time and attention on therapy participants rather than the technical equipment. Through our interviews, prototyping and field evaluations with RT facilitators and therapy participants, we have designed a novel, easy-to-use and, above all, useful system to facilitate group RT.

Acknowledgements. This work is supported by Science Foundation Ireland under grant SFI/12/RC/2289 and Enterprise Ireland under grant CF/2011/1318.

References

1. Woods, B., Spector, A.E., Jones, C.A., Orrell, M., Davies, S.P.: Reminiscence Therapy for Dementia. Cochrane Database Syst. Rev. 2 (2005)
2. Kim, E., et al.: Evidence-Based Practice Recommendations for Working with Individuals with Dementia: Group Reminiscence Therapy. J. Med. Speech Lang. Pathol. 14, 23–34 (2006)
3. Bermingham, A., O'Rourke, J., Gurrin, C., Collins, R., Irving, K., Smeaton, A.F.: Automatically Recommending Multimedia Content for use in Group Reminiscence Therapy. In: 1st ACM MM Workshop MIIRH. ACM, Spain (2013)
4. Yasuda, K., Kuwabara, K., Kuwahara, N., Abe, S., Tetsutani, N.: Effectiveness of Personalized Reminiscence Photo Videos for Individuals with Dementia. Neuropsych Rehab. 19, 603–619 (2009)
5. Sarne-Flaischmann, V., Tractinsky, N.: Development and Evaluation of a Personalized Multimedia System for Reminiscence Therapy in Alzheimer's Patients. Int. J. Social and Humanistic Computing 1, 81–96 (2008)
6. Hallberg, J., Kikhia, B., Bengtsson, J., Sävenstedt, S., Synnes, K.: Reminiscence Processes Using Life-Log Entities for Persons with Mild Dementia. In: 1st International Workshop on Reminiscence Systems, Cambridge, UK, pp. 16–21 (2009)
7. André, P., Sellen, A., Schraefel, M.C., Wood, K.: Making public media personal: Nostalgia and Reminiscence in the Office. In: 25th BCS Conference on Human-Computer Interaction, Newcastle, UK, pp. 351–360 (2011)
8. Wallace, J., Thieme, A., Wood, G., Schofield, G., Olivier, P.: Enabling Self, Intimacy and a Sense of Home in Dementia: An Enquiry into Design in a Hospital Setting. In: SIGCHI Conference on Human Factors in Computing Systems, pp. 2629–2638. ACM, Texas (2012)
9. Astell, et al.: Involving Older People with Dementia and their Carers in Designing Computer Based Support Systems: Some Methodological Consideration. Univ. Access Inform. Soc. 8, 49–58 (2009)
10. O'Rourke, J., Tobin, F., O'Callaghan, S., Sowman, R., Collins, D.R.: 'You-Tube': A Useful Tool for Reminiscence Therapy in Dementia? Age and Ageing 40, 742–758 (2011)
11. Hesse, B.W., Shneiderman, B.: E-Health Research from the User's Perspective. American J. Prev. Med. 32, 97–103 (2007)

Visibility of Wearable Sensors as Measured Using Eye Tracking Glasses

Meggan King[1], Feiyan Hu[2], Joanna McHugh[3], Emma Murphy[1], Eamonn Newman[2], Kate Irving[1], and Alan F. Smeaton[2]

[1] School of Nursing & Human Sciences, Dublin City University
[2] INSIGHT: Centre for Data Analytics and School of Computing, Dublin City University
[3] Institute of Neuroscience, Trinity College Dublin
{meggan.king25,feiyan.hu4}@mail.dcu.ie, mchughje@tcd.ie,
{emma.murphy,eamonn.newman,kate.irving,alan.smeaton}@dcu.ie

Abstract. Sensor technologies can enable independent living for people with dementia by monitoring their behaviour and identifying points where support may be required. Wearable sensors can provide such support but may constitute a source of stigma for the user if they are perceived as visible and therefore obtrusive. This paper presents an initial empirical investigation exploring the extent to which wearable sensors are perceived as visible. 23 Participants wore eye tracking glasses, which superimposed the location of their gaze onto video data of their panorama. Participants were led to believe that the research entailed a subjective evaluation of the eye tracking glasses. A researcher wore one of two wearable sensors during the evaluation enabling us to measure the extent to which participants fixated on the sensor during a one-on-one meeting. Results are presented on the general visibility and potential fixations on two wearable sensors, a wrist-work actigraph and a lifelogging camera, during normal conversation between two people. Further investigation is merited according to the results of this pilot study.

Keywords: Eye-tracking Glasses, Wearable Sensors, Assistive Technology, Dementia, Fixations.

1 Introduction

Assistive technology has potential to support the functional requirements of people with dementia and enable independent living, delaying and perhaps eradicating the need for institutionalisation. Ambient assistive living and sensor technologies can help to keep people living independently in the home [1,2], by monitoring their behaviour and identifying points where support may be required [1-4]. A central difficulty in living with dementia is the associated stigma [6]. An important part of dementia care research, then, is to reduce the sources and impact of this stigma. However, assistive technologies may themselves constitute a source of stigma if they are considered obtrusive or even visible by the person with dementia or their caregiver [7,9]. This obtrusiveness is particularly relevant when exploring the

M.J. O'Grady et al. (Eds.): AmI 2013 Workshops, CCIS 413, pp. 23–32, 2013.
© Springer International Publishing Switzerland 2013

potential of wearable sensors to enhance independent living for people with dementia. One of the fundamental principles of responsible technology design for dementia is ensuring that sensors are not obtrusive in any way [9]. Hensel et al. [8] have defined obtrusiveness in this context as "characteristics or effects associated with the technology that are perceived as undesirable and physically and/or psychologically prominent". Therefore the visibility of wearable sensors may constitute obtrusiveness. As such, attempts have been made to minimise the visibility of sensors, including decreasing their size. One example is the development of the Vicon Autographer Memoto & Google Glass devices, in the form of the older SenseCam device, but smaller. However, these are still large enough to be visible to the naked eye and while these developments are ongoing, SenseCam is a popular choice for many health researchers [10]. In this study we investigate the extent to which relevant wearable sensors are perceived within dyadic interactions. Using eye-tracking technologies we can quantify the visual attention given to these sensors in a controlled experimental situation, and extrapolate about the visibility of these sensors. It is intended that the results from this experiment will inform the design of further research investigating the potential obtrusiveness of sensors which currently support people with dementia.

2   Wearable Sensors and the Dem@Care Toolbox Approach

The Dem@Care[1] project aims to develop a technological support and monitoring system for people with dementia. While the Dem@Care project also involves work in diagnostic laboratories and nursing homes, our focus is on the private home-based deployment of the Dem@Care system. This system uses sensor technologies and feedback to enable the individual to remain independently at home, and optimise wellbeing. The Dem@Care system stems from a person-centred, user-led philosophy [11]. We have defined a "toolbox" approach to the deployment of sensor technology for people with dementia. This approach constitutes a personalised system, built by the person with dementia from 'tools' and software components made available by the researchers, thus constituting an empowering, person-centred approach to care [11].

Part of the Dem@Care toolbox approach involves "wearable" sensors, which are fixed to the body or clothing of the individual. These include the SenseCam (Figure 1a), a camera which hangs by a lanyard around the neck, and the Philips DTI-2 sensor, an actigraphy device with accelerometer and galvanic skin response measures, which is worn as a wristwatch. We were particularly interested in evaluating these sensors in this present visibility investigation so that the results could directly inform our lead users in this project. As the Philips device (a research prototype) was not available at the time of testing, we have chosen to test a similar actigraphy device, the LARK wrist sensor (Figure 1b).

---

[1] http://www.demcare.eu

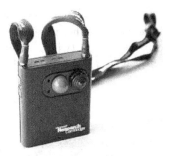
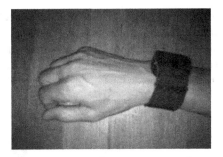

Fig. 1a. SenseCam   **Fig. 1b.** LARK Sensor worn on wrist

3   Visibility Experiment

We investigate, as our primary hypothesis, whether the sensors worn by the researcher are visible as defined by frequency of fixations made during dyadic interaction, as collected via eye tracker recordings made by the participant. In order to explore the visibility of both the neck-based SenseCam and the wrist-worn LARK sensor, we divided participants into two groups to test both sensors (10 participants in each condition). To explore general areas of fixation without a sensor we also ran a small control condition with no sensor (3 participants).

All participants wore Tobii eye tracking glasses (Figure 2a), which tracked the focus point of a subject's gaze and superimposed this onto video data of their panorama. The researcher comprised part of this panorama, while wearing one of the above sensors (either SenseCam or the LARK wrist sensor, or no sensor for control group), and analytics from the recorded gaze allowed us to investigate the extent to which the sensor is the subject of visual attention, if at all. The placement of infra-red (IR) markers on the sofa around the researcher (acting as location anchors) was crucial to accurately aggregate quantitative fixation data. All IR markers were placed in the same two-dimensional plane as the sensors to enhance accuracy, because the video does not contain depth information. We attached 6 IR makers to the sofa where the researcher sat for every evaluation session (see Figure 2b). Exploratory analyses (heat mapping, detailed video analysis, inferential statistics and follow-up questionnaires) were employed for the current pilot study to investigate the presence and degree of fixation on the sensors.

3.1   Participants

23 participants were recruited by email for this study from the student and staff population at Dublin City University. Researchers or students specialising in the area of sensor research were precluded from participating. Reported history of psychiatric disorders with a social dysfunctional component (schizophrenia, some personality disorders including autistic spectral disorder) precluded participation, since in many of these disorders, fixation upon the face of a stranger is impaired.

Participants wearing glasses were also precluded from taking part in the study, as it is difficult to calibrate and use the eye tracking glasses over another pair of glasses. 14 males and 9 females, all with normal or corrected-to-normal (with contact lenses) vision, volunteered to participate in the study, between the ages of 19 and 46 (M=28, SD=8).

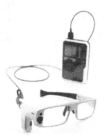
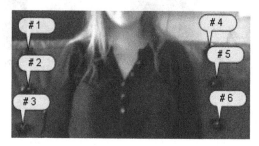

Fig. 2a. Tobii Eye tracking glasses   **Fig. 2b.** Placement of IR markers on sofa behind researcher

3.2   Protocol

At the time of recruitment and during the experiment, participants were told that the research was investigating the comfort and potential applications of the eye-tracking glasses. Before the participant was greeted, the researcher affixed the sensor to her person, in order to maintain visual environmental consistency throughout the experiment's duration. Path of entry to the experimental room, visual distractions in the room, seating arrangements, orientation, and researcher's appearance and conversation were all kept consistent throughout for all 23 participants. Following informed consent, participants were asked to complete a short visual task in order to calibrate the glasses. This involved standing 1 metre away from a yellow IR marker on a wall, and following this marker with their gaze as the researcher moved it around the wall. The researcher then invited participants to sit opposite her on a sofa. The researcher sat on the sofa opposite, with IR markers fixed around her, and proceeded to describe the Tobii glasses. The researcher then asked the participant a number of questions regarding the comfort of the glasses, how they found the calibration process and a number of open ended questions on potential benefits and uses for the glasses. The researcher engaged with the subject at all times during this period, during which the social norm would be not to stare at clothes, jewellery or anything out of the ordinary worn by the researcher, though when not being engaged in eye-to-eye contact, quick glances at something unusual would also constitute normal behaviour. Since the eye tracked sampled gaze at 25Hz, these quick glances would be measurable. Following this, participants were thanked and told that they would soon receive a debriefing email. In the debriefing e-mail participants were informed of the true aims of the study and asked a series of questions to determine the noticeability, and extent thereof, of the sensors worn.

4   Results

Data generated from heat map analysis revealed that the majority of participants for both sensor conditions and control group, fixated on the researchers face/head for the largest proportion of the evaluation time (figure 3 illustrates heat map data for each condition). The average time that participants spent in conversation with the researcher and having their gaze recorded was 256 seconds (SD=64s). Participants spent an average of 73% total time fixating on the researcher's face, in comparison to less than an average of 1% of the total time fixated on sensors. When we analysed the heat maps individually, 20 participants fixated primarily on the researcher's face/head and 3 participants fixated on other areas. Of these 3, one fixated on the researcher's shoulder, one on her neck and one participant fixated on their own reflection in a glass panel behind the researcher. Data generated from the heat map analysis also revealed that participants spent approximately 1% of the overall time fixating on the researcher's hands. The average percentage of fixation time recorded on the head/face for the SenseCam condition was 74.24% (SD = 16.14%). For the LARK condition, participants fixated on the head/face 71.98% (SD = 27.60%) of the total evaluation time. The average proportion of fixation time recorded on each sensor was 0.78% for the SenseCam (SD = 1.12%) and 0.37% for the LARK (SD = 0.79%).

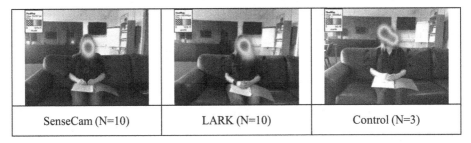

| SenseCam (N=10) | LARK (N=10) | Control (N=3) |

Fig. 3. Heat map data for each condition

4.1   Detailed Video Analysis

To investigate in more detail the actual frequency of fixations on sensors and the researcher's hands, we conducted a fine-grained analysis of fixations on both sensors and hands in all conditions by manually analysing each participant video. Each video was played in slow motion and was paused at every point of fixation on the sensor or the hands and the time of fixation was recorded. This was repeated to reduce the chance of error. For the SenseCam condition, fixations were recorded on the SenseCam and the hands (as one score). For the LARK condition, fixations were recorded on the LARK and on the hands (as three scores: one for the hands, one for the left hand and one for the right hand). The analyst also recorded relevant comments or particulars in fixation data that were made during the videos.

Data were frequency of fixations on the sensors, as well as fixations on a secondary point in the visual field (hands). The manipulated variable was sensor type with two levels (SenseCam or LARK). Data were screened for outliers and assessed for normality of distribution. There were no outliers and both the kurtosis and skewness test indicated no serious departures from normality (all coefficients resulted in absolute values of less than 1). Levene's test for homogeneity of group variance was also non-significant. The Shapiro-Wilk test was conducted to test for normality, due to having a small sample size, and found to be non-significant, indicating normality of distribution [SenseCam: D_{10}= 1.90, p<0.05; LARK, D_{10} = 2.54, p<0.05].

Number of fixations on each sensor was recorded for every participant. A mean of 5 fixations for the LARK (SD = 4.62) and of 2.87 fixations for the SenseCam (SD = 2.89) were recorded, and an independent samples t-test was then conducted, which found that there was no significant difference between fixations on the two sensor types (t_{18} <1).

A 2 x 2 ANOVA was used to investigate potential effects of gender and sensor type on frequency of fixations (see Table 1). There was no statistically significant interaction effect ($F_{1,18}$<1), nor was there a main effect for gender ($F_{1,18}$<1), nor sensor type ($F_{2,18}$=2.247, p>0.05). Female participants in the SenseCam condition (M=5.0, SD=2.65) had a higher mean frequency of fixations than the males in the SenseCam condition (M=3.14, SD=3.18), d=0.6 (See Figure 4a).

Table 1. Means and standard deviations for sensor fixation scores

Condition	Gender	Mean	Std. Deviation	N
SenseCam	Male	3.1429	3.18479	7
	Female	5	2.64575	3
	Total	3.7	3.0203	10
LARK	Male	3	2.88675	7
	Female	2.6667	3.05505	3
	Total	2.9	2.76687	10
Control	Female	0	0	3
	Total	0	0	3
Total	Male	3.0714	2.92112	14
	Female	2.5556	2.96273	9
	Total	2.8696	2.88104	23

Independent t-tests were conducted to determine whether or not participants fixate on the hands in a similar way across each of the three sensor type conditions (SenseCam, LARK and control). Hands were fixated on with lower frequency when the SenseCam was worn, (M=4.2, SD=3.29), than when the LARK was worn (M=7.3, SD=5.14). However, no significant difference was found (t_{18}= -1.6, p>0.05, d=0.7). Hands were fixated upon more frequently when SenseCam was worn (M=4.2, SD=3.29) than in the control condition when no sensor was worn (M=0, SD=0) and this difference was not significant (t_{11}= 2.142, p> 0.05). In the LARK condition

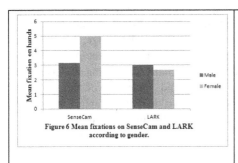

Figure 6 Mean fixations on SenseCam and LARK according to gender.

Fig. 4a. Mean fixations on SenseCam and LARK according to gender

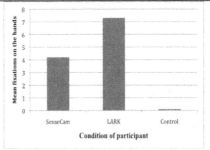

Condition of participant

Fig. 4b. Mean fixations on hands for each sensor condition

(M=7.3, SD=5.14), participants fixated significantly more often on the hands than in the control condition (M=0, SD=0), (t_{11}= 2.384, p>0.05). Frequency of fixations on the hands of the researcher are illustrated in Figure 4b.

To explore the possibility that the participant might fixate on one hand more than the other, independently of presence of the wrist-worn LARK (worn on the right wrist), the frequency of fixations on each hand was also recorded for the control group in which no sensors were worn. An independent samples t-test was conducted to investigate if participants fixated on each hand in a similar way, regardless of the researcher wearing the LARK. Frequency of fixations on the left hand were compared between the LARK condition (M = 4.3, SD = 3.16) and the control condition (Mean = 3, SD = 2.65), and no significant difference was found (t_{11}=0.642, p>0.05). Frequency of fixations on the right hand were also compared between the LARK condition (M = 3, SD = 2.54) and the control condition (M = 2.67, SD = 2.89), and again no significant difference was found (t_{11}<1).

4.2   Post Study Questionnaires

Table 2. Participants who reported noticing sensor vs. actual fixations on sensor

Sensor	Gender	Noticed Sensor	Fixations on sensor
SenseCam	M	N	0 fixations
SenseCam	M	N	0 fixations
SenseCam	F	N	4 fixations
SenseCam	M	N	0 fixations
SenseCam	M	N	6 fixations
SenseCam	M	N	3 fixations
LARK	M	N	1 fixation
LARK	F	N	2 fixations
LARK	M	N	5 fixations
LARK	M	N	0 fixations
LARK	F	N	6 fixations
Control	M	N	N/A

None of the 12 respondents to the post-study questionnaire reported seeing the sensor as worn by the researcher. 9 participants ranked the sensor as not noticeable at all. 1 participant in the wrist sensor condition reported seeing an ID badge, 1 participant mistook the IR markers for sensors and 1 participant reported that she perceived the glasses (spectacles) worn by one researcher as potentially containing a sensor. All participants responded yes when asked if they would wear one of the wearable sensors if they thought it would be of some benefit to their life. Table 2 highlights that, even though potential fixations were identified in the manual video analysis for many of the participants, they did not report noticing a sensor after the study.

5   Discussion

This investigation concerned the fixation of participants' gaze upon sensors worn by the researcher, in two conditions. Our primary aim was to ascertain whether the sensors were fixated upon at a rate significantly higher than any other area, and we conclude that they were not. The sensors do not appear to constitute a particularly visible or obtrusive item even in direct face-to-face conversations, at least with reference to the number of fixations made upon them. Further, neither type of sensor was differentially more or less visible than the other, indicating that both sensor types explored in the current analysis can be said to be non-obtrusive as measured by eye tracker fixation metrics. The sensors are worn on the wrist and around the neck on a lanyard respectively, potentially drawing attention to two different body parts. It was suspected that gender may impact area of fixation (the researcher was female). As such we investigated frequency of fixations on the sensors as a function of gender and no such relationship was found; it appears that male and female participants fixated equally upon the two sensor types. Thus the data remained pooled for the duration of the analyses.

We also investigated whether the wrist-worn sensor attracted more fixations to the hands, but there was no difference across sensor conditions in the frequency of fixations to the hands. Nor was there a difference found in fixations to the left or the right hand, indicating that the LARK sensor (worn on the right hand throughout) did not attract increased levels of fixation. The hands were nevertheless a region of significant fixation across participants, which may reflect the adaptive importance of perception of hand-related action from others. This area is responsible for the majority of instrumental actions carried out by others and is therefore an important area to accurately and sufficiently monitor [12].

There are limitations to the heat map analyses performed. While this data shows overwhelmingly that participants spent a relatively small proportion of the time fixating on both wearable sensors in comparison to the head area, the snapshots used to generate heat maps are only assumed to be representative of the eye tracking video rather than being totally accurate, as the area that we are investigating moves relative to the IR markers. In this case, it is likely that the researcher moved her head or torso or used gestural language. The more the researcher moves, the less accurate the fixation time. As we cannot presently quantify the movements of researcher and resultant artefact in the video data, further analyses are necessary to accurately determine actual fixations on the sensors, as well as to detect quick glances.

There are a number of limitations to report in the current study, namely, sampling and environmental issues. The current study included a limited sample size, a restricted pool of participants and was not gender-balanced which means that the sample does not constitute generalisable data and could result in reduced power. Future research should include a larger sample size to determine more conclusive findings. Furthermore, environmental background noise was notable in the current study. The presence of infrared (IR) markers attached to the seat surrounding the researcher during the study, may have been a distraction, as several participants remarked on the IR markers after the study, fixated on them during the study or mistakenly reported them as the sensors in the follow-up questionnaire. Also, due to changes in natural daylight, reflections off the glass panelling behind the interviewer varied across participants, with one participant primarily fixating on their reflection throughout the study. These limitations related to the experimental set up are important issues to highlight for future experiments using the eye tracking glasses to explore a physical environment. A similar investigation could ensure internal validity by means of more naturalistic settings (i.e. a set-up in which the IR markers would not be obviously visible). Furthermore, the issues identified in the results section in relation to the accuracy of the automated heat map data analysis are also a worthwhile area of further investigation.

6   Conclusion

As this study was intended as a pilot for further research, it succeeded to identify several important limitations of the study design and physical set-up, which will aptly inform the design of a similar study with a larger cohort of participants. In spite of the limitations identified above, the data produced in this experiment overwhelming illustrates that participants spent a very small proportion of the evaluation time fixating on wearable sensors, in comparison to lengthy fixations on the researcher's face or other areas of the room. While the more detailed annotated video analysis revealed that some participants fixated a number of times in the areas of both wearable sensors, none of the participants reported having noticed the sensors in post study questionnaires. This is a positive result to report in the context of promoting wearable sensors to enable independent living for people with dementia. Wearable sensors can provide such support without constituting an additional source of stigma for the user. This study has revealed that while observers did minimally fixate on the two wearable sensors evaluated in this experiment, sensors were not consciously noticed by observers and therefore can be considered unobtrusive.

Acknowledgements. This research is supported by the European Community 7th Framework Programme (FP7/2007- 2013) under grant agreement 288199 (Dem@Care) and by Science Foundation Ireland under grant SFI/12/RC/2289 (INSIGHT). We would also like to thank all participants for their time and effort in taking part in this study.

References

1. Drennan, J., Treacy, M.P., Butler, M., Byrne, A., Fealy, G., Frazer, K., Irving, K.: Support networks of older people living in the community. International Journal of Older People Nursing 3(4), 234–242 (2008)
2. Favela, J., Alamán, X.: Special theme: ambient assisted living for mobility: safety, well-being and inclusion. Personal and Ubiquitous Computing 17(6), 1061–1062 (2013)
3. Hoof, J., van, K.H., Rutten, P., Duijnstee, M.: Ageing-in-place with the use of ambient intelligence technology: Perspectives of older users. International Journal of Medical Informatics 80, 310–331 (2011)
4. Orpwood, R., Gibbs, C., Adlam, T., Faulkner, R., Meegahawatte, D.: The design of smart homes for people with dementia: user-interface aspects. Universal Access Information Society 4, 156–164 (2005)
5. Biswas, J., Tolstikov, A., Jayachandran, M., Foo, V., Wai, A.A.P., Phua, C., Huang, W., Shue, L., Gopalakrishnan, K., Lee, J., Yap, P.: Health and wellness monitoring through wearable and ambient sensors: exemplars from home-based care of elderly with mild dementia. Annals of Telecommunications - Annales Des TéléCommunications 65(9-10), 505–521 (2010)
6. Batsch, N.L., Mittelman, M.S.: Alzheimer's Disease International: World Alzheimer Report 2012: Overcoming the stigma of dementia. Alzheimer's Disease International, London (2012)
7. Demiris, G., Hensel, B.: "Smart homes" for patients at the end of life. Journal of Housing for the Elderly 23(1), 106–115 (2009)
8. Hensel, B.K., Demiris, G., Courtney, K.L.: Defining obtrusiveness in home telehealth technologies: A conceptual framework. Journal of the American Medical Informatics Association 13, 428–431 (2006)
9. Orpwood, R., Faulkner, R., Gibbs, C., Adlam, T.: A design methodology for assistive technology for people with dementia. In: Craddock, G.M., McCormack, L.P., Reilly, R.B., Knopps, H.T.P. (eds.) Assistive Technology: Shaping the Future (2003)
10. Hodges, S., Berry, E., Wood, K.: SenseCam: A Wearable Camera that Stimulates and Rehabilitates Autobiographical Memory. Memory 19(7), 685–696 (2011)
11. McHugh, J.E., Smeaton, A.F., Irving, K., Newman, E.: The Dem@Care Toolbox Approach. Position paper presented at the SIGCHI 2013 Workshop on Designing for and with Vulnerable People, CHI, Paris, France (April 2013)
12. Grezes, J., Costes, N., Decety, J.: Top down effect of the strategy on the perception of human biological motion: a PET investigation. Cognitive Neuropsychology 15, 553–582 (1998)

Towards a Transfer Learning-Based Approach for Monitoring Fitness Levels

Michiel Van Assche, Arun Ramakrishnan,
Davy Preuveneers, and Yolande Berbers

iMinds-DistriNet, KU Leuven, 3001 Leuven, Belgium

Abstract. The mobile ecosystem is rife with applications that aim for individuals to persue a more active and healthier lifestyle. Applications vary from simple diaries that track your weight, calorie intake or blood glucose values towards more advanced ones that offer health recommendations while monitoring your fitness levels during workouts and throughout the day. Leveraging machine learning techniques is a popular approach to recognize non-trivial activities, such as different types of sports. However, such applications face a time consuming training phase before they become practical. In this work, we report on our feasibility analysis of transfer learning as a way to apply learned models from one individual on another, and report on various feature variabilities that may jeopardize the applicability of transfer learning.

Keywords: activity recognition, transfer learning, accelerometer.

1 Introduction

The evolution of mobile phones and corresponding advancements in functionality has often been paired with the introduction of new sensors in the phone. Smartphones have sensors to observe acceleration, location, orientation, ambient lighting, sound, imagery, etc. [8]. Accelerometer-based activity recognition has applications in healthcare to assess physical activity [3] and to aid cardiac rehabilitation [2]. For example, the Samsung Galaxy S4 smartphone ships with the *S Health* application. This personal wellness application features a pedometer, a food and exercise tracker that uses the accelerometer and possibly other sensors. Furthermore, machine learning is a popular approach to infer human activities.

For monitoring fitness levels, we are interested in discriminating activities that include certain degrees of motion. However, many applications, such as S Health, are built for one particular device only. Targeting different devices and brands, we aim to explore the effects of the variability in the accelerometer (e.g. sensitivity and sampling rates) on activity recognition schemes.

Transfer Learning [9] is known as the practice to use knowledge from a related task that has already been learned, to improve learning in a new task. In the context of simple activity recognition, this means using a model trained with data from one particular person, to monitor fitness levels on another person.

M.J. O'Grady et al. (Eds.): AmI 2013 Workshops, CCIS 413, pp. 33–43, 2013.
© Springer International Publishing Switzerland 2013

The contributions in this work are twofold: (1) we explore the effects of sensor specific characteristics on the accuracy of accelerometer-based activity recognition, and (2) we explore the feasibility of using transfer learning techniques to mitigate the time consuming and error-prone individual training process.

The next section provides an overview of related work on accelerometer-based activity recognition. The general methodology towards accelerometer-based activity recognition is discussed in section 3, with adjustments required to transition to a transfer learning scheme. These adjustments are put into practice as part of our experimental evaluation in section 4. We conclude this paper with some final thoughts and topics for future work in section 5.

2   Related Work

Before we dive into the contributions of our work, we first discuss existing approaches that use accelerometers as key building blocks for activity recognition, and challenges that other researchers have investigated. Accelerometer data helps to analyze the human behavior in an effective way. With proper processing of this raw data, a variety of human activities can be inferred [10,7].

In [11], Lin et al. present an activity recognition approach using a mobile phone. All the data is collected on the same phone (Nokia N97) and the data coming from 6 different persons is not specifically treated. The data from all test subjects is used to build an SVM-classifier. Five types of features are employed in this work, including *mean, variance, correlation, FFT-energy* and *frequency-domain entropy*. One of the main factors that can influence the recognition rate is the position where a user is carrying his device. This position can either be in the pocket near the hip, in the front pocket or just in his hand. The influence of this position on the accuracy of predictions is researched in this work. In our work, we assume that the user is carrying his phone is his pocket, near the hip.

In [6], the focus is on the fact that the activity recognition approach should work in real-time. The authors claim that frequency domain features work best, but that these require too much computation to be feasible in a real-time scenario. Today's smartphones are significantly faster than a few years ago and performance issues are not really a concern anymore. Benchmark testing is carried out with data coming from one specific accelerometer. While not further elaborated on, they note that the specific set of used features makes the approach more person dependent. In their multiple-subject scenario, data coming from multiple persons is used to train the classification algorithm. They use this input from multiple subjects irrespective of the physique of the persons, but do note that adding some subjects decreases the performance. In our opinion, it would make more sense to only use subjects with similar physique.

3   Transfer Learning for Activity Recognition

The approach to activity recognition is achieved by using a classical supervised learning technique. It is conceived as a classification problem. Beforehand, the learner is presented with training examples to train a classifier that is capable of classifying new, unseen data. Normally recognition is carried out in three steps:

1. Collect small time segments (or windows) of the sensor signal
2. Extract features that describe general characteristics of each window
3. Infer the activity with a classification algorithm

We have chosen to use Decision Tree Classifiers, as they have proven to give good accuracy in the activity recognition problem [13,12]. The embedded triaxial accelerometer inside a mobile phone can continuously produce 3-D acceleration readings $A = (a_X, a_Y, a_Z)$, which are measures of the acceleration experienced in the three orthogonal axes: X-axis, Y-axis and Z-axis.

3.1 Data Collection

The Human Activity Sensing Consortium [5] (HASC) is an organization that aims at *achieving the recognition and understanding of human activity through sensing*. HASC aims at constructing a large scale database that is available for developers to test their algorithms. We used their Hasc-Logger[1] application to collect accelerometer-data at both 50 Hz and 100 Hz on a iPod Touch 3g device, and at 50 Hz on a Huawei Ascend G615 Android smartphone.

3.2 Extracting Features

Each training example consists of a target label and a number of features that are representative for this training instance. The choice of features is critical for the performance of a machine learning algorithm. Various kinds of features of the accelerometer sensing data have been investigated in previous activity recognition work, including *mean, variance, correlation, energy, frequency-domain entropy, cepstral coefficients, log FFT frequency bands*, etc. [13,12]. Using more features may be beneficial for the recognition accuracy, but will also result in higher power consumption. For our experiments, the chosen features include the FFT-coefficients and the FFT-energy (which is basically the sum of a number of coefficients over a certain time window). These are features that haven proven to be successful in activity recognition [4,1].

3.3 Ensuring FFT-Coefficient's Correct Meaning

When using FFT-coefficients (or the FFT-energy based on these coefficients) as input for transfer learning, one must take into consideration that these features are not independent of the sampling rate of the accelerometer. The supported sampling rates are mostly fixed because of hardware constraints. As a consequence, we need to adapt the FFT-size depending on the used sampling rate to ensure that the coefficients correspond with the same frequencies when the accelerometer is sampled at a different sampling rate.

---

[1] http://hasc.jp/hc2012/hasclogger-en.html

For example, assume a sampling rate of 100 Hz is used for sampling the accelerometer and that the chosen FFT size is 128 samples. The computation of this FFT results in 128 coefficients or frequency bins. The frequency bin width is Fs/N ($100/128 \approx 0.8$ Hz) where Fs is the sampling rate and N is the FFT size. The bins of interest will be those from 0 to $N/2 - 1$. Because of the Nyquist sampling theorem, only half of the coefficients contribute useful information when the input signal only consists of a real-valued part and no imaginary part.

The ratio Fs/N should be the same in the training phase and the online recognition phase. Suppose a classifier is trained on data from a person that was sampled at 100 Hz with an FFT size of 128 samples. This classifier is then used on another person which was sampled at 50 Hz. To make sure that each frequency bin reflects the same frequency boundaries), the FFT size has to be halved to 64 samples in the online recognition phase:

$$Fs/N = 100/128 = 50/64 \approx 0.8 Hz$$

Choosing the FFT size that results in the smallest difference in frequency bin size seems appropriate, although this will probably only result in good performance when the bin size difference is small.

3.4 Number of Usable FFT-Coefficients for Different Sampling Rates

The number of coefficients used for classification has to correspond between the training phase and the online prediction phase. Assume that training is carried out at 100 Hz with an FFT size of 128 samples, and online prediction is done at 50 Hz. As argued previously, the FFT size should be 64 samples to ensure the same meaning for the FFT coefficients. However, the maximum number of coefficients that can be used as features in this case is 32, as this is the number of coefficients that is available in the shortest FFT. Furthermore, these 32 coefficients do not span the same frequency range as the 100 Hz FFT. As a result, higher frequency coefficients obtained through training cannot be used for classification purposes when sampling at lower frequencies during the online prediction phase.

3.5 Accelerometer Sensitivity

Accelerometer values are internally usually represented in 8, 10 or 12 bits. A more expensive accelerometer will typically deliver a higher resolution (using more bits), and come with user selectable sensitivity scales of $\pm 2g / \pm 4g / \pm 8g$. The practical importance of these accelerometer specifications lies in the fact that exposing two different accelerometers to the same movements can result in different acceleration values, causing some activity recognition approaches to no longer work when directly using these accelerometer values with trained threshold values. We *normalized the obtained acceleration forces* by dividing all acceleration forces by the maximum acceleration force measured. This is the most simple adjustment that can be made to account for amplitude range and sensitivity effects without knowing the exact specifications of the accelerometers.

Table 1. Recognition accuracy on the iPod Touch at 50 Hz using *FFT-coefficients*

FFT size Coefficients	64	128	256
16	99.8 %	100.0 %	95.0 %
32	99.3 %	100.0 %	98.3 %
64	-	100.0 %	98.3 %
128	-	-	98.3 %

Table 2. Recognition accuracy on the iPod Touch at 50 Hz using the *FFT-energy*

FFT size Coefficients	64	128	256
16	93.8 %	94.3 %	78.6 %
32	98.6 %	95.7 %	96.7 %
64	-	98.5 %	100.0 %
128	-	-	100.0 %

4 Experimental Evaluation

Several experiments were set up to establish the performance of the activity recognition in a variety of scenarios. At first, the performance of the activity recognition is tested when using a device in the pocket near the hip and one particular person. When it is clear that this approach works quite good, we turn our attention to the more interesting cases where transfer learning is used. This includes scenarios involving several devices and different sampling rates for the accelerometer. All results are obtained using ten-fold cross validation.

In the first experiment, we use $9/10^{th}$ of the collected data as training data, while the other $1/10^{th}$ is used as test data. For the other experiments involving transfer learning with different people, we use all the data from one person and $1/10^{th}$ of the data from another person is used as test data. This process is then repeated ten times (a.k.a. 10 fold cross-validation).

4.1 Experiment 1: Same Person, Same Sensor, Same Sampling Rate

The variable parameters in this setting are: the FFT-size and the number of coefficients used (either as pure features or after calculation of the FFT-energy value being the sum of the coefficients over the time window). The performance of correctly classifying walking and running can be deduced from Tables 1 and 2. These tables show the results when an iPod Touch was used to collect data at a sampling rate of 50 Hz. Both using the FFT-coefficients and the FFT-energy value as features result in very similar recognition rate results.

The critical aspect lies in the fact that the chosen combination of FFT-size and number of coefficients results in capturing frequencies no lower than approximately 10 Hz. The results for the same person using the iPod Touch at 100 Hz and using the Huawei Ascend Android device are extremely similar.

Table 3. Recognition accuracy for the iPod Touch at 50 Hz and 100 Hz in a Transfer Learning scheme using the FFT-coefficients as features

Training Data − Test Data	FFT-adaptation	No FFT-adaptation
iPod Touch: 50 Hz − 100 Hz	99.0 %	98.8 %
iPod Touch: 100 Hz − 50 Hz	99.3 %	84.5 %

Table 4. Recognition accuracy for the iPod Touch at 50 Hz and 100 Hz in a Transfer Learning scheme using the FFT-energy value as feature

Training Data − Test Data	FFT-adaptation	No FFT-adaptation
iPod Touch: 50 Hz − 100 Hz	94.6 %	85.6 %
iPod Touch: 100 Hz − 50 Hz	98.6 %	84.3 %

These results also show that reducing the number of coefficients used as features does not really deteriorate the recognition rates. This is important, as we will adapt the FFT-size according to the sampling rate used by the accelerometer. As a result, the number of coefficients will also change. These results show that this is not a problem, as long as these coefficients have the same meaning (i.e. the frequency bins describe the same frequency boundaries).

4.2   Experiment 2: Same Person and Sensor, Different Sampling Rate

To show the influence of the sampling rate and changing the FFT-size a small experiment is set up. The FFT-size is set to ± 1 second. This size worked good for the previous experiment. Using the same iPod Touch device, data is sampled at both 50 Hz and 100 Hz. First, the 50 Hz data is used for training and the 100 Hz data for testing. The results are shown in Tables 3 and 4, using the FFT-coefficients and the FFT-energy value as features respectively.

When comparing the results, the attentive reader may have noticed there is something strange going on when the FFT-coefficients are used as features. One would expect that not changing the FFT-size according to the sampling rate would lead to significantly worse results. However, this does not seem to be the case. This can be explained by the fact that the main feature that is selected by the decision tree classifier is the DC-component of the used Fourier Transformation, i.e. the average acceleration magnitude over the window. The fact that this value is not frequency dependent explains why the results are surprisingly good when the FFT-size is maintained. The confusion matrix in

Table 5. Confusion matrix with the recognition accuracy for the walking and running classes. The Transfer Learning scheme is from the iPod at 50 Hz to the iPod at 100 Hz, with the FFT-size not adapted according to the sampling rate.

	Walking	Running
Walking	75.5 %	4.0 %
Running	24.5 %	96.0 %

Table 6. Recognition accuracy for the iPod Touch and Huawei Ascend device at 50 Hz in a Transfer Learning scheme using the FFT-coefficients as features

Training Data – Test Data	Normalization	No normalization
50 Hz: iPod Touch – Huawei Ascend	50.5 %	49.5 %
50 Hz: Huawei Ascend – iPod Touch	47.6 %	37.6 %

Table 7. Recognition accuracy for the iPod Touch and Huawei Ascend device at 50 Hz in a Transfer Learning scheme using the FFT-energy value as a feature

Training Data – Test Data	Normalization	No normalization
50 Hz: iPod Touch – Huawei Ascend	100.0 %	50.2 %
50 Hz: Huawei Ascend – iPod Touch	92.8 %	51.7 %

Table 5 shows that although the results are still quite good when the FFT-size is not adapted, the errors are mostly located in one class, which gives a slightly too positive impression. The recognition rate has dropped more than the overall recognition rate suggested.

4.3   Experiment 3: Same Person and Sampling Rate, Different Sensor

In this section we explore how the activity recognition behaves when a different device (and thus accelerometer) is used. The model is trained using data collected on the Huawei Ascend Android device and then tested on data collected with an iPod Touch. This process is then repeated with the iPod Touch data as training data and the Android data as test data. Because we are now entering a scenario with two different devices, we also have to take care of the hardware differences between those two devices. As argued earlier, we will use normalization to cope with sensitivity differences.

The FFT-size and used coefficients parameters are fixed at ± 1 second. This means an FFT-size of 128 samples at 100 Hz and 64 samples at 50 Hz. The number of used coefficients is then 32 (because that is the maximum that is available in the FFT-64 case because of the Nyquist sampling theorem). As can be seen in Tables 6 and 7, our approach only works well when the FFT-energy value is used as a feature and when the normalization is used. This is in line with our expectations that the FFT-energy value is a more stable measure than the coefficients themselves. It is also not a surprise that the normalization helps in alleviating the accelerometer sensitivity problem. It should also be noted that in this setting, being successful means that the recognition rates should be particularly high. As can be seen from the confusion matrix in Table 8, a recognition rate of 50 % can be achieved by always predicting one class.

4.4   Experiment 4: Different Person, Same Sensor and Sampling Rate

In this last scenario we want to test whether our approach will generalize when doing Transfer Learning between two different persons (with similar physique) using an iPod Touch device sampled at the same sampling rate (see Figure 1).

Table 8. Confusion matrix with the recognition accuracy for the walking and running classes. The Transfer Learning scheme is from the iPod Touch to the Huawei Ascend device both at 50 Hz, using the FFT-coefficients as features.

	Walking	Running
Walking	0 %	0 %
Running	100 %	100 %

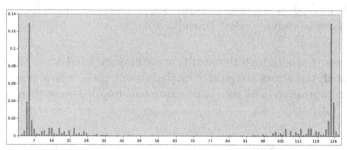

Frequency domain: Power spectrum excluding DC component for male 1

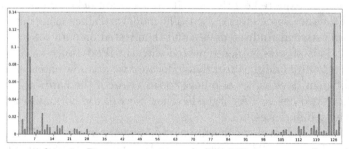

Frequency domain: Power spectrum excluding DC component for male 2

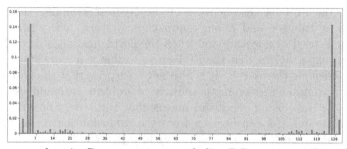

Frequency domain: Power spectrum excluding DC component for male 3

Fig. 1. 128 samples captured by an iPod Touch at 100 Hz for three males running

The data of three male persons (P1, P2, P3) is used during testing. All persons are of comparable length and weight. Each persons' data is used as training data and as test data in different experiments. In one setting, the vice versa test in both directions is used to get an idea of whether the approach would generalize. As a result of previous results, only the FFT-energy value is used as a feature, and the FFT-size is ± 1 second.

The results in Table 9 show moderate results. As noted in previous sections, the somewhat lower recognition rates are obtained by having 100% accuracy in one class, which gives a slightly too positive impression.

Table 9. Recognition accuracy for the iPod Touch at 50 Hz in a Transfer Learning scheme between several persons

Training Data − Test Data	Recognition rate
iPod Touch 50 Hz: P1 − P2	71 %
iPod Touch 50 Hz: P1 − P3	89 %
iPod Touch 50 Hz: P2 − P1	73 %
iPod Touch 50 Hz: P3 − P1	72 %

5   Conclusion

We found that our activity recognition approach works very good when using a particular person uses a specific device. The approach is not too dependent on small parameters like FFT-size (number of samples per window) and the used accelerometer sampling rates. The most important parameter is the person itself, or the way that he walks and runs.

We explicitly excluded other types of activity recognition, such as fall detection, sleep analysis, step counting, and many others, as we aimed to investigate the effect of feature differences in accelerometer sensors and variability in human behavior, and not so much any misclassifications due to any limitations of the learning algorithms themselves. Furthermore, the training phase of walking and running activities is fairly simple to be carried out with minimal risks for mislabeling. The transfer learning approach taken in this paper can be considered partly successful, as it is not guaranteed to generalize across all types of persons and devices. Overall, one must say that the measured acceleration depends quite heavily on the hardware and the way someone performs the activities.

As future work, it will be beneficial to look into extracting new accelerometer features that are more tolerant for differences in the measured acceleration forces. The main contribution of our approach is that it has proven to be very successful using a limited amount of training data. The training data of three minutes for each activity results in very good recognition rates. Therefore, when high precision is important collecting this limited data is preferential instead of using our transfer learning. Also, to recognize more activities (like jumping, cycling, ...) additional features should be used, as our simple features are not be able to discriminate these. In the future, sensor fusion (combining the input of other sensors like GPS or light sensors) will be explored to improve our activity recognition approach.

In our work, we explained the use of the J48 decision tree algorithm to classify different activities, though other learning algorithms have been tested with different degrees of success. To leverage the best of all approaches, we will further investigate the use of meta-learning, i.e. automatic learning algorithms on meta-data about machine learning experiments to improve the performance of activity recognition.

Acknowledgments. This research is partially funded by the Research Fund KU Leuven.

References

1. Bao, L., Intille, S.S.: Activity recognition from user-annotated acceleration data. In: Ferscha, A., Mattern, F. (eds.) PERVASIVE 2004. LNCS, vol. 3001, pp. 1–17. Springer, Heidelberg (2004)
2. Bidargaddi, N., Sarela, A., Klingbeil, L., Karunanithi, M.: Detecting walking activity in cardiac rehabilitation by using accelerometer. In: 3rd International Conference on Intelligent Sensors, Sensor Networks and Information, ISSNIP 2007, pp. 555–560 (2007)
3. Bouten, C.V., Koekkoek, K.T., Verduin, M., Kodde, R., Janssen, J.D.: A triaxial accelerometer and portable data processing unit for the assessment of daily physical activity. IEEE Trans. Biomed. Eng. 44(3), 136–147 (1997), http://view.ncbi.nlm.nih.gov/pubmed/9216127
4. Huynh, T., Schiele, B.: Analyzing features for activity recognition. In: Proceedings of the 2005 Joint Conference on Smart Objects and Ambient Intelligence: Innovative Context-Aware Services: Usages and Technologies, sOc-EUSAI 2005, pp. 159–163. ACM, New York (2005), http://doi.acm.org/10.1145/1107548.1107591
5. Kawaguchi, N., Watanabe, H., Yang, T., Ogawa, N., Iwasaki, Y., Kaji, K., Terada, T., Murao, K., Hada, H., Inoue, S., Sumi, Y., Kawahara, Y., Nishio, N.: Hasc2012corpus: Large scale human activity corpus and its application, pp. 10–14 (April 2012)
6. Khan, M., Ahamed, S.I., Rahman, M., Smith, R.O.: A Feature Extraction Method for Real time Human Activity Recognition on Cell Phones. In: isQoLT 2011 (2011), http://www.mridulkhan.com/pdf/khan-QoL10.pdf
7. Kwapisz, J.R., Weiss, G.M., Moore, S.A.: Activity recognition using cell phone accelerometers. SIGKDD Explor. Newsl. 12(2), 74–82 (2011), http://doi.acm.org/10.1145/1964897.1964918
8. Lane, N.D., Miluzzo, E., Lu, H., Peebles, D., Choudhury, T., Campbell, A.T.: A survey of mobile phone sensing. Comm. Mag. 48(9), 140–150 (2010), http://dx.doi.org/10.1109/MCOM.2010.5560598
9. Pan, S.J., Yang, Q.: A survey on transfer learning. IEEE Trans. on Knowl. and Data Eng. 22(10), 1345–1359 (2010), http://dx.doi.org/10.1109/TKDE.2009.191
10. Ravi, N., Dandekar, N., Mysore, P., Littman, M.L.: Activity recognition from accelerometer data. In: Proceedings of the 17th Conference on Innovative Applications of Artificial Intelligence, IAAI 2005, vol. 3, pp. 1541–1546. AAAI Press (2005)

11. Sun, L., Zhang, D., Li, B., Guo, B., Li, S.: Activity recognition on an accelerometer embedded mobile phone with varying positions and orientations. In: Yu, Z., Liscano, R., Chen, G., Zhang, D., Zhou, X. (eds.) UIC 2010. LNCS, vol. 6406, pp. 548–562. Springer, Heidelberg (2010),
    http://dl.acm.org/citation.cfm?id=1929661.1929712
12. Wu, J., Pan, G., Zhang, D., Qi, G., Li, S.: Gesture recognition with a 3-d accelerometer. In: Zhang, D., Portmann, M., Tan, A.-H., Indulska, J. (eds.) UIC 2009. LNCS, vol. 5585, pp. 25–38. Springer, Heidelberg (2009),
    http://dx.doi.org/10.1007/978-3-642-02830-4_4
13. Yang, J.: Toward physical activity diary: motion recognition using simple acceleration features with mobile phones. In: Proceedings of the 1st International Workshop on Interactive Multimedia for Consumer Electronics, IMCE 2009, pp. 1–10. ACM, New York (2009), http://doi.acm.org/10.1145/1631040.1631042

Unsupervised Learning in Ambient Assisted Living for Pattern and Anomaly Detection: A Survey

Francisco Javier Parada Otte, Bruno Rosales Saurer, and Wilhelm Stork

FZI Research Center for Information Technologies
Embedded Systems and Sensors Engineering Karlsruhe, Germany
parada@fzi.de

Abstract. Population ageing is an issue that has encouraged the development of Ambient Intelligence systems to support elderly people to live autonomously at home longer. Some key aspects of these systems are the detection of behavior patterns and behavior profiles in their daily life. The information we can infer from these patterns could prove to be very valuable for monitoring the health status of a person, like to control deterioration of diseases or to provide personalized assistive services. In this paper we focus on the unsupervised learning techniques in health monitoring systems for elderly people, which has the advantage of not needing annotations. Collecting these is a tedious job and sometimes difficult to accomplish. We discuss the different existing approaches, identify some limitations and propose possible challenges and directions for future research.

Keywords: Ambient Assisted Living, unsupervised learning, behavior profiling, health monitoring.

1 Introduction

Ambient Assisted Living (AAL) is the application of Ambient Intelligence (AmI) to support elderly people to live at home longer. Population ageing has become a very important fact in our society due to the social and economic implications that it entails [1].

An AmI system can be dissected in three main parts [2], as seen in Fig. 1: sensing, reasoning and acting. *Sensing* is the ability to capture or record any type of context information that is relevant for the system. This could be any information about the user and his environment. This information is collected mostly through sensors, which provide a wide variety of data, but there could also be user interfaces to get user input or some predefined information. Sensors could be environmental like cameras, microphones, motion, contact, brightness, and temperature sensors, or wearable like accelerometers and vital parameters sensors.

The second part, *reasoning*, consists in obtaining more abstract or higher level information from the sensor data in order to acquire valuable and useful information for the system. The process is based on the application of some inferring techniques to the context data to obtain the information. There are mainly two most extended types;

M.J. O'Grady et al. (Eds.): AmI 2013 Workshops, CCIS 413, pp. 44–53, 2013.
© Springer International Publishing Switzerland 2013

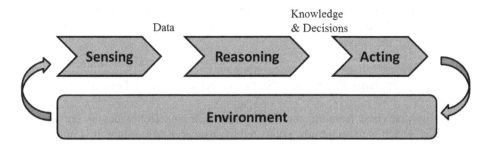

Fig. 1. Structure of AmI Systems [2]

on the one hand, we have specification-based systems, where some domain knowledge is reflected in defined rules for inferring the information. On the other hand, we have machine learning, which explores the relationships between the context data and the information to be inferred. Machine learning can be divided as well into two subcategories, supervised and unsupervised. The difference lies in the usage or not of labeled data for the learning process respectively. Supervised learning needs annotations or references in order to train the system to learn the relationship model. But the process of collecting the annotations is very tedious and time consuming. Sometimes it is very difficult to carry out such tasks, for example, in large installations, in long-term studies and with people who have cognitive problems. In these cases unsupervised learning can be applied.

The third part, *acting*, basically defines the application or goal of the system. Here the system reacts to the information inferred in a proper way. It could present the information to the caregiver in case of health monitoring systems, provide a service if it is an assistive system, or inform the responsible person in case of emergency detections.

The analysis and detection of behavior patterns belong to the reasoning part and is a cornerstone in AmI systems, and especially relevant in AAL. The behavior patterns, how they evolve, and the detection of deviations from expected behavior can provide very valuable information about a person's health status. The main applications in the home environment are the health status monitoring over time, for detecting depression, control early stages of dementia or chronic diseases like diabetes. Secondly, it is possible to monitor the progress of patients after surgery, in rehabilitation or under treatments like for multiple sclerosis. Then, it could also work as a supporting tool for caregivers as backup for assessments like the Barthel index [3] and other documentation. The system is also useful for emergency detections like an inactivity period after a fall. And the last application to remark is the provision of personalized services in assistive systems, such as lighting control at night.

In this paper we examine the work performed in the field of monitoring systems for behavior patterns, activity recognition and anomaly detection, centering on the unsupervised learning techniques for AAL. In the next section we cover the other main alternatives to the unsupervised learning, the ones just mentioned above. We explain and discuss them compared to unsupervised learning. In the third section we discuss the current work based on unsupervised learning. We classify and comment the differences among them. Finally in the last section we discuss the current status of the research in this field and what might be interesting challenges and future directions for research for the community.

2   Specification-Based and Supervised Learning Techniques

Besides unsupervised learning, there are other reasoning techniques as previously mentioned, which we present now compared to unsupervised learning. It is important to acknowledge, that depending on what the goal of the system is, or what information is needed, different techniques can fit the requirements better.

Specification-based systems apply expertise knowledge in a domain in form of logic rules. Reason engines then infer the situations from the sensor data. Bikakis et al. provide an extended survey describing the work carried out in this direction [4]. They distinguish among three main types and some minor solutions. The first one is ontological reasoning, where an ontology represents the data model and the systems benefit from the tools already available like query languages and reasoning tools. Secondly, they mention the rule-based reasoning, where logic rules define policies, constraints and preferences applied to the context data in order to retrieve higher level information. Then the third model is distributed reasoning, where different reasoning components interact together. These components may have different reasoning, storage and computing capabilities, and may deal with data from different sources and different formats. These systems perform well when using small datasets, but they have limited computational capacity. The rapid development of pervasive devices increases the use of a more diversity of sensors, thus, the datasets increase as well, becoming more incomplete and uncertain. The efficiency and the capacity of retrieving information are considerably reduced in this case. A second drawback is the lack of adaptability of such systems. Different people will generate different behavior patterns and will also change over time, while these systems cannot learn from the changes. This technique is limited as a stand-alone system, but combined with learning algorithms, it could provide very interesting results.

Supervised learning deals better with the huge datasets and with the incompleteness and uncertainty. These techniques explore associations between the sensor data and the situations to be inferred. There is a lot of work in this field and Aztiria, Izaguirre and Augusto have surveyed these techniques centered on pattern learning in Ambient Intelligence [2]. Neural networks, classification techniques like decision trees or Bayesian networks, and sequence discovery are examples of the most extended algorithms. The main drawback of these systems is the need of labeled data for a training phase. The collection of annotations is a very laborious and time-consuming task and sometimes impossible to achieve. It also might not be reliable when elderly people annotate their own activities as they may become forgetful or have difficulties. There have been some works improving the collection, gathering them electronically via a PDA [5] or taken them from a recorded video [6]. However, doing this for each new installation would be arduous for large-scale evaluations or when bringing such systems to the market. For the matter of research of new algorithms, it is helpful to do a training phase with labeled data, but when considering real-world conditions, it would become hard to collect the annotations. Unsupervised learning could fit in these cases.

There exist two more approaches lying in between supervised and unsupervised learning. First, semi-supervised learning uses both labeled and unlabeled data for the learning process, reducing the amount of labeling data needed. They use the labeled data to label automatically the unlabeled data with some classifier, incrementing the labeled set for the model. There is some work in behavior modeling [7] and detecting unusual events [8]. This system is proper when only a few annotations are available, but these are still needed. The second alternative is reinforcement learning, where the learning process is supported by a feedback function, indicating how well the system operates. Thus, the model adapts itself according to the feedback received. Reinforcement learning works well for adaptive systems, like light control systems, using the user actions (switching on/off) as feedback [9]. In our case, focusing on finding outliers, we cannot rely on the feedback from the sensors, but the concept is interesting to apply adaptability to the system.

3   Unsupervised Learning

There is an active work in pattern recognition and outlier detection and the work in unsupervised learning is not less. It is difficult to classify the different current solutions, as the algorithms differ from each other. Most of them are based on cluster techniques, which are the most extended unsupervised techniques, but there are some others as we will see. Other solutions are combinations of two algorithms, where clustering techniques are often also involved. We have categorized them in clustering-based solutions and mixed solutions.

3.1   Clustering Techniques

Clustering consists mainly in dividing a dataset in subsets by grouping them with some similarity criteria. There are two different clustering techniques, partitional and hierarchical. In the former, clusters are found at once while in the latter, clusters are found iteratively based on previous clusters. Some concrete algorithms are density models, where clusters are the densest regions, distribution models based on statistical distributions, or centroid models, where all clusters are mean vectors and the belonging relationship is some distance parameter to the center value. K-means is a well-known centroid algorithm based on the partition of a dataset into k clusters in which each observation belongs to the cluster with the nearest mean. The term nearest is based on a metric, as it could be the Euclidean distance. Although clustering is the most common, it is often combined with other techniques to achieve better results and is not used as a stand-alone.

Monekosso applies unsupervised learning to find out routines based on daily activities [10]. She uses clustering techniques, concretely k-means, k-medoids, agglomerative clustering and EM (expectation-maximization) clustering. Then she built a behavior model based on a hidden Markov model (HMM), defining behavior as a sequence of clusters. For the evaluation she collected data from one household for several alternate weeks, and then applied them to the algorithm. It is a good start, but validation of this work in real-time and with more subjects would be desirable, as these systems should work in real-world conditions. It is quite interesting, that she evaluates all four algorithms for pattern detection with HMM and different hidden states, and then for anomaly recognition. Results vary depending on the number of hidden states and the length of the sequence. This addresses the difficulty of choosing the best algorithm, as the performance varies depending on several factors. Behavior not recognized with the model is tagged for informing caregivers and they receive some information to make decisions. This information is the probability of an anomalous behavior, and the behavior itself, like a lack of activity in a room. This output would result in useful information for a monitoring system.

Barger and the group at the University of Virginia study how to obtain behavioral patterns for a monitoring system in a Smart House by applying mixture-models [11]. The so-called mixture models combine the k-means clustering technique and self-organizing maps, which is a sort of neural network, as a method for event estimation. For their study they use real motion data from a Smart Home collected discontinuously during 65 days, 25 for training and 40 for the tests. They make the distinction in their system between work and days off by activity level, thus, the amount of sensor firings, which helped to reduce the uncertainty when classifying the observations. It also allows for the possibility of finding different patterns in work and days off. The evaluation is then performed offline including the unsupervised training phase. A user log was available as well, allowing them to compare the patterns to the activities performed by the user. They could identify many of the recorded patterns as activities such as sleep behavior, changing clothes or bathroom use. The output of the system would be sequences of motion sensor firings, which are hard to interpret by the end user.

The MavHome group is a very active working group in pattern recognition and behavior prediction in intelligent environments [12]. Regarding clustering techniques, Rao and Cook use the task-based Markov model which consists of the combination of clustering and HMM [13]. The system aims to predict a person's behavior in an intelligent environment, in order to provide assistance and adaptation to the inhabitant's needs. They divide the sensor data in groups based on some heuristic rules, then apply clustering to these sequences to represent tasks, and finally the HMM is applied for the behavior prediction. This group validated their system offline with simulated and real data, which provided different results. This fact emphasizes the importance of using real data. One positive aspect is that they compared their algorithms with a simple Markov model, showing a better performance for certain datasets. They state that the choice of the algorithm parameters (number of clusters, sequence length and allowable time difference) is important for the algorithm performance and they vary for concrete datasets. This issue shows the algorithms are closely dependent on several factors such as the configuration parameters or the data format and completeness, implying the difficulty of finding a universal algorithm that best fits all situations. The output information is a set of patterns of sensor data, which are usable for the system itself, but difficult to interpret by non-technical experts.

Fuzzy logic is also used as an unsupervised technique in the smart environment iDorm [14]. Their end goal is to provide an automatic control of the intelligent environment based on the user's behavior. They propose an online adaptive framework for extracting fuzzy membership functions and rules representing the behavior of persons. These functions are extracted directly from the sensor data by applying a double clustering approach. The system adapts to change behaviors thanks to a loopback module. They performed an online and offline evaluation with data collected from the iDorm during 5 consecutive days. The offline experiment consists of the performance comparison among their solution and 3 more algorithms, namely GP (genetic programming), ANFIS (adaptive-neuro fuzzy inference system), and the MLP (multiplayer perceptron), a neural network. Although their solution is the second in results after GP, it provides a lighter computation than the other ones and it is better suited for online operation. The online evaluation showed during 2 days, after 3 of learning, that the system can learn the functions and respond appropriately with the control rules. Again, the output is based directly on sensor data, hard to interpret by non-technicians, as would be expected for a monitoring system.

3.2   Other Unsupervised Solutions

Besides clustering techniques, there are several different solutions that perform unsupervised learning that apply a variety of algorithms for discovering behavior patterns.

Wyatt and Intel Research people were pioneers in activity recognition based on unsupervised learning [15]. They focused on labeling and learning sensor data from information obtained by web mining processes without human intervention to recognize activities but not behavior patterns. They mined from the web activities description to get a correlation of appearance of objects usage. Their experiments were offline with real data from 9 subjects, each subject only performing activities for 20 to 40 minutes in an equipped home. Nevertheless, this solution works only when every object is tagged, which would result in a very complicated process, especially for long-term studies. It would also be interesting to test it with ambient sensors, although the mining process should be adapted to this sensor input. It is also dependent on how good, quantitative and qualitative, the available descriptions are, and there is no possible personalization. However, it is a very interesting work, as it provides a completely different perspective when avoiding human intervention. The output presented is already at an activity level instead of a sensor level, thus easier to understand by non-experts.

Robben has some recent work on pattern discovery for health status monitoring. This group presents the possibility of predicting functional health status from ambient sensor data [16]. They applied expert knowledge for extracting important features for the caregivers and then looked for mapping the features to the functional status by linear regression and Gaussian processes. The feature extraction is matched to the

AMPS (assessment of motor and process skill), a functional health metric [17], which was performed and collected by caregivers. They carried out an offline experiment with data from 9 subjects at an assisted living facility and different time lengths between one and five weeks. They have found that some features can be detected, but individual differences are very influential and should be taken into account. Results are quite interesting and show that at this early stage it is not possible to generalize and results vary among the participants. They also present a visualization model of deviations in ADLs [18], which is a key aspect in monitoring systems. This information shown here is still sensor based and can be abstracted to a more understandable format for caregivers.

Virone works on detecting long-term activity patterns based on the circadian activity rhythm (CAR) [19]. The study of temporal structures called chronobiology, has demonstrated that human behavior is ruled approximately by a 24-hour fluctuating rhythm, known as the circadian rhythm. He uses statistical software called SAMCAD for detecting behavior patterns. He estimates the average time spent in each room and the average number of motion events per room, named as activity, in 24-hour periods. Anomalies result from comparing the behavior of the current day and the habitual behavior estimated on the basis of the CAR. These might be indicative of a problematic situation or a change in the person's health status. Results are sensor data estimations which could lead to very helpful information. Nevertheless, it is still presented in graphics of activity, as seen in Fig. 2, difficult to understand by non-experts. The detection is done in an offline process, although he aims to evaluate it in real-time for further work.

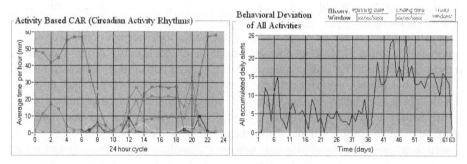

Fig. 2. Application for caregivers [16]

There are some more works using similar algorithms. A combination of HMM and a Viterbi algorithm is applied to analyze motion sensor data to model elderly persons' behavior and find unusual activities to inform caregivers [20]. Then, unsupervised neural networks have been applied as well, to find patterns in the Adaptive Home, a Smart Home environment, for improving comfort by home automation [21]. Rivera also explored adaptive neural networks for anomaly detection again in the iDorm intelligent environment [22].

4   Discussion and Research Challenges

There is a lot of work going on in pattern recognition and unsupervised learning is a very interesting technique, especially for anomaly detection, which might prove to be very useful for monitoring elderly people at home. No need for labeled data is also an advantage for large-scale evaluations or bringing a system to the market. However, there is still some work ahead to get full functional monitoring systems.

One of the limitations of unsupervised learning is the absence of the interpretation of the outputs. This is of special interest in monitoring systems, where readable information should be presented to the caregivers or the person responsible for the monitoring. The results and information that we get for such algorithms are not understandable for the end user. A pattern of sensor events or a deviation of this pattern is far from what a caregiver could expect. That is why many works combine two different techniques, so they can identify activities and apply the algorithm to an activity level and not only to the sensor level. One approach that could be interesting is to apply some semantic knowledge in order to interpret the results of the algorithms and to provide valuable information. Thus, when an outlier is detected due to a lot of motion at night time in contrast to the normal behavior, which is just light motion in the bedroom, the system could report some sleeping problems on a concrete date. However, there could be a large difference in the outliers and people also have different behaviors, which would complicate this approach. One option would be to implement algorithms that provide a readable output, or as said before, combine different techniques. We consider there is a lot of work in interpreting and visualizing the information, in order to provide a useful system for the end users.

On the other side, every work presents different algorithms and there is a wide variety of solutions. Each work uses their own data, real or simulated, and performs the tests and evaluation with it. This makes it very hard to make comparisons among the different systems. A good example to follow is the Artificial Intelligent community, where they make datasets available, allowing other techniques to be evaluated with these same datasets. There already are some public datasets, but still not really extended and used. Another proposal that would help to work in this direction is to standardize the sensor data format. This would facilitate sharing datasets and comparing solutions so everybody could benefit. Currently there are not any standards extended in the community.

Another aspect of the evaluation is the time when it is performed. Most of these evaluations are carried out offline. This means the data is collected for a specific time period or even using simulated data, and then the complete dataset is passed to the algorithm. In any case, the main purpose of these systems is to run independently and be able to work and respond in real-time. Simulated data is also good for a first evaluation, but this system should be validated both with real data and in real-time. We have seen in one work before, how different the results are when using simulated or real data [13]. Currently it is difficult to have the opportunity to perform such an evaluation, but infrastructures, like smart home environments, which are increasing quickly, and investment in this field, are making these studies become a reality.

Another issue when evaluating the systems is the duration of the datasets. So far only short time periods have been used, with a maximum of a few days or even a few hours. From this data, some is also used for training, leaving even less data for the evaluation. However, health monitoring systems aim to provide behavior patterns which should be recognized for long-term periods. Thus, some studies or datasets for longer time periods, for instance from one month in advance, would be desirable in order to validate such techniques. Secondly, online studies should be performed as well, as we addressed before. Although it is hard to make such studies and get subjects for a long-term period, there are already some institutions that allow carrying out these studies and there is an increasing interest for actors involved in eldercare like public administrations and healthcare organizations.

Finally, we also encourage the implementation of adaptive systems. A system should not only learn at the first stage and then keep working with the learnt model, but it should also keep learning over the time, as a person's behavior can change easily. This is already present in some works, but we think it is an essential feature for such systems.

There is still some work to be done and we propose here some directions for future research, but each contribution brings the community some advance in the field. This evolution will allow us to get improved AmI systems to support elderly people and everyone else involved in their care.

References

1. Bloom, D.E., Canning, D., Fink, G.: Implications of population ageing for economic growth. Oxford Review of Economic Policy 26(4), 583–612 (2010)
2. Aztiria, A., Izaguirre, A., Augusto, J.C.: Learning patterns in Ambient Intelligence environments: A Survey. Artificial Intelligence Review 34(1), 35–51 (2010)
3. Mahoney, F.I., Barthel, D.: Functional evaluation: the Barthel Index. Maryland State Medical Journal 14, 56–61 (1965)
4. Bikakis, A., Patkos, T., Antoniou, G., Plexousakis, D.: A Survey of Semantics-based Approaches for Context Reasoning in Ambient Intelligence. In: Mühlhäuser, M., Ferscha, A., Aitenbichler, E. (eds.) AmI 2007 Workshops. CCIS, vol. 11, pp. 14–23. Springer, Heidelberg (2008)
5. Stumpp, J., Anastasopoulou, P., Sghir, H., Hey, S.: Sensor Chest Strap Wirelessly Coupled with an e-Diary for Ambulatory Assessment of Psycho-Physiological Data. In: 2nd Biennial Conference of the Science of Ambulatory Assessment, Ann Arbor, Michigan (2011)
6. Tolstikov, A., Biswas, J., Tham, C.K., Yap, P.: Eating activity primitives detection - a step towards adl recognition. In: 10th IEEE International Conference on e–Health Networking, Applications and Service, HEALTHCOM 2008, pp. 35–41 (2008)
7. Hoey, J., Poupart, J., Boutilier, C., Mihailidis, A.: Semi-supervised learning of a POMDP model of Patient-Caregiver Interactions. In: International Joint Conference in Artificial Intelligence, Workshop on Modeling Others from Observations, pp. 101–110 (2005)
8. Zhang, D., Gatica-Perez, D., Bengio, S.: Semi-supervised adapted HMMs for unusual event detection. In: Conference Computer Vision and Pattern Recognition, CVPR 2005, pp. 611–618 (2005)

9. Sandhu, J.S., Agogino, A.M., Agogino, A.K.: Wireless Sensor Networks for Commercial Lighting Control: Decision Making with Multi-agent Systems. In: Association for Advancement of Artificial Intelligence Conference, Sensor Networks Workshop, San Jose, pp. 88–92 (2004)
10. Monekosso, D.N., Remagnino, P.: Anomalous behaviour detection: supporting independent living. In: Monekosso, D.N., Remagnino, P., Kuno, Y. (eds.) Ambient Intelligence Techniques and Applications, Advanced Information and Knowledge Processing, pp. 33–48. Springer, London (2009)
11. Barger, T.S., Brown, D.E., Alwan, M.: Health-status monitoring through analysis of behavioral patterns. IEEE Transactions on SMC-A 35, 22–27 (2005)
12. Cook, D.J., Youngblood, M., Heierman III, E.O., Gopalratnam, K., Rao, S., Litvin, A., Khawaja, F.: MavHome: An Agent-Based Smart Home. In: First IEEE International Conference on Pervasive Computing and Communications, PerCom 2003, pp. 521–524 (2003)
13. Rao, S., Cook, D.J.: Predicting Inhabitant Actions Using Action and Task Models with Application to Smart Homes. International Journals of Artificial Intel. Tools 13(1), 81–100 (2004)
14. Doctor, F., Hagras, H., Callaghan, V.: A fuzzy embedded agent-based approach for realizing ambient intelligence in intelligent inhabited environments. IEEE Transactions on Systems, Man, and Cybernetics, Part A 35(1), 55–65 (2005)
15. Wyatt, D., Philipose, M., Choudhury, T.: Unsupervised activity recognition using automatically mined common sense. In: 20th National Conference on Artificial Intelligence, Pittsburgh, Pennsylvania, pp. 21–27 (2005)
16. Robben, S., Krose, B.: Longitudinal Residential Ambient Monitoring: Correlating Sensor Data to Functional Health Status. In: 7th International Conference on Pervasive Computing Technologies for Healthcare, PervasiveHealth, pp. 244–247 (2013)
17. Fisher, A.G.: Assessment of Motor and Process Skills, 6th edn. Development, Standardization, and Administration Manual, vol. 1. Three Star Press Inc., Fort Collins (2003)
18. Robben, S., Boot, M., Kanis, M., Kröse, B.: Identifying and Visualizing Relevant Deviations in Longitudinal Sensor Patterns for Care Professionals. In: 7th International Conference on Pervasive Computing Technologies for Healthcare, PervasiveHealth, pp. 416–419 (2013)
19. Virone, G., Sixsmith, A.: Monitoring activity patterns and trends of older adults. In: 30th IEEE Engineering in Medicine and Biology Society, Microtechnologies in Medicine & Biology, pp. 2071–2074 (2008)
20. Yin, G., Bruckner, D.: Daily activity model for ambient assisted living. In: Camarinha-Matos, L.M. (ed.) DoCEIS 2011. IFIP AICT, vol. 349, pp. 197–204. Springer, Heidelberg (2011)
21. Mozer, M.C.: Lessons from an Adaptive Home. In: Cook, D.J., Das, S.K. (eds.) Smart Environments: Technologies, Protocols, and Applications. John Wiley & Sons, Inc., Hoboken (2005)
22. Rivera-Illingworth, F., Callaghan, V., Hagras, H.A.: Neural Network Agent Based Approach to Activity Detection in AmI Environments. In: IEE International Workshop on Intelligent Environments, pp. 92–99 (2005)

Correlating Average Cumulative Movement and Barthel Index in Acute Elderly Care

Michael Walsh[1], Brendan O'Flynn[1], Cian O'Mathuna[1], Anne Hickey[2], and John Kellett[2]

[1] Tyndall National Institute, University College Cork, Cork, Ireland
[2] Mid-Western Regional Hospital, Nenagh, County Tipperary, Ireland
{michael.walsh,brendan.oflynn,cian.omathuna}@tyndall.ie

Abstract. Functional status is a major determinant of clinical outcomes. The Barthel Scale or Barthel Index (BI) is an ordinal scale used to measure performance in activities of daily living. A higher BI is associated with reduced length of stay in hospital and a greater likelihood of being able to live at home with a degree of independence following discharge from hospital. Currently on admission to hospital the BI is assessed subjectively by nursing staff. This work explores the possibility of using wearable wireless inertial measurement as a means of automating and detecting changes in BI. Preliminary findings for a study comprising of 16 patients suggest a correlation (0.7613) between average cumulative movement over 24 hours and variance in BI over the same period.

Keywords: Barthel Index, Activities of Daily Living, Wireless Inertial Measurement.

1 Introduction

The importance of early ambulation to recovery in patient populations is well established [1], [2]. This can in turn be a predictor of complications such as prolonged length of stay (LOS) [3] particularly in older adults [4]. Indeed level of ambulation during the first 48 hours after admission has been directly linked to LOS in geriatric patients [5]. While there have been some recent attempts to establish a basis for therapeutic guidelines regarding ambulation (walking about) in older adults hospitalized for acute illness [6] this work has not encompassed the significant percentage of admissions that are partially or completely bed bound.

Currently upon admission to hospital the mental and functional status of patients are assessed subjectively by nursing and medical staff. In order to make this process more objective and quantifiable several scoring systems to measure these parameters are employed. One such scale the Barthel Index (BI) is an ordinal scale used to measure performance in activities of daily living (ADL) [7]. BI is calculated for each patient considering presence or absence of fecal and urinary incontinence as well as the level of help required with grooming, toilet use, feeding, transfers (e.g. from chair to bed), walking, dressing, climbing stairs and bathing. Usually the patient's performance over the preceding 24-48 hours is important, but longer periods may be relevant.

M.J. O'Grady et al. (Eds.): AmI 2013 Workshops, CCIS 413, pp. 54–63, 2013.
© Springer International Publishing Switzerland 2013

WIMUs have played an important role in inferring metabolic energy expenditure [8-10], measuring gait parameters [11], [12], predicting falls [13], post stroke assessment [14] and detecting activities of daily living [15], [16]. Their extensive uptake is mainly due to the small size, relatively low cost, as well as their ease of integration with existing platforms for sensor networks. The potential therefore exists to employ WIMUs in the clinical setting to measure and track functional status. Introduction of this technology is currently limited mainly because not enough is known about its reliability and robustness in "real life" clinical practice.

Currently all patients admitted to the Elderly Care Unit in Nenagh Hospital are assessed using multiple scoring systems, and all the parameters of these scores are being entered into a computer database. This score is subsequently used to determine the intensity of care required. This work proposes the attachment of a wireless inertial measurement unit (WIMU) to each patient for the first 24 hours following admission. The devices transmit all movement recorded during this time. These continuous streams of data are subsequently analyzed to determine if average cumulative patterns of movement can be correlated with changes in BI recorded upon admission and taken again after 24 hours.

2   System Architecture

This section provides a description of the hardware and software employed for the clinical study along with an outline of how average cumulative movement and BI are recorded.

2.1   Infrastructure Description

In the first instance WIMUs were designed and manufactured. The WIMU is comprised of two separate modular components. The data processing and communications module consists of the Atmega1281 microcontroller (Atmel Corp.) and the EM2420 (Ember Corp.) 802.15.4 compliant transceiver. The inertial module has onboard circuitry for battery recharging and signal conditioning. It includes the ADXL330 (Analog Devices, Inc) low power, complete 3-axis accelerometer. This component was selected as it can capture dynamic movement as well as static acceleration of gravity in tilt-sensing applications. The WIMU is programmed using the TinyOS embedded operating system. Sampling frequency for this study was set to 200Hz. Care was given when selecting communications channel so as to avoid interference from the Wifi. The WIMU forwards time stamped data to the base station unit shown in Fig. 1 which in turn sends data via USB to a PC.

Wireless networks are inherently lossy due mainly to the propagation environment in which they operate. While most non-safety critical applications will ignore that some data will inevitably be lost this attribute is less acceptable in the clinical environment. To overcome this limitation a custom multi-hopping protocol was developed for this work. To illustrate how the protocol works the elderly care unit at Nenagh hospital, where the trial is ongoing, is shown in Fig. 2(a). The base station unit is located in the nurses office. There are two mains powered repeater nodes which relay data from the WIMUs to the base station. Rather than establishing a route to the central access point based on link quality or network traffic as is generally the case in multi-tier networks, this protocol allows the data travelling through the network to arrive at the base station via multiple paths.

Packaging the WIMUs so that they are deployable in the clinical setting is a key element to the adoption of this type of wearable technology. A number of enclosures were designed ensuring the devices would be as user friendly as possible while also adhering to the stringent hygiene requirements of hospital use. Fig. 2(b) illustrates the custom made plastic enclosure selected for use in the trial which exposes an on/off switch and a mini USB connection for recharging the device.

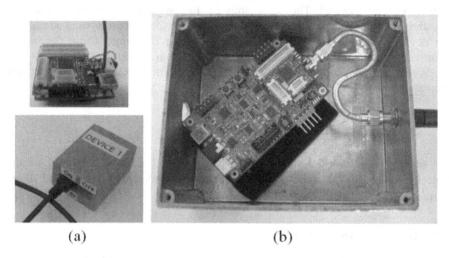

(a)   (b)

Fig. 1. (a) WIMU Technology (top), Packaged and charging (bottom), (b) Shielded base station unit

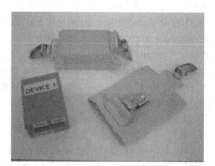

Fig. 2. (a) Network topology for the Elderly Care Unit (b) Cloth enclosure for WIMU ensuring the devices remain sterile while minimising artefact introduction

2.2   Graphical User Interface

A user friendly GUI has been developed as part of this work and is shown in Fig. 4. The GUI is designed with nursing needs in mind and following further consultation with the nursing staff the following functionalities were included. The 'Add Patient' button allows a patient to be added to the system. Once pressed the nurse is required to input patient name, patient hospital number and the number of the WIMU to be attached. The 'Remove Patient' button allows a patient to be removed from the system following 24 hours of assessment. If an event of importance occurs while the patient is instrumented an 'Add Note' button allows the nurse to input details of the event. For instance if a patient were to have a fall, become unresponsive or exhibit agitation this would be recorded. These events are later correlated with WIMU data to determine if the event has been flagged by the system. A 'Device Active' LED light indicates that the device is functioning as it should. If the device is switched off, running low on battery or out of wireless communications range this light switches off.

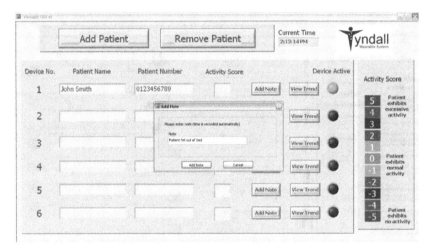

Fig. 3. Labview Graphical User Interface

2.3   Calculating Average Cumulative Movement over 24 Hours

Data is captured in real-time and forwarded to the base station as illustrated in Fig. 2(b). Information is then sent via USB to the GUI (Fig. 4) where it is parsed and stored for analysis. Raw accelerometer is employed to calculate cumulative movement σ on a per minute basis as follows:

$$\sigma = \sum_{k=1}^{n} \sqrt{(x_k - x_{k-1})^2 + (y_k - y_{k-1})^2 + (y_k - y_{k-1})^2} \tag{1}$$

where k is the sample number, n is the number of samples per minute, x_k, y_k and z_k are the x-axis, y-axis and z-axis accelerometer readings at sample k. This simple approach measures cumulative movement overtime including all three axes. As it is singularly the variation between subsequent samples that is measured this makes the score independent of acceleration due to gravity and calibration as well as more robust to sensor drift over prolonged periods of measurement. The score is finally averaged over a 24 hour period to determine average cumulative movement.

2.4   Barthel Index Calculation

As mentioned previously upon admission to the Mid-Western Regional Hospital in Nenagh currently all patients are assessed using multiple scoring systems and all the parameters of these scores are entered into a computer database. The medical assessment input screen for calculating BI is illustrated in Fig. 5 below. This user interface allows the medical care giver to subjectively access the patient in terms of the presence or absence of fecal and urinary incontinence as well as the level of help required with grooming, toilet use, feeding, transfers (e.g. from chair to bed), walking, dressing, climbing stairs and bathing. The care giver is immediately presented with the resulting BI calculation along with a falls risk score.

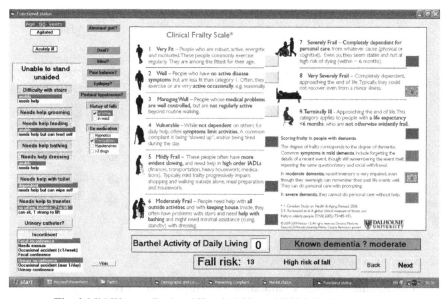

Fig. 4. Mid-Western Regional Hospital, Nenagh BI Medical Assessment

3   Results and Discussion

For the purpose of this work this assessment is carried out upon admission and following 24 hours of the patient being instrumented with a WIMU. Data from 16 patients has been gathered and analysed extensively. All subjects involved in the study were over 80 years of age at the time of data capture. Fig. 6 illustrates average cumulative movement for the 16 patient cohort. The WIMUs were placed in the torso of each patient for the data capture. Fig. 7 illustrates BI for 16 patients recorded immediately following admission (green line) and again measured 24 hours later (dashed blue line) employing the computerised system shown in Fig. 5. BI ranging from values of 0 to 20 are present in the data indicating a sample cohort with widely varying functional status. Fig. 8 illustrates the variation in BI for each of the patients over the 24 hour period ranging from a decrease in BI by as much as 3 to an increase in BI by 3 also again indicating a widely dispersed sample.

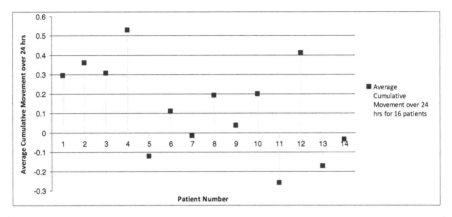

Fig. 5. Average cumulative movement over 24 hours for 16 patients

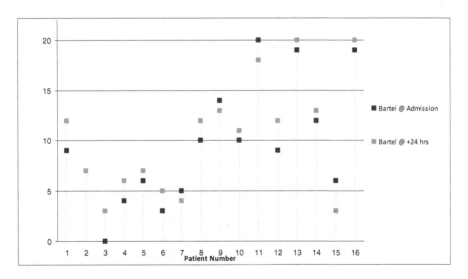

Fig. 6. BI recorded following admission and again 24 hours later for the 16 patient cohort

Fig. 9 illustrates average cumulative movement recorded over a 24 hour period for 16 patients plotting versus variations in BI for that same period. There is a clear correlation between increased negative BI and lower average cumulative movement and increased positive BI and higher average cumulative movement. The indication is that there is a relationship, quantifiable as a correlation value of 0.7613, between variations in BI and average cumulative movement for the cohort of patients.

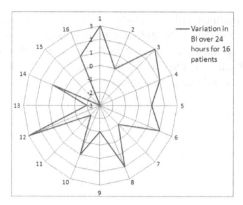

Fig. 7. Variation in BI over a 24 hour period for 16 patients

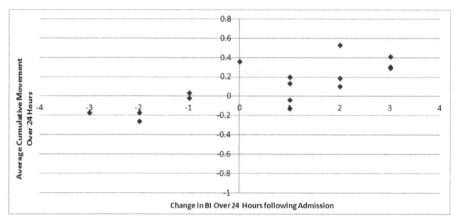

Fig. 8. Average cumulative movement recorded over 24 hours compared with variations in BI over the same period for 16 patients

3.1   Analysis Breakdown by Gender

The question then arises if the relationship is gender biased and while the sample cohort is small a breakdown of the results is useful. Of the 16 subjects involved in the study 7 were male and 9 were female. Fig. 10 (a) and (b) illustrate the variation in BI for male and female subjects respectively over the 24 hour period and in both cases the data sets range from a decrease in BI by as much as 3 to an increase in BI by 3 also again indicating a well dispersed sample.

Fig. 11 illustrates average cumulative movement recorded over a 24 hour period for 7 male patients plotting versus variations in BI for that same period. There is a clear correlation between increased negative BI and lower average cumulative movement and increased positive BI and higher average cumulative movement. The indication is that there is a relationship, quantifiable as a correlation value of 0.8354, between variations in BI and average cumulative movement for the male cohort of patients. Fig. 12 illustrates that there is a relationship, quantifiable as a correlation value of 0.6359, between variations in BI and average cumulative movement for the

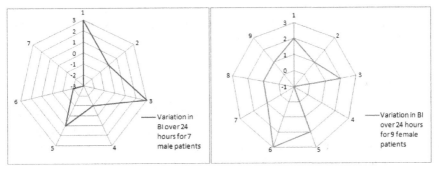

Fig. 9. Variation in BI over a 24 hour period for (a) 7 male patients and (b) 9 female patients

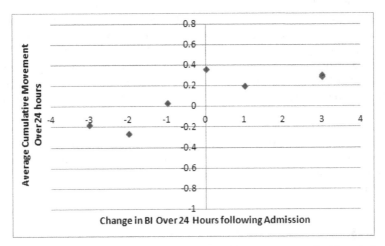

Fig. 10. Average cumulative movement recorded over 24 hours compared with variations in BI over the same period for 7 male patients

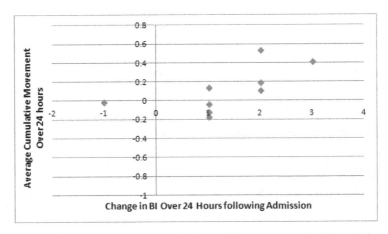

Fig. 11. Average cumulative movement recorded over 24 hours compared with variations in BI over the same period for 9 female patients

female cohort of patients. There is clearly a bias toward a stronger correlation for the male component of the patient cohort which requires further study and a larger sample group to validate and begin to understand.

4   Conclusion

This paper has provided a system description and preliminary results for a preliminary clinical study carried out at the Mid-Western Regional Hospital, Nenagh, Ireland. The system was designed in consultation with the medical staff in the Elderly Care Unit to be as user friendly as possible and deployable in a real clinical setting.

The study involving a 16 patient cohort was designed to explore the relationship between variations in Barthel Index (BI) and average cumulative movement over a 24 hour period following admission. A statistically significant correlation was shown to exist between variations in BI and average cumulative movement. This relationship was shown to be biased toward the male subjects in the patient cohort.

This phase of the research will be followed by a further trial involving a larger cohort of patients where attempts will be made to validate the findings of this preliminary study. In addition the bias toward the male component of the patient cohort will be studied in more detail.

Automating BI, which has been shown to have portability and has been used in a diagnostic capacity, by capturing average cumulative movement employing wearable technology could allow for earlier intervention and provide a stepping stone toward the automation of patient electronic medical records reducing what is a significant draw on medical staff's time.

References

1. Mundy, L.M., Leet, T.L., Darst, K., Schnitzler, M.A., Dunagan, W.C.: Early mobilization of patients hospitalized with community-acquired pneumonia. Chest 124(3), 883–889 (2003)
2. Harpur, J.E., Conner, W.T., Hamilton, M., et al.: Controlled trial of early mobilisation and discharge from hospital in uncomplicated myocardial infarction. Lancet 2(7738), 1331–1334 (1971)
3. Kamel, H.K., Iqbal, M.A., Mogallapu, R., Maas, D., Hoffmann, R.G.: Time to ambulation after hip fracture surgery: relation to hospitalization outcomes. J. Gerontol. A Biol. Sci. Med. Sci. 58(11), 1042–1045 (2003)
4. Fisher, S.R., Kuo, Y., Graham, J.E., Ottenbacher, K., Ostir, G.V.: Early ambulation and length of stay in older adults hospitalized for acute illness. Arch. Intern. Med. 170(21), 1942–1943 (2010)
5. Brown, C.J., Friedkin, R.J., Inouye, S.K.: Prevalence and outcomes of low mobility in hospitalized older patients. J. Am. Geriatr. Soc. 52(8), 1263–1270 (2004)
6. Fisher, S.R., Graham, J.E., Brown, C.J., Galloway, C.V., Ottenbacher, K.J., Allman, R.M., Ostir, G.V.: Factors that differentiate level of ambulation in hospitalised older adults. Age Ageing 41(1), 107–111 (2012)
7. Mahoney, F., Barthel, D.: Functional evaluation: the Barthel Index. Maryland State Med. Journal 14, 56–61 (1965)

8. Choi, J.H., Lee, J., Hwang, H.T., Kim, J.P., Park, J.C., Shin, K.: Estimation of activity energy expenditure: Accelerometer approach. In: 27th Annual International Conference of the Engineering in Medicine and Biology Society, IEEE-EMBS 2005, pp. 3830–3833 (2005)

9. Swartz, A., Strath, S., Bassett, D., O'Brien, W., King, G., Ainsworth, B.: Estimation of energy expenditure using CSA accelerometersat hip and wrist sites. Med. Sci. Sports Exer. 32, S450–S456 (2000)

10. Crouter, S., Clowers, K., Bassett, D.: A novel method for using accelerometer data to predict energy expenditure. J. Appl. Physiol. 100, 1324–1331 (2006)

11. Ramachandran, R., Ramanna, L., Ghasemzadeh, H., Pradhan, G., Jafari, R., Prabhakaran, B.: Body sensor networks to evaluate standing balance: interpreting muscular activities based on inertial sensors. In: HealthNet 2008: Proceedings of the 2nd International Workshop on Systems and Networking Support for Health Care and Assisted Living Environments, pp. 1–6. ACM, New York (2008)

12. Mayagoitia, R., Lotters, J., Veltink, P.H., Hermens, H.: Standing balance evaluation using a triaxial accelerometer. Gait and Posture 16(1), 55–59 (2002)

13. Bourke, A., O'Brien, J., Lyons, G.: Evaluation of a thresholdbased tri-axial accelerometer fall detection algorithm. Gait and Posture 26(2), 194–199 (2007)

14. Wade, E., Parnandi, A.R., Mataric, M.J.: Automated administration of the wolf motor function test for post-stroke assessment. In: 2010 4th International Conference on Pervasive Computing Technologies for Healthcare, PervasiveHealth, pp. 1–7. IEEE (2010)

15. Atallah, L., Yang, G.: The use of pervasive sensing for behaviour profiling – a survey. Pervasive and Mobile Computing 5(5), 447–464 (2009)

16. Yang, J.Y., Wang, J.S., Chen, Y.P.: Using acceleration measurements for activity recognition: An effective learning algorithm for constructing neural classifiers. Pattern Recognition Letters 29(16), 2213–2220 (2008)

Object Tracking AAL Application and Behaviour Modelling for the Elderly and Visually Impaired

Dimitris M. Kyriazanos, George E. Vastianos, Olga E. Segou,
and Stelios C.A. Thomopoulos

NCSR "Demokritos", Institute of Informatics and Telecommunications, Athens, Greece
{dkyri,gvastian,osegou,scat}@iit.demokritos.gr

Abstract. Different degrees and types of visual impairment have become a common condition among the elderly, as aging inevitably affects the health and lifestyle of individuals. Partial or complete lack of sight is often accompanied by other ailments and conditions which further hinder the individual's activities. In this work, a novel Ambient Assisted Living (AAL) platform is proposed, aiming to support the functional capabilities of the elderly and visually impaired, thus ameliorating their lifestyle. This platform is based on indoor tracking of commonly used objects, such as medication packages. Accompanied by a proposed behavioural modeling methodology, the application also offers valuable observations that may indicate developing ill-health conditions in an early stage. The proposed platform was tested and evaluated by end-users in Spain, Greece and Finland.

Keywords: AAL applications, object tracking, indoor localisation, behaviour modelling.

1 Introduction

As time passes and old age further progresses, the physiology of an individual's eyes manifests significant changes. Eye tissue is susceptible to losing its flexibility, suffering from damages caused by everyday life, other health conditions (such as diabetes or blood pressure) and gravity.

While our capability to prevent vision impairment with technology is very limited, there are promising solutions aiming to support the visually impaired elderly in better managing their everyday lives with the help of modern information and communication technology. The authors' research explores the possibilities for improving the quality of life by providing service access for the visually impaired elderly using services related to (a) medication and medicine related information and services, and (b) health monitoring. Other AAL applications for the visually impaired, focus on object inspection via RFID-enabled pens or smartphones that allow the user to record an audio description of tagged objects [3-5] without offering object tracking services. Object tracking via visual recognition and 3D modeling has also been proposed, aiming more at obstacle recognition and navigation rather than tracking of small packets

M.J. O'Grady et al. (Eds.): AmI 2013 Workshops, CCIS 413, pp. 64–77, 2013.
© Springer International Publishing Switzerland 2013

[6]. Moreover, visual tracking systems are considered to be less respectful of the individual's privacy and inadequate in this context.

RFID technology has been applied in relevant research in AAL scenarios, confirming our selection of UHF RFID technology as a most promising for future AAL applications as also [7] states. However where other studies apply smart tags and more complex body monitoring analytic procedures, our study relies solely in passive RFID technology for object tracking, imposing constraints in terms of performance and functionalities on the one side, having however the advantages of energy, cost efficiency and enhanced privacy – since we track specific objects on demand and not track people constantly.

Other object tracking technologies that have been proposed outside the AAL context [8-11], utilize more complex and bulky sensors which would add weight to the medication packages and require an external power source; thus, they were not considered to be appropriate for use. However, the platform described herein, is based on passive RFID tags that do not require a power source and feature a minimal size and weight. Moreover by applying UHF RFID technology, more capabilities in medication and object tracking are offered due to the increased range, compared to touch and very short range radio technologies like NFC [12].

In the context of interacting with the user, relevant research on audio sensing technology [13] for a voice-commanded smart home could offer a suitable User Interface (UI) for severe visual impairments. The current UI is mostly adapted to common visual impairments found among the elderly. Object tracking service however is designed to interface with both text/visual and audio UIs.

Taking into account user feedback collected from elderly homes and national blind people associations in Spain, Finland and Greece, a medication and object tracking application was developed, and an appropriate UI was designed based on the extracted guidelines. The application aims to offer people with visual impairments assistance with finding their medication and other personal objects in indoor environments, all of which are tagged with passive RFID tags, featuring multimodal interaction and indoor tracking services.

The medication or any object tracking service request is initiated on demand by the user, when he realizes he can't find a specific object. The system receives the request and retrieves the [x,y] location for the specific object provided the localization service is operating normally or the last known [x,y] location for the object in case of RFID tag "invisibility". The estimated location of the object is correlated with other objects in the indoor environment taking into account mobility and physical parameters of all objects involved. The result of this correlation is a user friendly and understandable description of where the object should be. The description is provided as text to the multi-modal UIs for presentation to the user. If required (e.g. in unknown environments) navigation instructions can also be included based on an initial reference point. The system can receive an optional acknowledgment by the user that the object was found or a new request indicating that the object was not found in the initially specified location. In the case where the object is not actually tracked the system can offer alternative potential suggestions on where the object could be based on the tracking history.

The RFID setup for this application includes an RFID reader connected with 8 antennas all of which are mounted on the ceiling of the indoor area covered. Regarding User Interface and Use Case Scenario, the application was integrated into an integrated Medication Planning application, offering large readable prompts on a touch screen, while a clear voice also announces text that appears on screen. The system presented in this application was installed and tested inside Tecnalia's Homelab [1] at Bilbao, Spain, as shown in Fig. 1.

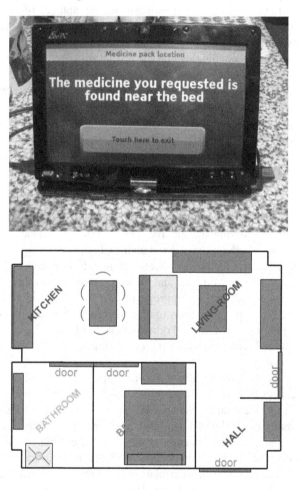

Fig. 1. Medication Tracking Service UI (up) and map of Tecnalia Homelab (down)

The complete scenario as it was implemented and tested at Bilbao, along with the UI detailed paper prototype, is provided in the following section. Section 3 presents the enabling framework for object tracking, including the software and hardware architecture descriptions. In Section 4 the authors present a methodology for mapping behaviour observations and a behavioural model based on the tracking of everyday objects, enhancing in this way the system presented to detect changes that may help indicate health complications.

2   Scenario and UI Prototype

In this section, we go through the use case scenario for medication package tracking inside the user's home. After each screen the corresponding scenario step is described, along with all interaction modalities offered to the user.

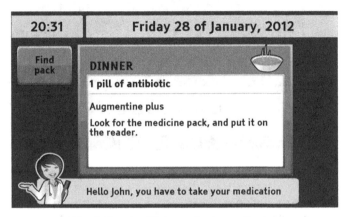

Fig. 2. Step 1 – Time to take the medication

STEP 1: In the above screen (Fig. 2), a beeping sound is heard as it is time for the user (here named John) to take his medication. Once the user taps on the screen, the user can see the screen above and a synthesized yet natural sounding human voice announces "Hello John (User profile name here), it is time to take your medication". The user can't find the medication so he touches the "Find Pack" button on the screen.

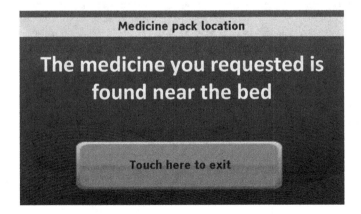

Fig. 3. Step 2a – Medication found

STEP 2a: the application has searched for and found the medicine near the bed. The above screen (Fig. 3) appears almost immediately informing the user with the message above. The voice announces: "The medicine you requested is found near the bed". The user goes and searches on the bed, founds the medicine and then touches on the "Touch here to exit" button to return to the previous screen.

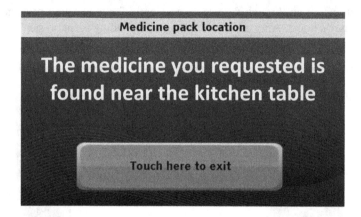

Fig. 4. Step 2b – Medication found (alternate location)

STEP 2b: (alternate location) the application has searched and found the medicine near the kitchen table. The above screen appears (Fig. 4) almost immediately informing the user with the message above. The voice announces: "The medicine you requested is found near the kitchen table". The user goes and searches on the kitchen table, founds the medicine and then touches on the "Touch here to exit" button to return to the previous screen.

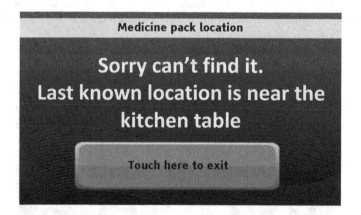

Fig. 5. Step 2c – Last known location feature

STEP 2c: the application can't find the medicine right now but remembers where it was the last time it could find it. The above screen appears (Fig. 5) almost immediately informing the user with the message above. The voice announces: "Sorry can't find it. Last known location is near the kitchen table". The user goes and searches on the kitchen table and then touches on the "Touch here to exit" button to return to the previous screen.

3   Evaluation Results

Besides on-site evaluation and following the release of the prototype application, end user paper prototyping evaluation interviews were also conducted in Finland, Spain and Greece, including caregivers, health professionals as well as care center residents. As key results from general and usability findings, the following have been selected:

- In general, the usefulness of the service was successfully validated. Besides medication packages, help to find any other objects like glasses, keys, TV remote control, and so on should be more demanded by elderly users at home, and more often than medication packages. As the application and system is designed to support tracking of any kind of object (except liquids and metal objects that can interfere with the RFID efficiency) this is a feature already supported.
- A challenge was identified in reaching the user group and making them to realize how useful the service would be (marketing). Price vs. quality should be good, and the system should be easy to manage. If also the relatives could add reminders, it would have business potential.
- When targeting users suffering from dementia, improved guidance and navigation instructions would be required.

Proceeding to more usability and evaluation findings, caregivers participating in the evaluation mentioned that they would probably be able to learn to use this system by themselves. Also older people who don't suffer from severe problems with cognitive skills and memory and who have some experience of technology could use this (at least after the proposed changes and improvements).

Older people, who have some memory problems and are not experienced with technology, could be able to use this, but they would need a lot of training and support. People with severe memory problems and those who are not willing to take their medicine could not use this.

This would be suitable for a person who is living independently, who has only some problems with his/her eyesight, who have medicine dispenser and who is still able to take medicines by himself/herself.

System use would have potential benefits for nurses. Reminder –functionality could bring more flexibility for nurses' schedules, because they could postpone the visits half an hour or so (many older people take their medicines at the same time, which is problematic for the nurses who visit them).

The following difficulties and risks in the system use were identified from the group interview:

- The older person is not present when the system reminds him/her -should it be in a mobile phone also?
- With the current user interface, the user might not understand that it is time to take the medicines.
- How power failure would influence on the system use? mobile phones usually alarm also when the power is off, how about computers?
- People could get dependent on the technology. It is typical is care work that when people are provided with some help, they'll take less independent initiatives to do things afterwards.
- If the person is near the system and the system works, it could help to find the medicine package.
- If a person with severe memory problems would use this how we could be sure that he/she takes his/her medicines and the correct amount?
- If a person would like to cheat with his/her medication taking, it would be easier to do. And who would be responsible about the possible consequences?
- There's a risk if relatives of an older person would buy this and think that now the older person can manage at home independently. Care professionals should always evaluate the situation (using e.g. memory test) and then consider if the service is suitable.

There are some groups of people who suffer from difficulty of taking initiatives by themselves. They have difficulties "to get things done" without personal advisor and support. These groups involve people with minor memory loss, people with disabilities and people with some neurological diseases. They would benefit from reminder - not just medicine reminder, but a more general "life instructor".

Home care customers typically suffer from severe memory loss or they are not willing to take their medicines without help. Thus, they would not benefit from ICT based medicine reminder that much. The potential user group includes people who don't yet have difficult cognitive and memory problems. In practice, the reminder service would be useful for anybody, such as people who are still in work life. The difficulty is in reaching this user group and making them to realise how useful the service would be (marketing). Price vs. quality should be good, and the system should be easy to manage. If also the relatives could add reminders, it would have business potential.

4   The Framework for Object Tracking in Indoor Environments

The proposed framework consists of the software architecture, the hardware platform and the ontology and reasoning models, described each in the following sub-sections.

4.1   System Architecture

The overall architecture of the Indoor Object Tracking Solution is depicted in Fig. 6, consisting of two main, interconnected components: the Object Tracking Information

Management Server and the RFID Localization Module. The former encapsulates the main application logic, handling HMI feedback and requests, and extracting valuable rulings and conclusions based on the information stored in the repository. The latter is the module enabling the localization of RFID-tagged objects based on location determination algorithms and RFID infrastructure, providing location information to the Server and receiving information regarding its operation. A short description of each subcomponent follows, along with specifications for each interconnecting interface, shown in the picture as ia, ib, ic, id and ie.

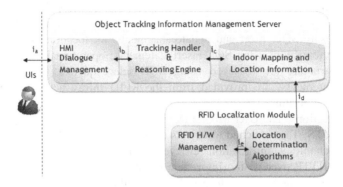

Fig. 6. Indoor Object Mapping & Tracking Solution - Overall Architecture

HMI Dialogue Management: here requests and responses from and to the UIs are managed. Multi-modal UIs may exist as described based on the type and level of user accessibility requirements. This component is responsible for receiving and parsing requests, forwarding extracted information to the reasoning, receiving feedback and finally preparing the reply "package" for the corresponding UI.

Tracking Handler & Reasoning Engine: this is the engine responsible for managing information stored in the repository in order to extract valuable conclusions for the user regarding the location of the object the user wishes to track. The [x,y] of the object is not understandable by the user. Instead this component compiles a user-friendly description of the estimated location of the object. The engine is also responsible for configuring and fine-tuning the operation of the RFID Module by checking and updating appropriate fields on the repository. This is also connected with the location determination reasoning: e.g. in case of RFID technology shortcoming, tracking history as well as indoor map and object correlations will be consulted from the repository.

Indoor Mapping and Location Information: this is the repository where relevant information and ontology models are implemented and populated. More details on the ontology and reasoning modeling are provided in the following section.

Location Determination Algorithms: here the location determination algorithms are implemented in order to determine and provide to the repository the [x,y] of the RFID-tagged objects based on input from the RFID infrastructure.

RFID H/W Management: the component managing the RFID hardware, namely the operation of RFID readers and of the array of antennas based on the operational requirements stored in the repository (i.e. frequency of RFID tag scanning and intervals). The main tasks are to collect the data from "visible" RFID tags and feed the algorithms in order to determine the [x,y] of the RFID-tagged objects.

Interface Analysis: ia: provides to the Object Tracking IMS the request with the id of the object the user wishes to track; returns to the UIs a "packaged" response with the text with a user-friendly description of the location of the object. The interface is standardized to support multiple UIs (XML and SOAP). ib: provides the id of the object to be located as parsed information element to the tracking handler and reasoning component; returns the text information containing a user-friendly description of the location of the object. ic: extracts information from the repository using SQL select queries; updates information regarding localization history and RFID operation parameters using SQL insert and update statements. id: location of objects [x,y] is stored in the repository using SQL insert statements; operational parameters for the RFID infrastructure are retrieved using SQL select queries. ie: RFID tag data (RSSI measurements) are provided from the RFID infrastructure to the location determination algorithms

Communications: The User Mobile Device access Web Services, either over wi-fi or GPRS/UMTS. Tags attached to objects communicate with the appropriate Reader via RFID technology. Information retrieved by Readers is sent to the Application Server over HTTP over wi-fi. Information sent over HTTP will follow a standard format, defined using the SOAP format. Privacy will be safeguarded, via use of secure channels in case of Wi-Fi and Bluetooth (SSL) and privacy enhanced tags in case of RFID.

4.2   RFID Hardware Platform

RFID Hardware Platform is an in-house developed cost-effective solution by NCSR Demokritos for object localization using passive UHF RFID tags and a single reader with up to nine multiplexed antennas. Localization of objects is achieved either using the cell-id of the specific multiplexed antenna or based on the combined received signal strength at the antennas. Detailed description of the platform along with testing results and performance evaluation can be found in [2].

5   Extracting Behaviour Observations and Modelling Methodology

The process of assisting people with visual impairments to locate their medication and everyday activity objects (e.g. glasses, keys, TV remote control, books and dvd/cd cases) allows for the collection of behavioral data. This fact motivated the research, whose concept and methodology is presented in this section.

Users' duration of activities, their habits as well as their reactions to the system's assistance, are queues that can be used as input for a behavior model. Our hypothesis is that by monitoring subtle changes in user behavior and by mapping these changes to a representation of the user's mood, we can detect changes that may help indicate health complications.

5.1   Proposed Methodology

The authors wish to investigate the user modeling possibilities offered by the existing HMFM system and establish a plan for future work and research. In particular we wish to develop a model of the patient's affective state and use it to detect abnormalities and study long term behavior trends non intrusively. In order to do so, first we need to identify three key parameters: i) what user states are deemed relevant in the context of the application, ii) based on which methodology could the observed behavior be associated with these states, iii) what would be the added value of such an approach.

5.2   Behavior Tracking

The existing system allows for the observation of user behavior while locating and taking their daily prescribed medication. For the purposes of this study, the system needs to enhance its tracking methods. Parameters such as the types of requests the user makes, the frequency of certain requests and the speed in which the patient responds to the system's advice need to be carefully monitored. Moreover, on a higher level observation of forgetfulness patterns or context information associated with the occurrence of specific events (i.e. the patient tends have slower responses in the evening etc) is of particular interest.

5.3   Choosing an Affective State Representation

According to state of the art research on modeling user affect there exist three coarse affective state representations - namely: categorical representations, dimensional descriptions and appraisal representations. The selection of any one depends on the application at hand [14].

Categorical representations are the simplest and most wide-spread, using a word to describe an emotional state. Such category sets have been proposed on different grounds, including evolutionarily basic emotion categories [15][16]; most frequent everyday emotions [21]; application-specific emotion sets; or categories describing other affective states, such as moods or interpersonal stances.

Dimensional descriptions capture essential properties of emotional states, such as arousal (active/passive) and valence (negative/positive). Emotion dimensions can be used to describe general emotional tendencies, including low-intensity emotions. There exist several dimensional representations of emotion either in two [20][23] or three dimensions i.e. pleasure-arousal-dominance by Mehrabian [18]. According to a recent cross-cultural study by Fontaine et al (2007) the number of dimensions adopted is closely related to the research question at hand.

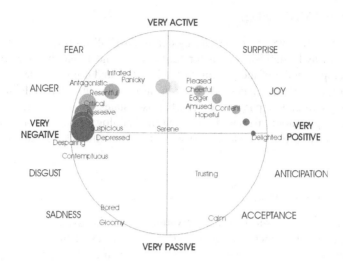

Fig. 7. Whissel's dimensional representation of emotion and the Feeltrace tool [24]

Appraisal representations characterize emotional states in terms of the detailed evaluations of eliciting conditions, such as their familiarity, intrinsic pleasantness, or relevance to one's goals. Such detail can be used to characterize the cause or object of an emotion as it arises from the context, or to predict emotions in AI systems [19][22]

Based on the results of a preliminary evaluation study of the current system we propose the use of a two dimensional representation of the user's affective state. The nature of the data collected does not allow for deeper reasoning on the user's affective state beyond the dimensions of activation/arousal (active, passive) and evaluation/valence (positive, negative) at this point. Results from this approach could feed into a more complicated future study, using appraisal representations based on specific patient goals and interpretations of events. The patient's activation/arousal will be monitored on a daily basis, with a frequency that will derive from his/her medication schedule.

5.4   Ground Truth

In addressing question (ii) and associating this behavioral input with specific affective states or values on the dimensions of valence and arousal, ground truth data needs to be collected. In order to do so a pilot study is advisable. This study should comprise of patients using the system on a daily basis and participating in short interviews at the end of each day. The interviews will aim to collect feedback on the patient's mood during the day. This feedback will be used as input and create associations between the collected data on the patient's behavior and her affective state. In this context there is insufficient data for drawing conclusions on the user's affective state every instant. Thus her affective state over a given period of time will be observed – her mood state. These periods can be selected based on daily activities such as meals and nap/sleep/active times.

5.5   Model Output

The collected ground truth will be used as input for the process of training a Sugeno type neuro-fuzzy neural network in order to classify user behavior to affective states - expressed in dimensions of arousal and valence. This type of neural network performs well both approximation and generalization wise. Training of the network will produce a set of rules and membership functions that will be used as a tool for automatically annotating novel patient behavior.

5.6   Evaluation of Model Performance

In order to test the performance of the proposed behavior model, more data needs to be collected keeping in mind the guidelines put forward. The performance can then be evaluated using the four typical performance measures of a confusion matrix.

5.7   Added Value in Healthcare

The added value of the suggested approach is the automated monitoring of the user's mood. This allows for the quick identification of abnormal mood swings that could be signaling changes or anomalies in the user's health. Furthermore, the user's mood states are inferred through her actions without the use of intrusive sensors.

6   Conclusions and Future Work

The authors presented in this paper the scenario and UI prototype for an AAL application offering medication tracking capabilities for the elderly and visually impaired people. The application was evaluated in the challenging usability requirements environment surrounding AAL applications, with key findings being also reported.

Moreover, the authors presented the enabling underlying framework which supports various novel applications for RFID-tagged object tracking in indoor environments. The framework's architecture design allows adaptation to different levels of geographic abstraction and location estimation accuracy, meeting requirements for a wide range of object tracking applications.

As the system monitors and tracks objects in an unobtrusive for the user way, the authors were motivated to explore the value of observation data in the area of behavioural modeling,   analyzing activity, health and mood levels in the process, and with the potential beneficial capability of identified developing disorders or diseases. Concepts and proposed methodology were presented, which expect to bear interesting results in the near future.

Future work includes (i) applying the behavioural modeling methodology for the user's activity, health and mood level in real conditions and using actual data and (ii) evaluating the model's performance.

Acknowledgments. This work is partially funded by (a) "HMFM" (HMFM-FP7-AAL-2008-1/ET: 13591-07/07/2009); "TASS" (TASS-FP7-SEC-2010-241905) and "DITSEF" (DITSEF-FP7-ICT-SEC-2007-1-225404) research projects funded by the European Commission and, in part, by the General Secretariat of Research and Technology (GSRT) of the Ministry of Education, Greece; (b) a Ph.D. Fellowship of NCSR "Demokritos" and the Hellenic Ministry of Education; The authors would like to acknowledge the Tecnalia (Health and Quality of Life Unit) and its research staff for the use of its HomeLab facilities as testbed and demonstrator of the Passive RFID localization system in the context of the HMFM project, and the permission to use the floor layout of the HomeLab shown in Figure 1. The authors would also like to cordially thank their HMFM colleagues from VTT and Technalia for conducting end user interviews in Finland and Spain.

References

1. Tecnalia, Health and Quality of Life Unit,
   http://www.tecnalia.info/sect_salud_calidad.php?lang=en&PHPSESSID=kv1bf2a4s94m11s7vk0rrqbp41
2. Vastianos, G.E., Kyriazanos, D.M., Segou, O.E., Mitilineos, S.A., Thomopoulos, S.C.A.: Indoor Localization Using Passive RFID. In: Proceedings of SPIE Defense, Security, and Sensing, Orlando, Florida, USA, April 25-29 (2011)
3. IDBLUE RFID Stylus, http://idblue.com/products
4. U-SPEAK Voice Recording Pen,
   http://nlcco.co.jp/english0/products.html
5. SeeingEyePhone, http://mocs.vtt.fi/resource_center/videos.html
6. Hub, A., Hartter, T., Ertl, T.: Interactive Tracking of Movable Objects for the Blind on the Basis of Environment Models and Perception-Oriented Object Recognition Methods. In: ASSETS 2006, Portland, Oregon, USA, October 22-25 (2006)
7. Álvarez, J.A., Pérez, C., Angulo, C., Antonio Ortega, J.: Combining Smart Tags and Body Fixed Sensors for Disabled People Assistance. In: Apolloni, B., Howlett, R.J., Jain, L. (eds.) KES 2007, Part II. LNCS (LNAI), vol. 4693, pp. 10–17. Springer, Heidelberg (2007)
8. Priyantha, N.B., Chakraborty, A., Balakrishnan, H.: The Cricket Location-Support system. In: Proc. 6th ACM MOBICOM, Boston, MA (August 2000)
9. Mitilineos, S.A., Goufas, J.N., Segou, O.E., Thomopoulos, S.C.A.: WAX-ROOM: an indoor WSN-based localization platform. In: 2010 Symposium on Proceedings of the XIXth SPIE Conference on Signal Processing, Sensor Fusion and Target Recognition – SPIE Defense Security and Sensing 13, pp. 1–5, April 5-9 (2010)
10. Tüchler, M., Schwarz, V., Huber, A.: Location accuracy of an UWB localization system in a multi-path environment. In: IEEE International Conference on Ultra-Wideband, Zurich (September 2005)
11. Want, R., Hopper, A., Falcão, V., Gibbons, J.: The active badge location system. ACM Trans. Inf. Syst. 10(1), 91–102 (1992)
12. Isomursu, M., Ervasti, M., Tormanen, V.: Medication management support for vision impaired elderly: Scenarios and technological possibilities. In: 2nd International Symposium on Applied Sciences in Biomedical and Communication Technologies, ISABEL 2009, November 24-27, pp. 1–6 (2009)

13. Vacher, M., Portet, F., Fleury, A., Noury, N.: Development of Audio Sensing Technology for Ambient Assisted Living: Applications and Challenges. IJEHMC 2.1 (2011), 35-54. Web (October 11, 2013), doi:10.4018/jehmc.2011010103

14. Cowie, R.: Emotion-oriented systems: the Humaine handbook. Springer-Verlag New York Inc. (2011)

15. Ekman, P., Friesen, W.V.: Pictures of facial affect (1976)

16. Izard, C.E., Ellis, C.: The face of emotion. Appleton-Century-Crofts, New York (1971)

17. Fontaine, J.R.J., Scherer, K.R., Roesch, E.B., Ellsworth, P.C.: The world of emotions is not two-dimensional. Psychological Science 18(12), 1050–1057 (2007)

18. Mehrabian, A.: Pleasure-arousal-dominance: A general framework for describing and measuring individual differences in temperament. Current Psychology: Developmental, Learning, Personality, Social 14, 261–292 (1996)

19. Ortony, A., Collins, A., Clore, G.L.: The Cognitive Structure of Emotions. Cambridge University Press (1988)

20. Russell, J.A.: A circumplex model of affect. Journal of Personality and Social Psychology 39, 1161–1178 (1980)

21. Schröder, M., Pirker, H., Lamolle, M.: First suggestions for an emotion annotation and representation language. In: Proceedings of LREC, vol. 6, pp. 88–92 (2006)

22. Scherer, K.R.: Appraisal considered as a process of multilevel sequential checking. Appraisal processes in emotion: Theory, methods, research, pp. 92–120 (2001)

23. Whissell, C.M.: The dictionary of affect in language. The Measurement of Emotions: Theory, Research and Experience: The Measurement of Emotions, p. 113 (1989)

24. lCowie, R., Douglas-Cowie, E., Savvidou, S., McMahon, E., Sawey, M., Schroeder, M.: FEELTRACE: An instrument for recording perceived emotion in real time. In: ISCA Tutorial and Research Workshop (ITRW) on Speech and Emotion (2000)

System for Supporting Clinical Professionals Dealing with Chronic Disease Patients

Simon Kozina[1,2], Paolo Emilio Puddu[3], and Mitja Luštrek[1]

[1] Jožef Stefan Institute, Jamova cesta 39, 1000 Ljubljana, Slovenia
[2] Jožef Stefan International Postgraduate School, Jamova cesta 39,
1000 Ljubljana, Slovenia
[3] University of Rome "La Sapienza", Viale del Policlinico 155, Rome 00161, Italy
{simon.kozina,mitja.lustrek}@ijs.si, paoloemilio.puddu@uniroma1.it

Abstract. To deal with the large amount of data produced by telemonitoring of patients with chronic diseases, a decision support system (DSS) was developed. The DSS uses sensor data and the data from a patient's electronic health record as the input. It assesses the risk to the patient's health by exploiting the existing medical knowledge. The risk assessment can show the contribution of the individual monitored parameters to the risk, and can be tailored by the doctor to each patient.

Keywords: Decision support system, Expert knowledge, Risk assessment, Chronic diseases.

1   Introduction

The amount of data produced by telemonitoring solutions can be overwhelming, so using it for clinical decision-making is difficult. When telemonitoring data is combined with data obtained by traditional means, the problem becomes even larger. In a European project aiming to integrate telemonitoring into the clinical workflow, we tackle this problem by a decision support system.

In the CHIRON project [1], a patient is equipped with wearable ECG, temperature, sweating and activity sensors. The data produced by the sensors is sent to a user's mobile phone where the data is transformed into several parameters. These are then sent to a central server and are combined with the data from the patient's health record in order to be examined by the doctor. The DSS system uses all the data to automatically assess the risk to the patient's health and helps the doctor understand its assessment. It also offers personalization, allowing the doctor to tailor the risk assessment to each patient. For the most part, the DSS can support the management of any chronic disease. Our test case, however, is the congestive heart failure (CHF), and the choice of sensors and the expert knowledge contained in the DSS reflects that.

The architecture of the DSS is as follows: (i) the system input are sensor values from monitored parameters and electronic health records; (ii) in the risk assessment module, which is designed as an expert system, the input values are transformed to a risk; (iii) the risk value can be used to trigger alerts (e.g., if the

M.J. O'Grady et al. (Eds.): AmI 2013 Workshops, CCIS 413, pp. 78–85, 2013.
© Springer International Publishing Switzerland 2013

risk is too high, the doctor will receive a notification); and (iv) the configuration module can be used to tailor the risk assessment to each patient.

2   Related Work

Pocock et al. [2] conducted an analysis that included individual data on 39,372 patients with heart failure. Using multivariable piece-wise Poisson regression methods with step-wise variable selection, a final model included 13 highly significant independent predictors of mortality. Conversion from real parameter values to an easy-to-use integer-based model was done by translating mortality rate into a risk score. The score facilitates the identification of low-risk patients, e.g. score < 17 has an expected 90% 3-year survival, and very high-risk patients, e.g. score ≥ 33 has an expected 30% 3-year survival.

Yan et al. [3] presented a medical decision support system based on the Multilayer perceptron neural network architecture for heart disease diagnosis. They have identified the 40 input variables critical to the diagnosis of the heart diseases. A heart diseases database consisted of 352 cases in this study. Three assessment methods, cross validation, holdout and bootstrapping, were applied to assess the generalization of the system. The results showed that the proposed system can achieve very high diagnosis accuracy ($> 90\%$) and comparably small intervals ($< 5\%$), proving its usefulness in support of clinic diagnosis decision of heart diseases.

In the Chiron project an observational study is currently undergoing in Italy and United Kingdom and consists of 30 patients diagnosed with CHF. First difference with two above mentioned studies is that Chiron observational study targets only CHF patients. Second difference is that in this study more than 60 parameters will be collected and evaluated at the end of the study, which has not been done at such scale before. Hopefully this will improve above results.

3   Expert System for Risk Assessment

The expert system is a set of knowledge-based models for risk assessment, which attempts to exploit the large amount of existing medical knowledge. Its construction and the result is first presented in general terms suitable for a range of diseases, and then specifically for the CHF and the CHIRON project. The CHF/CHIRON models will be updated with the knowledge generated during the CHIRON observational study. This is of particular importance for the parameters that have not been studied at such a scale before (for example continuous monitoring of several ECG parameters).

3.1   Selection of Parameters

Parameter selection was made by a three-stage process. First a literature search was performed and a list of parameters was made available. There were more than 60 variables selected including clinical, angiographic, biological, pharmacological, local ambient and electrocardiographic items which were considered in previous published investigations in CHF patients and were deemed relevant as potential short- or long-term risk factors for complications including hospitalization or mortality. A medical expert (reference) initially subdivided all selected variables into baseline Information (for which an agreement exist on the capability of potential long-term predicting value) versus short- or very short-term potential predictors (on which CHIRON will specifically focus in this Expert system construction). The baseline parameters included: demographic and clinical variables including socio-economic status and activity parameters, results obtained from blood sample and electrocardiographic tests, comorbidities and ongoing drug regimen or devices. Short-term parameters included oxygen saturation, skin and ambient humidity and temperature, parameters to monitor movements, electrocardiogram and potassium blood content from high fidelity electrocardiogram. The same medical expert ranked all these variables by giving a synthetic probabilistic value to each potential risk factor, allocating a reliability code: L = low, M = average, H = high.

The second step was to perform a survey among European Opinion Leaders (OL) in cardiology as a means to obtain a comparative evaluation of the value of the selected variables. A questionnaire was constructed and the OL were asked to reply to the questions by giving a semiparametric coded series of responses to specific questions, made such to be adapted to the risk under evaluation. The questionnaire consisted of two parts. The first aimed at questioning on clinical elements not definitely proved in published studies (25 questions), whereas the second part addressed elements to be considered as more definitely proved (41 questions). The semiparametric responses might be given taking the probabilistic nature of the question into account. There were 32 OL respondents from Italy, Slovenia, Spain and UK.

4   Risk Modeling

We decided to use three risk models, since the risk within different time horizons is affected by different parameters:

- Long-term, which models static risk, and is mostly affected by the parameters that change rarely
- Medium-term, which primarily models risk with causes in the last three months, and is mostly affected by the parameters that change with a medium frequency
- Short-term, which primarily models risk with causes in the last three days, and is mostly affected by the parameters that change frequently

These three models are tailored to the CHF and the CHIRON observational study, although they are suitable for other settings as well. In principle one could use any number of models and any time horizons, as long as matching parameters are available. In order to include each parameter in one or more models, and assign the risk value to it, the following information is required:

- The importance, which was obtained through the surveys: low, medium, high
- The frequency at which the parameter changes, which roughly corresponds to the frequency at which it is measured: low fairly static (e.g., age); medium measured during regular visits to the doctor (e.g., blood pressure); high measured continuously using sensors (e.g., heart rate)
- The minimum and maximum expected value of the parameter p: p_{min}, p_{max}
- The relation between the parameter value and the risk: $(+)$ - the higher the value, the higher the risk; $(-)$ - the higher the value, the lower the risk; (U) - high risk at low and high values, low risk in between (for such parameters the lowest-risk value p_{mid} is needed in addition to the minimum and maximum expected value)
- The low threshold, which separates the parameter values corresponding to low risk (green) from those corresponding to medium risk (yellow), and the high threshold, which separates the parameter values corresponding to medium risk from those corresponding to high risk (red)

4.1 Parameter Value to Risk Transformation

The value of each parameter is transformed into a risk value, which lies in the $[0, 1]$ interval. If a given parameter p is numeric and has the $(+)$ or $(-)$ relation, this is straightforward:

$$risk(p) = (p - p_{min})/(p_{max} - p_{min}); \qquad p\text{'s relation is } (+)$$
$$risk(p) = 1 - (p - p_{min})/(p_{max} - p_{min}); \qquad p\text{'s relation is } (-)$$

Computing the thresholds on the risk scale is also straightforward. If p_l and p_h are the low and high threshold in terms of parameter values, then the thresholds in terms of risk values are $risk(p_l)$ and $risk(p_h)$, computed using the equations above. If the parameter p has the (U) relation, computing the risk is somewhat more complicated. Each such parameter has two low and two high thresholds in terms of parameter values, one on the left and one on the right side of the U-shaped curve: $p_l^{(left)}$, $p_h^{(left)}$, $p_l^{(right)}$ and $p_h^{(right)}$. Since we wish to have only one low and one high threshold in terms of risk, we assume that $risk(p_l^{(left)}) = risk(p_l^{(right)}) = 1/3$, and $risk(p_h^{(left)}) = risk(p_h^{(right)}) = 2/3$, and transform as follows:

$$risk(p) = \tfrac{1}{3} \cdot (p - p_{mid})/(p_l^{(right)} - p_{mid}); \qquad p_{mid} < p \leq p_l^{(right)}$$
$$risk(p) = \tfrac{1}{3} + \tfrac{1}{3} \cdot (p - p_l^{(right)})/(p_h^{(right)} - p_l^{(right)}); \qquad p_l^{(right)} < p \leq p_h^{(right)}$$
$$risk(p) = \tfrac{2}{3} + \tfrac{1}{3} \cdot (p - p_h^{(right)})/(p_{max} - p_h^{(right)}); \qquad p_h^{(right)} < p$$
$$risk(p) = \tfrac{1}{3} \cdot (p_{mid} - p)/(p_{mid} - p_l^{(left)}); \qquad p_l^{(left)} < p \leq p_{mid}$$
$$risk(p) = \tfrac{1}{3} + \tfrac{1}{3} \cdot (p_l^{(left)} - p)/(p_l^{(left)} - p_h^{(left)}); \qquad p_h^{(left)} < p \leq p_l^{(left)}$$
$$risk(p) = \tfrac{2}{3} + \tfrac{1}{3} \cdot (p_h^{(left)} - p)/(p_h^{(left)} - p_{min}); \qquad p \leq p_h^{(left)}$$

The transformation is illustrated in Figure 1. If the risk is never high on one side and thus $p_h^{(left)}$ or $p_h^{(right)}$ is not given, we assume that $p_h^{(left)} = p_{min}$ or $p_h^{(right)} = p_{max}$.

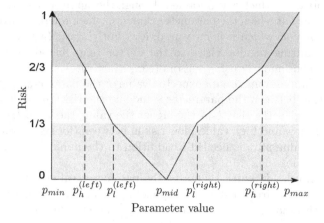

Fig. 1. The graph of the risk with respect to the parameter value

The parameters with only two values (0 and 1, e.g., gender) also require special treatment. For these, one value is always assigned low risk (0), and the other may be assigned medium risk ($1/2$) or high risk (1). The thresholds in terms of risk values are $risk(p_l) = 1/3$ and $risk(p_h) = 2/3$.

All above formulas are experimental as there is currently not enough data to evaluate them, but they are still derived from the current medical knowledge about congestive heart failure and use principals for designing clinical decision support system [4]. At the end of the observational study the parameter thresholds and risk thresholds will be evaluated and the model will be updated accordingly.

4.2   Construction of the Models

We propose simple additive models, which means that the risk values are added up to the overall risk. In risk modeling, various exponential models are more common [5], but their parameters are typically computed from data. Since we are using expert knowledge, and the risk values are only rough estimates, we believe the transparency and simplicity of additive models is preferable.

Let N be the number of parameters, and let each parameter be associated with weight. The formula for a model is then as follows:

$$risk = \frac{1}{\sum_{i=1}^{N} w(p_i)} \cdot \sum_{i=1}^{N} w(p_i) \cdot risk(p_i)$$

The weight of a parameter depends on its importance (w_I) and model-specific properties (w_M):

$$w(p_i) = w_I(p_i) \cdot w_M(p_i)$$

The importance weights were set to $1/3$ for low-importance parameters, 1 for medium-importance parameters and $3/2$ for high-importance parameters by the reference expert. The model-specific weights are 1 by default; the exceptions are specified in the following three paragraphs.

Long Term. This model uses parameter values upon enrollment, which is a common point for all the patients.
- Low-frequency parameters: all are included with the enrollment values.
- Medium-frequency parameters: all are included with the enrollment values.
- High-frequency parameters: selected are included with the average values over the first month after the enrollment. The averaging is needed because the impact of the exact time of measurement could otherwise be too large.

Medium Term. This model uses recent parameter values, and deemphasizes the low-frequency parameters in order to give a greater weight to the more frequently-changing ones.
- Low-frequency parameters: all are included with the last known values and the model-specific weight of $1/3$.
- Medium-frequency parameters: all are included with the averages over the last three months. For those with numeric values, the slope of a linear approximation over the last three months is also included.
- High-frequency parameters: selected are included with the average values over the last month.

Short Term. This model also uses recent parameter values and deemphasizes both the low-and the medium-frequency parameters.
- Low-frequency parameters: all are included with last known values and the model-specific weight of $1/9$.
- Medium-frequency parameters: all are included with the averages and in some cases slopes over the last three months, and the model-specific weight of $1/3$.
- High-frequency parameters: all are included with the averages and slopes over the last three days. For those measured continuously, the standard deviations are also included.

As mentioned before, these three models are tailored to the CHF and the CHIRON observational study. For other purposes, one could modify the selection of the attributes (e.g., include all the high-frequency attributes in the medium-term model, or exclude some of the low-frequency attributes from the short-term model) and the model-specific weights ($1/3$ and $1/9$).

5   Prototype

The prototype of the expert system is implemented in Java as a stand-alone PC application, and shown in Figure 2. The upper left window allows the selection of the patient, model and parameter, the upper middle window shows the

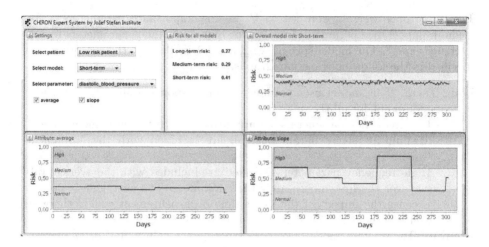

Fig. 2. Prototype of the expert system

short- medium- and long-term risk, and the upper right window shows the selected risk over time. The lower two windows show the selected parameters over time.

The expert system prototype is fully configurable. Essentially, all parameters are stored in an XML file that can be changed at any time. Parameters (and their averages, slopes and standard deviations) can be removed or added to any of the three models. When the prototype is started, the XML file is loaded and the system configured. Only adding a new type of parameter would require modifying the prototype itself.

To test the prototype, the reference expert defined static parameter values for three imaginary patients: one with low, one with medium and one with high risk. Since data at multiple time points are needed for the models, a year's worth of data was generated by adding normally distributed noise to the static values.

In order to improve user experience and provide data about patients' risks to the medical experts during the observational study, Advanced Medical Expert Support Tool (A-MEST) [6] was developed. It is a step towards achieving the patient-centric approach by incorporating the health information into the Electronic Health Record (EHR). Risk values produced by presented decision support system are also recorded to EHR and therefore made available for use by A-MEST. It also has a Graphical User Interface which shows the visualization of the health status of the patients providing meaningful information to the cardiologists. Furthermore, alert system is incorporated into A-MEST to facilitate the medical experts by prioritizing patients with higher risks and alert them when a certain patient has a critical risk value. Due to the use of EHR by A-MEST, it could also be used by any Hospital Information System using European standard ISO/EN 13606.

Conclusion

In this paper we presented a DSS for the management of chronic diseases using telemonitoring. Since the DSS was designed with CHF in mind, the sensors used for telemonitoring (ECG, temperature, sweating and activity) are suitable for CHF patients, and the expert knowledge contained in the system also pertains to CHF. The DSS is otherwise general.

The main module of the DSS deals with risk assessment. It is designed as an expert system which provides the risk assessment from sensor data values and electronic health record. The risk assessment module is supported by a configuration module which can be used to meet the requirements of a specific patient. The correctness and the accuracy of the risk assessment module proposed in this paper will be evaluated at the end of the observational study. The thresholds will be updated accordingly and the system will hopefully be ready for deployment in real-life environment.

Acknowledgments. This research described in this paper was carried out in the CHIRON project, which is co-funded by the ARTEMIS Joint Undertaking (grant agreement no. 2009-1-100228) and by national authorities.

References

1. Chiron project, `http://www.chiron-project.eu`
2. Pocock, S.J., Ariti, C.A., McMurray, J.J.V., Maggioni, A., Krber, L., Squire, I.B., Swedberg, K., Dobson, J., Poppe, K.K., Whalley, G.A., Doughty, R.N.: Predicting survival in heart failure: a risk score based on 39 372 patients from 30 studies. European Heart Journal 34, 1404–1413 (2013)
3. Yan, H., Jiang, Y., Zheng, J., Peng, C., Li, Q.: A multilayer perceptron-based medical decision support system for heart disease diagnosis. Expert Systems with Applications 30(2), 272–281 (2006)
4. Berner, E.S.: Clinical Decision Support Systems: Theory and Practice, 2nd edn. Health Informatics Series. Springer (2007)
5. Puddu, P.E., Brancaccio, G., Leacche, M., Monti, F., Lanti, M., Menotti, A., Gaudio, C., Papalia, U., Marino, B.: Prediction of early and delayed postoperative deaths after coronary artery bypass surgery alone in Italy. Italian Heart Journal 3(3), 166–181 (2002)
6. Barca, C.C., Rodríguez, J.M., Puddu, P.E., Luštrek, M., Cvetković, B., Bordone, M., Soudah, E., Moreno, A., de la Peña, P., Rugnone, A., Foresti, F., Tamburini, E.: Advanced Medical Expert Support Tool (A-MEST): EHR-Based Integration of Multiple Risk Assessment Solutions for Congestive Heart Failure Patients. In: Roa Romero, L.M. (ed.) XIII Mediterranean Conference on Medical and Biological Engineering and Computing 2013. IFMBE Proceedings, vol. 41, pp. 1334–1337. Springer, Heidelberg (2014)

The Integration of ZigBee with the GiraffPlus Robotic Framework

Michele Girolami[1,2], Filippo Palumbo[1,2], Francesco Furfari[1],
and Stefano Chessa[1,2]

[1] ISTI-CNR, Via G.Moruzzi, 1 Pisa, Italy
{michele.girolami,filippo.palumbo,francesco.furfari}@isti.cnr.it
[2] Dipartimento di Informatica Largo B. Pontecorvo, 3 Pisa, Italy
{girolami,palumbo,ste}@di.unipi.it

Abstract. Robotic ecologies often comprise a large number of environmental sensors and actuators, that, on the other hand, operate by
means of their proper standards, among which ZigBee is one of the most
widely used. Being designed to build autonomous sensor networks, the
use of sensors based on ZigBee requires a deep knowledge of its logic
and protocols. In order to facilitate interoperability between ZigBee sensors and external applications we designed ZB4O, an application-level
gateway that exports ZigBee services in external networks. This paper
describes the experience of integration of ZB4O and ZigBee networks
within the robotic ecology GiraffPlus which is being developed within
the EU project GiraffPlus.

Keywords: ZigBee, robotic ecology, interoperability.

1 Introduction

After about a decade from its first specification, ZigBee [3] has become a successful standard for wireless sensor and actuators networks that found application in many fields, ranging from home automation to consumer electronic
and healthcare, and it is now considered an important building block of smart
environments. In this context it is not surprising the interest for interoperability between robotic ecologies and environmental sensors and actuators running
ZigBee. On the other hand, interacting with a ZigBee network requires prior
knowledge about the ZigBee protocol, in particular the messages (frames) format and its interaction paradigm. Accessing to a ZigBee network without such
prior-knowledge represents a challenge since this requires the design and implementation of gateways able to export the ZigBee services to different target
networks, and this may prevent its wider adoption. For this reason, we designed
an application-level gateway (called ZigBee for OSGi - ZB4O[1]) [10] that provides seamless integration of ZigBee nodes i.e. ZigBee nodes become accessible
from external networks without any prior knowledge about the specific technology (message format, hardware features, interaction paradigm, network topology

---

[1] http://zb4osgi.aaloa.org/

M.J. O'Grady et al. (Eds.): AmI 2013 Workshops, CCIS 413, pp. 86–101, 2013.
© Springer International Publishing Switzerland 2013

etc.) and service interoperability i.e. services exposed by ZigBee nodes cooperate by adopting a service-oriented model.

The problem of interacting with a Wireless Sensor Network is a challenging task that attracted researchers and industrials from at least a decade. Several solutions have been proposed such as the node-centric approach or the data-centric approach [2]. Moreover, the integration between WSN (and in particular ZigBee) with an existing robotic ecologies has been subject of several projects as discussed in [19]. Some notable examples are the Robot-ERA project [5] the RUNES middleware [8] and the PEIS system [4].

In this paper we discuss how we used ZB4O to integrate ZigBee wireless sensor and actuator networks into the robotic ecology of GiraffPlus, an ecology whose main component is the telepresence robot Giraff. The paper gives first an overview of the GiraffPlus project and of the ZB4O framework, then, in Section 4, it provides details of the integration of ZB4O within the GiraffPlus architecture, and Section 5 draws the conclusions by discussing the achieved benefits and the perspectives of this integration.

2   The GiraffPlus Project

The prolongation of independent living for promotion of a healthier society is a social and economic challenge and several issues need to be addressed. One is early detection of possible deterioration of health so that problems can be remediated in an early stage and timely involvement of health care providers and family can be assured. A second issue is to provide adaptive support which can offer services to assist in coping with age-related impairments. Third, ways of supporting preventive medicine must be found as it has been increasingly recognized that preventive medicine can contribute to promoting a healthy lifestyle and delay the onset of age-related illnesses. The GiraffPlus² system is developed in the GiraffPlus FP7 project and addresses the above challenges. The system consists of a network of home sensors that measure e.g. blood pressure or temperature, or detect e.g. whether somebody occupies a chair, falls down or moves inside a room. The data from these sensors are interpreted by an intelligent system in terms of activities, health and wellbeing: e.g. the person is exercising or the person is going to bed, or a fall has occurred [17]. These activities can then trigger alarms or reminders to the primary user or his/her caregivers (secondary users), or be analyzed off line and over time by a health professional (secondary users). The system should automatically adapt to perform specific services such as checking the persons night activities [16]. The main component of the system is a telepresence robot, the Giraff robot, which can be moved around in the home by somebody connected to it over Internet, e.g. a caregiver. The Giraff robot is an example of mobile robotic telepresence technology [13] and is effectively a mobile communication platform, equipped with video camera, display, microphone and speakers, and a touch screen, and it helps the user to maintain

---

² http://www.giraffplus.eu/

his/her social contacts. When a remote visitor uses the Giraff robot as a communication tool, what has happened in the home in terms of activities and the physiological measurements of the person can be seen and discussed. Both the remote visitor and the person in the home have access to the information and the system can be modified to assess other aspects with the agreement of the primary user. Figure 1 illustrates graphically the main components of the system. On the left the Giraff telepresence robot is shown. The robot uses a Skype-like interface to allow caregivers to virtually visit an elderly person in the home. The Giraff robot is enhanced with semi-autonomy in order to increase safety and ease-of-use. The GiraffPlus system also includes a network of sensors. Data from these sensors are processed by an advanced context recognition system based on constraint-based reasoning which both detects events on-line and can perform inference about long term behaviors and trends. Personalized interfaces for primary and secondary users are developed to access and analyse the information from the context recognition system for different purposes and over different time scales. An important feature of the system is an infrastructure for adding and removing new sensors seamlessly, and to automatically configure the system for different services given the available sensors. This is done using planning techniques. These features provide an adaptive support which facilitates timely involvement of caregivers and allows monitoring relevant parameters only when needed.

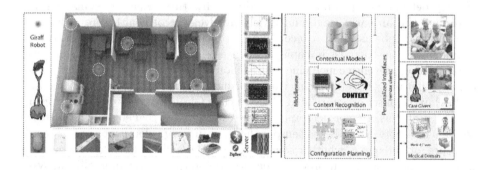

Fig. 1. The GiraffPlus system overview

2.1   The GiraffPlus Architecture

This section describes the general architecture of the GiraffPlus system. In particular, we present the specification of the system in terms of components, functionalities and interfaces among components. Also, here it is described how the components are integrated and interfaced with the rest of the system. Figure 2 shows an abstract component diagram of the GiraffPlus system. In particular, three main components can be identified: (a) the Physical Environment and Software Infrastructure, (b) the Middleware Infrastructure and (c) the Service Layer.

The Physical Environment and Software Infrastructure coupled with the Middleware Infrastructure represent the basic level of functionalities of the GiraffPlus system. Indeed, all the data services are grounded on the functionalities of this part of the system and these modules that are also in charge of providing the common and interoperable communication service. In particular, the Middleware Infrastructure constitutes a gateway shared among all the system components. Then, the Sensor Network, composed by both Physiological and Environmental sensors, gathers the information generated in the home environment as well as provides the collected data. Finally, the Telepresence Robot provides the Giraff-Plus social interaction functionalities enabling remote access in the environment through a Pilot software embedded in the visualization and interaction services. The Long-Term Data Storage component is responsible for providing a general database service for all the data generated by parts of the system and providing data access functionalities. Specifically, the main role of this component is to manage a database containing all the data collected through the Middleware Infrastructure and generated by the Sensors Network. The Context Recognition and Configuration Planning is the component responsible for context/activity recognition and system configuration planning, i.e., two high-level reasoning systems in charge of respectively implementing the monitoring activities by means of context/activity recognition [21] and providing suitable configuration settings for the Sensors Network according to the requested monitoring activities [15][7]. Finally, the Data Visualization, Personalization and Interaction Service is the part of the system responsible for creating user-oriented service. A broad way to summarize the module is to provide different end-users with suitable interaction modalities for the available services [6].

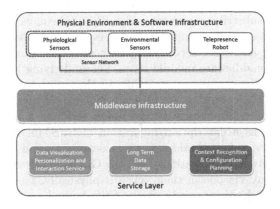

Fig. 2. The GiraffPlus components

2.2   The Middleware Infrastructure

In the GiraffPlus system, a crucial role is played by the Middleware Infrastructure as it provides the central connection point that is shared by all the
components according to the needed information exchanges. In fact, given the
inner context-aware nature of the GiraffPlus system, the presence of a pervasive
solution that provides any kind of information about the interaction between
the user and the surrounding environment becomes a key aspect for its effectiveness. The sensors, the services, and the components integrated in the GiraffPlus
system need a software infrastructure based on a middleware that hides heterogeneity and distribution of the computational resources in the environment. To
this aim, an AAL middleware solution well suited to the GiraffPlus context is
proposed. Within the proposed AAL ecosystem, hardware as well as software
components can be able to share their capabilities. The proposed platform facilitates the sharing of two types of capabilities: Service (description, discovery
and control of components) and Context (data based on shared models). Therefore, connecting components to the platform is equivalent to using the brokerage
mechanism of the middleware in these two areas for interacting with other components of the system. The GiraffPlus middleware is inspired by the concrete
architecture of the universAAL [18] middleware and partially derived from the
PERSONA [20] project. The universAAL[3] project is the most recent european
initiative aimed at delivering a software platform for AAL, which started to consolidate the architecture and software developed in recent research projects like
PERSONA[4], SOPRANO[5], OASIS[6], and mPOWER[7]. One of the main goals of
the GiraffPlus middleware is to be compatible at the level of reference architecture with universAAL-based systems. It means that with some simple adapter,
the components used in GiraffPlus will be able to run in a universAAL-based
system. The concrete middleware architecture is made up of two layers: a module
layer, containing the core middleware API modules, and a connector layer that
includes a publish/subscribe connector and a RESTful connector (Figure 3). A
generic service built upon the middleware can discover which sensors are present
in the environment and other services together with their functionalities using
methods from the middleware module layer. The underlying layer fulfills these
requests exploiting the connectors available. In the connector layer an MQTT
[12] and a RESTful [9] connector are present. By mean of these connectors, the
middleware realizes, transparently to the upper services, a publish/subscribe
mechanism as well as a description/invocation of RESTful APIs. Two buses
form the heart of the proposed middleware: a context bus and a service bus. All
communications between applications (i.e., the GiraffPlus services) can happen
in a round-aboutway via one of them, even if physically, the applications are
located on the same hardware node. Each of the buses handles a specific type

---

[3] http://universaal.org/

[4] http://www.aal-persona.org/

[5] http://www.soprano-ip.org/

[6] http://oasis-project.eu/

[7] http://www.sintef.no/Projectweb/MPOWER/

of message/request and is realized by different kinds of topics. The aim of the middleware is to provide a publish/subscribe mechanism for accessing the context information about the physical environment and physiological data. This information will be exposed as different topics: topics for describing and discovering devices and services that form the service bus and topics for publishing and retrieving data from devices and services that form the context bus. The middleware is in charge of presenting the available devices and services in the system implementing an announce mechanism on the service bus. These resources are presented with a message on the relative topic in the service bus. The message is a descriptor file containing an id, a description, a type (i.e exporter or service), a set of resources (i.e. sensors or components), a message format for the result data, and a set of methods. Once a resource has been announced on the service bus a generic service can search for it filtering on the descriptor fields and use it. The topics used for announce and discovery of devices and service, the so called service bus, has this format:

`<<location>>\serviceBus\<<serviceID>>`

where location identifies, e.g., the room in the assisted persons apartment, serviceBus is the keyword to identify the topic as a service bus topic and serviceID is the unique identifier of the service. The message of this topic is a JSON [8] descriptor file serialized as a string. The middleware takes care of dispatching information about the state of the resources among services by means of a context bus. Any service that wants to make available his data (sensors readings and events or data analysis results) can use the middleware API to publish it. Any service interested of monitoring these data can subscribe to the relative context bus topics indicated in the descriptor using the middleware API. The topics used for gathering data from devices and service, the so called context bus, has this format:

`<<location>>\contextBus\<<serviceID>>\<<subtreefield>>`

where location identifies the room, contextBus is the keyword to identify the topic as a context bus topic, serviceID is the unique identifier of the service and the subtreefield identifies all the resources of that service that can be monitored. For each resource there will be a dedicated context bus sub-topic. The message of these topics is a JSON message serialized as a string containing the service's result data formatted accordingly to the descriptor file directives.

3   The ZB4O Framework

3.1   The ZigBee Stack

The ZigBee specification defines low-power wireless networks based on the IEEE 802.15.4 standard. The network layer supports star, trees, and peer-to-peer

---

[8] http://www.json.org/

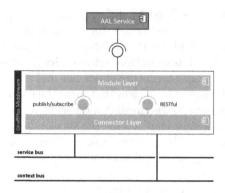

Fig. 3. The GiraffPlus middleware architecture

topologies, and it provides services for the initialization of the network, multi-hop routing, packet forwarding and management of connections and disconnections of nodes. The application layer comprises the Application Framework, the Zig-Bee Device Object (ZDO) and the Application Support Sublayer (APS). The APS offers transport layer functionalities. The Application Framework contains a number of user-defined Application Objects (APO) that implement ZigBee applications. The ZDO provides services that allow the APOs to organize themselves into a distributed application. Each APO is univocally identified by the network address of the hosting network-level device (ZigBee node) and by an EndPoint number (EP). Hereafter we refer to hardware devices as ZigBee nodes, and to APO as ZigBee devices. To enable interoperability of nodes from different manufacturers, the ZigBee alliance defines application profiles and clusters. The application profile is a collection of device descriptions that form a cooperative application. For instance, in the Home Automation Profile there exist descriptions for the Thermostat, Pump, and Pump controller devices. A device is described as the set of clusters (that are specification of messages) that it can manage. Clusters are defined in the ZigBee Cluster Library (ZCL) [1].

3.2   The ZB4O Architecture

The ZB4O gateway has been designed keeping in mind some guidelines.

Dynamic Discovery of Nodes: ZB4O makes use of the the discovery mechanisms of ZigBee. ZB4O registers a new OSGi services for evey new ZigBee device discovered in the network.

Abstraction of ZigBee Devices: ZB4O recognizes ZigBee devices adhering to the ZigBee profiles (some notable examples are: On/Off Switch device, Remote Control device, Light Sensor device) and it abstracts them. This allows external applications to ignore how to build clusters and how to send messages to the ZigBee device.

Extension Mechanisms for ZigBee Devices: The ZigBee Cluster Library [1] defines an extended set of clusters to be used with the ZigBee devices. Moreover, the ZCL allows to define custom clusters for proprietary devices. ZB4O implements this feature with a mechanism that allows to extend the set of available clusters.

Modular Integration Mechanisms: ZB4O maps the ZigBee devices to several OSGi services, which may expose the access to ZigBee applications with high-level protocols.

The ZB4O gateway is based on a three layered architecture [11], namely the Access, Abstraction and Integrations layer (see Figure 4). The Access Layer directly communicates with the ZigBee network by means of a network adapter (for instance a USB ZigBee dongle). According to the OSGi Device Access Specification, the component implementing the Access Layer is called Base Driver (in this work ZigBee Base Driver), whereas the components of the upper layers are called Refinement Drivers. The proxy services registered by the Access Layer are gradually refined by means of the upper layers. In particular, the Access Layer registers a ZigBee service proxy that does not implement any cluster. Such proxy provides simple methods that accept a ZigBee frame as parameter and injects the frame into the ZigBee network. The Abstraction Layer provides a more refined version of the proxy services registered by the Access Layer. The Abstraction Layer registers the refined services according to the ZigBee profile implemented by the remote ZigBee devices. For this reason the Abstraction Layer registers ZigBee services that are profile based (i.e. Light devices, Thermostat devices). Note that, although the Abstraction Layer is designed as a generic layer, it should include a specific refinement driver for each ZigBee profile in use in the ZigBee network. Currently we implement the Home Automation (HA) profile, but we plan to implement other refinement drivers such as the healthcare profile. The Integration Layer maps the profile-based ZigBee services to an application-level protocol. (note that Figure 4 only reports a general-purpose exporter). The Integration Layer follows the standard OSGi event mechanism: as soon as the Abstraction Layer registers new services, they are exported with one or more protocols. The Integration Layer comprises a set of exporters that detect the registration of profile-based ZigBee services. As soon as a new event occurs, the exporters act as protocol translator by injecting the ZigBee devices into the appropriate network. For example, in a UPnP network the ZigBee devices can appear as virtual UPnP devices or as end-points of a Web-Services based on RESTful or SOAP technologies. The rest of this section describes the three layers of the ZB4O architecture.

The Access Layer. The core component of the Acess Layer is the ZigBee Base Driver (ZBD), which implements the ZigBeeDevice API. The ZBD uses the Simple Driver API (that provides an abstraction of the ZigBee hardware).

The ZigBeeDevice API provides a model for the ZigBee nodes and EndPoints (EP). A ZigBee node is described in terms of network attributes such as IEEE address, network address, node type and pan ID. An EP is described in terms

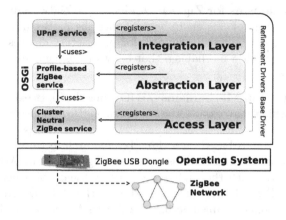

Fig. 4. The ZB4O architecture

of attributes such as profile ID, input cluster ID, output cluster ID, endpoint ID
and device category. The ZBD implements the ZigBee Device API by instanti-
ating OSGi services as soon as it discovers a new EP in the ZigBee network. For
each EP, the ZBD creates and registers an OSGi service called ZigBeeDevice.
The ZigBeeDevice service acts as proxy for the EPs. In particular, when an application interacts with a ZigBeeDevice service, the ZBD forwards the messages
to the corresponding EP on the ZigBee network. Vice versa, messages from the
EPs are forwarded to the applications waiting for them; in our case ZBD forwards the message to the Abstraction Layer that, in turns, forwards the message
to the high-level application by means of the Integration Layer.

The Abstraction Layer. The Abstraction Layer is composed by a number of
refinement drivers (generally one for every ZigBee profile), the ZigBee Cluster
Library and by other components used in order to register non-standard clusters
or devices. Figure 5 gives a view of the Abstraction Layer with the Home Automation Profile Refinement Driver (HA Driver). The HA Driver defines a set of
hierarchical Java classes modeling the Home Automation devices(HA Devices).
Some notable examples of HA Devices are the On/Off Switch, Remote Control,
Door Lock. The HA Driver monitors the ZigBeeDevice services that are registered by the Access Layer, ans it selects the proper device factory that, in turn,
installs a proxy instance of the remote ZigBee EP. To this end, the Abstraction
Layer provides a registry for the device factories. The registry is used in order
to keep device factories for both standard and non-standard profiles. The HA
Driver registers all its device factories during the start-up phase. In turn, every device factory checks that the ZigBeeDevice implements all the mandatory
clusters defined by the respective ZigBee profile. To this purpose, it checks that
the remote ZigBee endpoint implements the *Basic* and *Identify* clusters, and
the compliance of the remote device with the mandatory clusters of the specific
HA device. The ZigBee Alliance defines the ZigBee Cluster library (ZCL) in order to ease the interoperability among ZigBee devices. To this purpose, all the

devices adhering to a specific ZigBee profile should reuse clusters already defined in the ZCL. We adopted an similar approach in the Abstraction Layer. The HA devices make use of the clusters defined by the ZCL library, whose factories are registered at the start up. The development of new profiles is simplified because they can reuse the ZCL clusters. Moreover new versions of the ZCL library can either be upgraded or extended by registering only the missing clusters with the proper registry.

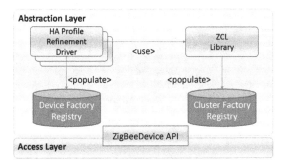

Fig. 5. The Abstraction Layer

The Integration Layer. The role of the Integration Layer is to export the Zig-Bee devices (refined by the Abstraction Layer) into different networks in order to provide a simpler way for interacting with the ZigBee hardware. ZB4O implements a general-purpose solution, without introducing any specific constraint for the target networks. With the term *exporter* we refer to the OSGi bundles implementing the business logic for the exporting routine. Currently, we have implemented the GiraffPlus exporter and the UPnP exporter. The rest of this section describes the UPnP[14] exporter (widely used in the Home Automation scenarios), while Section 4.1 describes the integration Layer for the GiraffPlus ecosystem. Figure 6 depicts the sequence diagram for mapping a ZigBee OnOff Light device as an UPnP BinaryLight device. The figure shows the role of the OSGi Framework service registry for the OSGi bundles involved. The starting point is the announce cluster sent by the ZigBee OnOff Light. The Access Layer receives the announce cluster and reacts by registering, in the OSGi framework, a ZigBee Device. The Home Automation refinement driver detects such service, and it registers a ZigBee OnOff Light Device that refines the ZigBee Device. At the end, the UPnP exporter wraps the ZigBee OnOff Light Device as UPn-PDevice. Such object models a general-purpose UPnP device as a Java objects. The model reflects all the features of the UPnP devices in a set of Java classes. In particular we modeled the UPnPDevice, UPnPService, UPnPAction and UP-npStateVariable. The role of the UPnPDevice is to translate the behavior of an UPnP device in the respective ZigBee Device. In particular the invocation of a UPnP action is associated to a ZigBee cluster and, similarly, it translates the UPnP state variables as ZigBee attributes. The final step is performed by the

UPnP Base Driver[9] whose role is to detect all the UPnPDevice and to announce them with the UPnP protocol. In this way, a UPnP Control Points can discover new UPnP devices, and it can interact with them via the UPnP protocol. The UPnP Exporter will translate the UPnP commands in the respective ZigBee ones.

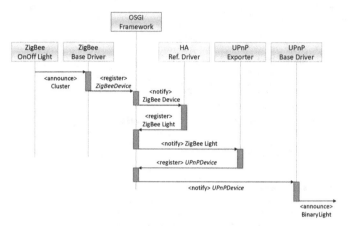

Fig. 6. The Integration Layer

4   Integration of ZB4O with the GiraffPlus Project

The aim of the proposed work is to combine the benefits arising from the use of a pervasive installation of ZigBee devices in a Smart Home with the presence of the GiraffPlus ecosystem in the ambient. This combination makes the ambient more suitable for an Ambient Assisted Living (AAL) scenario like the one proposed in the GiraffPlus project. Thanks to the integration of the ZB4O module on the GiraffPlus robot, a better context-awareness can be achieved.

4.1   The Integrated Architecture

In the proposed scenario, a GiraffPlus exporter implemented in the ZB4O Integration Layer interacts with the GiraffPlus middleware instance installed on the robot. Figure 7 shows how the exporter exploits the functionalities provided by the middleware in order to let GiraffPlus components to use the information from the ZigBee devices installed in the ambient. The exporter uses a subset of methods from the API exposed by the middleware to announce the presence of a new device and to publish status readings. The integration is made easier by the OSGi framework shared by the two architectures. When the ZB4O stack notifies the exporter of a new device turned on or installed in the ambient, the exporter creates a descriptor compliant to the GiraffPlus formalism and calls the

---

[9] http://felix.apache.org/site/apache-felix-upnp.html

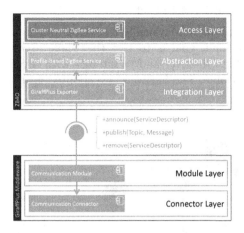

Fig. 7. The component diagram of the integrated architecture

announce method with that descriptor as argument. In this way the information is shared on the service bus with all the installed services. If a service subscribes or has already subscribed to that kind of service bus topic, it will be notified with the relative descriptor. Once the exporter has announced the devices it can start publishing messages regarding its readings and status changes. Each service subscribed to the relative context bus topic, listed in the descriptor, will receive the message. Figure 8 shows the sequence diagram of the described scenario. In the same way, when a device is turned off or uninstalled, the exporter calls the remove method with the relative descriptor as argument. In this way all the subscribers will be notified of the unavailability of that device.

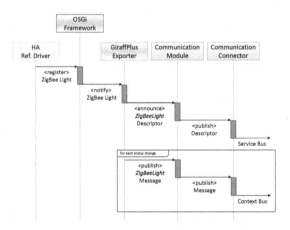

Fig. 8. The sequence diagram of the announcing and publishing mechanism for a sample device (ZigBee Light) in the integrated scenario

4.2   ZB4O and GiraffPlus in Action

This section describes how we physically tested the integration between ZigBee and GiraffPlus. The main goal is to test the whole architecture in order to let GiraffPlus be able to discover and to interact with several ZigBee networks installed in a Smart Home. The hardware we adopted is shown in Figure 9 and described below:

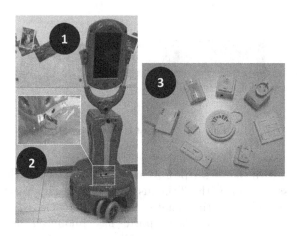

Fig. 9. The robot and the sensors used: 1) The GiraffPlus robot, 2) The ZigBee dongle connected to the robot, and 3) The environmental sensors

- the GiraffPlus robot equipped with the CC2531 USB ZigBee dongle. The USB dongle is used as access point for the ZigBee networks;
- a collection of ZigBee devices adhering to the Home Automation profile. In particular: *(i)* Generic devices such as On/Off switch, Remote Control, Door Lock, *(ii)* Lighting devices such as On/Off Light, Dimmable Light and Occupancy Sensor, *(iii)* HVAC devices such as Temperature Sensor and *(iv)*Intruder Alarm Systems such as IAS Zone device.

We tested GiraffPlus in a Smart Homes (see Figure 10). The environment is equipped with several ZigBee networks deployed in the bathroom, living room, bedroom and in the kitchen. The figure also shows the path followed by Giraff-Plus during the test. As soon as GiraffPlus moves close to a ZigBee network the ZB4O framework performs the following actions:

- the Access Layer discovers the new devices from the ZigBee network, for every newly discovered device it creates a ZigBeeDevice object that acts as a proxy for the device;
- the Abstraction Layer checks if the ZigBeeDevice implements the Home Automation Profile. If it is the case, the Abstraction Layer refines the proxy;
- the GiraffPlus exporter announces with the service bus, the existence of a new service.

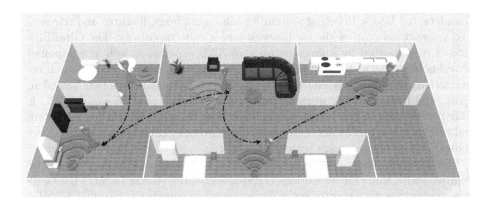

Fig. 10. The Integrated Scenario

5   Concluding Remarks - Achieved Benefits and Perspectives

This section describes the benefits achieved by the integration between the ZB4O framework and a the GiraffPlus framework.

Seamless Plug and Play. A new ZigBee device is installed at home, for instance a standard smart plug for monitoring the energy consumption. As soon as the user plugs the ZigBee device, the user is able to discover and to access it from all the DLNA-ready appliances installed at home (such as TVs, DLNA-enabled PCs, Smart Phones). The user is notified about the presence of the new devices and he can easily interact with the ZigBee device by using the UPnP protocol.

Multi-protocol Bridge. The user plugs a new ZigBee medical device. Similarly to the previous use-case, the device is easily integrated in the Smart Home. In this case it is also required that the device becomes available not only in the local UPnP network, but also remotely by means of standard protocols (such as IEEE 11073 and HL7 as advised by the Continua Health guidelines).

One Single Point of Control. A Smart Home is equipped by a number of heterogeneous devices. Some examples are: appliances (TV, refrigerator, HD camera, smart plug), smart sensors (temperature, humidity, gas detection) and health devices (blood pressure monitor, cardiovascular monitor, dosage sensor, glucose meter). The devices come typically from different vendors, each of them requires to install and configure a specific-custom gateway that allows the interaction with only a subset of the devices. The result would be a set of disjoint solutions not able to interact each other. The end-users require to access to all the home devices by means of one single point of control.

Community Support. Both projects have a wide and structured supporting community. The ZB4O project offers a very well organized software development model: mailing list, Steering Board Members, Administrators, Developers,

Founders and Users, ticketing system for managing bugs, features and releases, wiki pages, road map of the sw lifecylce and a code repository. The GiraffPlus project is supported by a large network of AAL experts, as well as companies as technology providers and systems integrators, service providers, research organizations and user associations from different European members (Sweden, Spain, and Italy). A close working relationship between the two communities is a big benefit both in the development of new features in the GiraffPlus ecosystem and bringing new technical requirements from primary (inhabitants of the smart homes) and secondary users (caregivers and relatives) to the ZB4O community.

The integration between ZigBee and the GiraffPlus robotic framework can be improved with some future works. *(i)* Extension of the Access Layer: ZB4O currently supports only a specific set of ZigBee dongles (namely CC480 and CC2530), *(ii)* adoption an IoT architecture: GiraffPlus could export the ZigBee devices recognized, to an IoT architecture. This allow to export the data gathered from the sensors also from Internet and *(iii)* implementation new ZigBee profiles: the Building Automation, Remote Control and Smart Energy profiles are more and more predominant in the ZigBee market. It will be necessary to extend ZB4O with these new profiles in order to recognized and integrate a wider number of sensors.

Acknowledgments. This work was supported in part by part by the European Commission in the framework of the FP7 project GiraffPlus (contract N.288173).

References

1. Alliance, Z.: Zigbee cluster library specification (May 2008)
2. Amato, G., Chessa, S., Vairo, C.: Mad-wise: a distributed stream management system for wireless sensor networks. Softw. Pract. Exper. 40(5), 431–451 (2010), http://dx.doi.org/10.1002/spe.v40:5
3. Baronti, P., Pillai, P., Chook, V.W.C., Chessa, S., Gotta, A., Hu, Y.F.: Wireless sensor networks: A survey on the state of the art and the 802.15.4 and zigbee standards. Comput. Commun. 30(7), 1655–1695 (2007), http://dx.doi.org/10.1016/j.comcom.2006.12.020
4. Bordignon, M., Rashid, J., Broxvall, M., Saffiotti, A.: Seamless integration of robots and tiny embedded devices in a peis-ecology. In: Proc. of the IEEE/RSJ Int. Conf. on Intelligent Robots and Systems (IROS), San Diego, CA (2007), http://www.aass.oru.se/~asaffio/
5. Cavallo, F., Aquilano, M., Carrozza, M., Dario, P.: Robot-era project: The vision of 3d service robotics. In: ISG ISARC2012 - 8th World Conference of Gerontechnology, vol. 2, p. 364 (2012)
6. Cesta, A., Coraci, L., Cortellessa, G., Benedictis, R.D., Orlandini, A., Palumbo, F., Stimec, A.: Steps toward end-to-end personalized aal services. In: Botía, J.A., Charitos, D. (eds.) Intelligent Environments (Workshops). Ambient Intelligence and Smart Environments, vol. 17, pp. 78–89. IOS Press (2013)
7. Coradeschi, S., Cesta, A., Cortellessa, G., Coraci, L., Gonzalez, J., Karlsson, L., Furfari, F., Loutfi, A., Orlandini, A., Palumbo, F., Pecora, F., von Rump, S., Stimec, A., Ullberg, J., Otslund, B.: Giraffplus: Combining social interaction and long term monitoring for promoting independent living. In: 2013 The 6th International Conference on Human System Interaction (HSI), pp. 578–585 (2013)

8. Costa, P., Coulson, G., Gold, R., Lad, M., Mascolo, C., Mottola, L., Picco, G.P., Sivaharan, T., Weerasinghe, N., Zachariadis, S.: The runes middleware for networked embedded systems and its application in a disaster management scenario. In: Proc. of the 5 th Int. Conf. on Pervasive Communications (PERCOM), pp. 69–78. IEEE Press (2007)

9. Fielding, R.T., Taylor, R.N.: Principled design of the modern web architecture. ACM Transactions on Internet Technology (TOIT) 2(2), 115–150 (2002)

10. Furfari, F., Girolami, M., Lenzi, S., Chessa, S.: A service-oriented zigbee gateway for smart environments. Tech. Rep. TR 2013-09-04, ISTI-CNR, Pisa (September 2013)

11. Girolami, M., Lenzi, S., Furfari, F., Chessa, S.: Sail: A sensor abstraction and integration layer for context awareness. In: 34th Euromicro Conference on Software Engineering and Advanced Applications, SEAA 2008, pp. 374–381 (2008)

12. Hunkeler, U., Truong, H.L., Stanford-Clark, A.: Mqtt-sa publish/subscribe protocol for wireless sensor networks. In: 3rd International Conference on Communication Systems Software and Middleware and Workshops, COMSWARE 2008, pp. 791–798. IEEE (2008)

13. Kristoffersson, A., Coradeschi, S., Loutfi, A.: A review of mobile robotic telepresence. Advances in Human-Computer Interaction 2013 (2013)

14. Li, C.S., Huang, Y.M., Chao, H.C.: Upnp ipv4/ipv6 bridge for home networking environment. IEEE Transactions on Consumer Electronics 54(4), 1651–1655 (2008)

15. Lundh, R., Karlsson, L., Saffiotti, A.: Autonomous functional configuration of a network robot system. Robotics and Autonomous Systems 56(10), 819–830 (2008)

16. Palumbo, F., Barsocchi, P., Furfari, F., Ferro, E.: Aal middleware infrastructure for green bed activity monitoring. Journal of Sensors 2013 (2013)

17. Palumbo, F., Barsocchi, P., Gallicchio, C., Chessa, S., Micheli, A.: Multisensor data fusion for activity recognition based on reservoir computing. In: Botía, J.A., Álvarez-García, J.A., Fujinami, K., Barsocchi, P., Riedel, T. (eds.) EvAAL 2013. CCIS, vol. 386, pp. 24–35. Springer, Heidelberg (2013), http://dx.doi.org/10.1007/978-3-642-41043-7_3

18. Ram, R., Baptist, J., Furfari, F., Girolami, M., Ibañez-Sánchez, G., Lázaro-Ramos, J.-P., Mayer, C., Prazak-Aram, B., Zentek, T.: universAAL: Provisioning Platform for AAL Services. In: van Berlo, A., Hallenborg, K., Rodríguez, J.M.C., Tapia, D.I., Novais, P. (eds.) Ambient Intelligence & Software & Applications. AISC, vol. 219, pp. 105–112. Springer, Heidelberg (2013), http://dx.doi.org/10.1007/978-3-319-00566-9_14

19. Sanfeliu, A., Hagita, N., Saffiotti, A.: Network robot systems. Robot. Auton. Syst. 56(10), 793–797 (2008), http://dx.doi.org/10.1016/j.robot.2008.06.007

20. Tazari, M.R., Furfari, F., Ramos, J.P., Ferro, E.: The persona service platform for aal spaces. In: Nakashima, H., Aghajan, H., Augusto, J. (eds.) Handbook of Ambient Intelligence and Smart Environments, pp. 1171–1199. Springer, US (2010), http://dx.doi.org/10.1007/978-0-387-93808-0_43

21. Ullberg, J., Pecora, F.: Propagating temporal constraints on sets of intervals. In: ICAPS Workshop on Planning and Scheduling with Timelines, pp. 25–32 (2012)

Temporal Issues in Teaching Robot Behaviours in a Knowledge-Based Sensorised Home

Joe Saunders, Maha Salem, and Kerstin Dautenhahn

Adaptive Systems Research Group, University of Hertfordshire, College Lane,
Hatfield, AL10 9AB, United Kingdomw
http://www.herts.ac.uk

Abstract. As part of the ACCOMPANY project we are researching the use of a companion robot for elderly people within a sensorised home. One of our goals is to give end users, such as care workers, relatives and the elderly persons themselves, the ability to create robot behaviours based on events within the home. We employ a knowledge-based approach in dealing with the creation of complex robot behaviours and need to have flexibility in dealing with events occuring at different times and in different timeframes and periods. In this paper we describe our overall approach to creating an environment where robot behaviours can be taught and focus especially on how we deal with the temporal aspects associated with this issue.

Keywords: Assistive technology, Robot Control Architectures, Robotic Companions, Smart Homes.

1   Introduction

It is predicted that the world is facing a demographics problem over the following decades. This is due to increasing life expectancy, leading to more elderly persons, combined with decrease in the size of the population of those providing support to the elderly. For example, it is predicted that in the European Union the number of people over 65 years will almost double (by 2060) and the number of people between 15-64 years will decrease by over 10% [5]. Health care costs are also rising [18], therefore there has been a focus on the further use of assistive and robotic technologies as one possible solution to this issue.

Various European projects have studied how such technologies can be used in this area[1]. These projects can be broadly categorised into two categeories: those which consider HRI (Human Robot Interaction) issues and those which focus on areas such as robotic ecology and system reliability. In the former category there are, for example, SRS: Multi-role Shadow Robotic System for Independent Living (srs-project.eu), CompanionAble (www.companionable.net), Hermes: Cognitive Care and Guidance for Active Ageing (www.fp7-hermes.eu), Florence: Multi Purpose Mobile Robot

---

[1] The list of projects shown is not exhaustive, but merely intended to show the commitment of research funding bodies to the issue of ageing populations.

M.J. O'Grady et al. (Eds.): AmI 2013 Workshops, CCIS 413, pp. 102–113, 2013.
© Springer International Publishing Switzerland 2013

for Ambient Assisted Living (`www.florence-project.eu`), KSERA: Knowledgable SErvice Robots for Aging (`ksera.ieis.tue.nl`). In the latter category there are, for example, Rubicon: creation of a self-learning robotic ecology (`http://fp7rubicon.eu/`) and ROBOT-ERA: Implementation and integration of advanced Robotic systems and intelligent Environments in real scenarios for the ageing population (`www.robot-era.eu`).

In the work described in this paper, which has been carried out in the European Framework 7 ACCOMPANY project [1], our focus is also on assistive technologies, and falls into the HRI category, where we emphasise the use of robotic *companions* focussing on co-learning and re-ablement [24] of the person within the home.

We investigate how a commercially available robot (Care-O-bot®) manufactured by Fraunhofer IPA [21] sited in a realistic, but sensorised, domestic environment (which we call the *robot house*) can be used to aid elderly persons [22]. The house itself, rather than being a modified scientific laboratory, is actually a normal British three bedroom house near the University of Hertfordshire which has been equipped with various sensing devices. The house is regularly used for Human-Robot Interaction experiments and is also often occupied and lived in by researchers and other persons [13].

1.1   Robot Behaviours within the Home

Part of our research concentrates on how robot behaviours can be built and coordinated to meet the needs of the elderly. We envisaged that these needs would change over time and that a flexible way of creating robot behaviours should be available. This behaviour creation and robot teaching facility should be capable of being used by non-technical persons, such as the elderly persons themselves, their relatives or carers. Clearly, the flexibility and ease of robot teaching needs to be based on facilities available both on the robot and supplied by the house sensors. However, as behavioural complexity increases, it would be no longer sufficient to base all behaviours simply on physical (robot or house) sensors. Instead, more abstract concepts are required, for example, rather than ask, "is the microwave in use?", we might ask "has the user had breakfast this morning?". By considering these more abstract concepts as sensory events, existing facilities which apply to sensory information, especially that based on sensory event periods, can then be applied to such 'abstract' sensors.

We define two types of abstract sensors, 'context' sensors and 'predicate' sensors. Context sensors are updated via a rule-based context analysis system derived from HRI experiments (see [4] for more details). This provides contextual information such as, for example, 'User Preparing Evening Meal'. Thus the sensor 'User Preparing Evening Meal' would be set 'on' if a given set of rules were true (for example, fridge has been opened recently, it is after 4pm, kitchen light is on etc.) and set 'off' otherwise. Predicate sensors are used in order to cope with ongoing events in the house which are not reflected by the physical environmental sensors, for example, a binary sensor with the label 'User has been reminded to turn off the TV' might be set if the robot has given such a reminder and would ensure that the reminder was not repeated.

This approach requires a number of pre-requisites, firstly a disciplined method of maintaining sensory information both current and historical, secondly, a way of creating 'abstract' sensors which can use existing facilities for sensor interrogation and finally, a way of dealing with temporal aspects of sensory information.

In the following sections we will describe our approach in meeting these challenges by describing the integration of house occupants, robot sensors and house sensors into one holistic system. This will be followed by a short description of how our behavioural components are constructed and how abstract sensory information can be created and used. We will then describe the approach we take in dealing with the temporal aspects of sensors, both real and abstract. Finally, we will present a short description of our ongoing experiments that are testing and evaluating the above ideas.

2   The Robot House, Its Occupants and the Robot

We consider a typical care environment to be one where a person or persons remain in their own home. Our physical home ontology is modelled within a mySQL database, and all information arising from robot, house sensors (including abstract sensors) and user or robot locations in the physical home causes a real-time update to the database (see Figure 1 for a partial view of the database). We also, however, appreciate that such an approach is only one method for encoding such complexity. Other approaches, such as, for example, the RACE project [20], encode semantic information using RDF (Resource Description Framework) and ontological information using OWL (Web Ontology Description Language). From our point of view, the use of a SQL database has the benefit of providing access to many tools for fast and relatively easy development, and is readily understood between project partners (who may not necessarily be experts in semantic web technologies). We model the home, the persons and the robot as one complete entity. The home itself consists of physical sensors, house locations and objects. In the University of Hertfordshire robot house there are over 50 'low level' sensors ranging from electrical (fridge door open, microwave on etc.), to furniture (cupboard door and drawers open etc.), to services (such as toilet flushing, taps running etc.) and pressure devices (sofa or bed occupied). House locations are encoded as map co-ordinates and organised hierarchically, for example, 'sofa location' is part of the 'living room' which is part of the 'robot house'.

The robot itself is the Care-O-bot® robot [21] (see picture in Figure 2) which has been especially designed for research in assistive environments. The Care-O-bot® uses ROS navigation (a form of SLAM) [19] using its laser range-finders to update a map of the house in real-time and can thus navigate to any given location whilst avoiding obstacles and replanning routes. Similarly the robot is equipped with high-level callable facilities for manipulating the arm, torso, 'eyes', robot LED's, tray and has a voice synthesiser to convert given text to

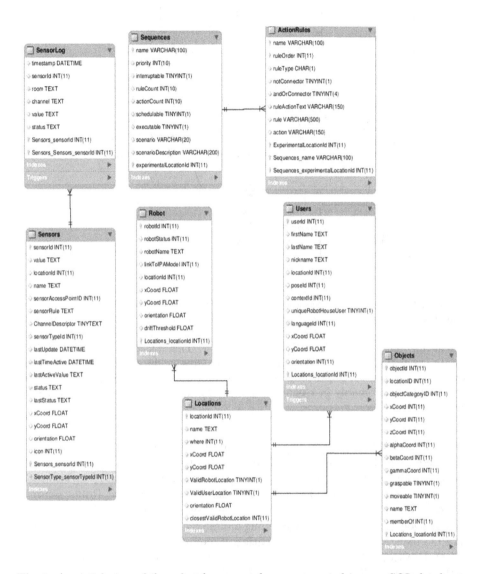

Fig. 1. A partial view of the robot house ontology represented in a mySQL database. Three sets of tables are shown. The first, shown on the left, is a sensor log and sensor table containing current and historical sensory information. The second, at the top, are the main tables used for behavioural encoding. The bottom set of tables show the relationships between robot, users, objects and locations. The actual database contains considerably more detail and complexity with around 50 tables in total.

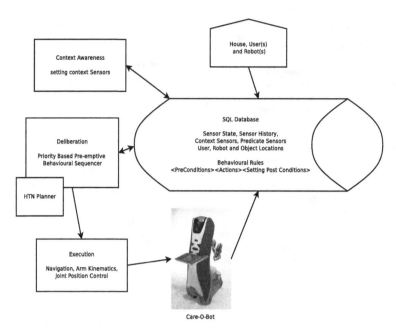

Fig. 2. A high level view of the control architecture for the Care-O-bot® within our robot house. The architecture is based on a typical three-layer approach comprising of deliberation, execution and reaction. The deliberative layer makes decisions based on real-time information from the central database. This information is composed of updates from the physical house sensors and updates made via the deliberation or context awareness rule-based programs to abstract sensors. The reactive layer (not shown) operates primarily in a tight control loop in areas such as navigation and arm kinematics.

speech. High level commands are sent via the ROS 'script server' mechanism and interpreted into low level commands by the robot software. Typical commands would be, for example, 'raise tray', 'nod', 'look forward', 'move to location x', 'grab object on tray', 'put object x at location y', 'say hello' etc. Robot sensors include its current location, the state of the tray, arms, torso and eyes. House occupant location is computed via ceiling mounted cameras [8] and robot location via ROS navigation [19]. The combination of hierachical location and person (or robot) detection allows for further behavioural rule generalisation, for example, 'is the user in the living room?' would be true if the user was at 'sofa location', similarly a question such as 'where is the robot?', might yield 'at the charging station, in the dining room, in the robot house'.

By describing the ontological characteristics of the house, robots and occupants together, we can then broadly consider the database as the memory of the whole. User and robot interaction events within the house we denote as 'episodic' memory, behavioural rules and behaviour execution on the robot we call 'procedural' memory, and the low and high level activities defined via both sensors and 'abstract' sensors together with the ontology as a whole, we define loosely as 'semantic' memory. In this paper we will focus on the procedural and semantic aspects of the memory, however our work on episodic aspects of memory is described in [7].

3   Procedural Memory - Behaviour Creation and Execution

One of our major goals was to be able to generate and execute behaviours on the robot. Generation of behaviours is considered a task that would be ongoing, due to changing living conditions, and be carried out by users of the system themselves. Behaviour encoding and behaviour execution are intimately tied and we have drawn inspiration from research on cognitive architectures (for a detailed survey see [11]) and especially behavioural control outlined in Freed [6] and Nilsson [16,17] together with work on Hierachical Task Planners (HTN's) (see, for example, [15]). Each of these approaches is based on what is sometimes called 'sketchy' planning', whereby outline plans for execution are generated with the details gradually being filled in as the behaviour executes.

Behaviour Creation. Each behaviour is 'taught' to the system via one of two GUI interfaces. The first is a semi-technical interface allowing for direct access to all types of sensors and all types of robot actions, the second interface is more restricted and generates behaviours based on templates. This latter facility trades behavioural generation complexity and expressiveness against ease of use and it is the interface which we would expect to be used by end users. Both of these GUI's are described in more detail in [22]. Behaviours that are generated follow the familiar pattern (similar to Nilsson's T-R formalism [16]) of evaluating pre-conditions, followed by execution of robot actions and updating of post-conditions (this is similar to the add/delete lists of planning systems). Physical sensors cannot be directly updated, however 'abstract' sensors can be modified. Pre-conditions here can be any form of sensory information, both real sensors (set by environmental changes) or context/predicate sensors (set by behavioural actions). An example of a behaviour would be as follows:

```
IF    the doorbell has rung in the last 20 seconds    (sensor pre-cond)
AND   the user has not yet been informed              (predicate sensor pre-cond)
THEN send the robot to the user location in the house  (action)
      make the robot say 'Someone at the door'         (action)
      update the database to signal
         that the user has been informed               (update predicate sensor post-cond)
```

If the set of preconditions are true, then the actions are executed. Actions, as well as being robot-based, can also be the setting of predicate and context sensors and the execution of other behaviours, which again can have pre-conditions and actions. Careful arrangement of behaviours allow the action of post-condition setting to fire sub-behaviours and thus 'fill in' the details of the sketchy plan. Some behaviours (although very few in our experience) may require detailed planning (for example, making the robot navigate through a series of rooms). In this instance we allow behaviours to call a HTN planner directly (we use

JSHOP2 [9]), and the results are sent back by the planner for subsequent execution[2]. Within each behaviour each pre-condition is automatically encoded into SQL statements by the teaching system as follows:

```
IF   the  doorbell has rung in the last 20 seconds        (sensor pre-cond)
AND  the user has not yet been informed                   (pred. sensor pre-cond)

resolves to the SQL statements...

SELECT * FROM Sensors WHERE sensorId = 302 AND lastStatus = "On"
     AND lastUpdate+INTERVAL 20 SECOND >= NOW()
SELECT * FROM Sensors WHERE sensorId = 701 AND value = 'notInformed'
```

Following execution of the SQL statements, if a row is returned, then that precondition is deemed to be true, otherwise false. The conjunction of statements (disjunction is also allowed), provides a final boolean decision. Typical robot actions, for example, calling the navigation system to move the base, making the robot say something and setting a predicate sensor, are shown below:

```
base,0,[4.329:0.837:51],999,wait    (moves the robot to the user position)
speak,0,Someone at the door         (makes the robot say 'someone at the door')
cond,701,informed                   (sets sensor 701 to the value 'informed')
```

These commands, depending on the command type (for example, if the move location was another room), would then be sent to the HTN planner, or directly sent to a lower level robot control module if planning was not required. A diagram of the overall system is shown in Figure 2.

Behaviour Execution. We use a priority-based pre-emptive scheduling system to control behaviour execution. Behaviours are created with a scheduling priority (as an integer) defined by the user. When the robot is running, the scheduling system checks all of the preconditions of all of the behaviours (in a manner similar to Nilsson [17]). If the combined (conjunction or disjunction) set of pre-conditions of a behaviour become true, then that behaviour becomes available for execution. Then, the highest priority behaviour is executed first. Priority ties result in a random choice of behaviour for execution. Note that due to continual checking of all behavioural pre-conditions, behaviours may become valid or invalid for execution as the currently executing behaviour operates. In this manner, the set of environment, context and predicate sensors drive behaviour execution. Some behaviours can also be set as non-interruptible, for example if a behaviour was reporting on a critical house event - such as the bathroom taps being on for a long time.

4 Semantic Memory - Temporal Reasoning

In this section we will explain how complex events can be constructed based both on discrete points in time and via intervals.

---

[2] Note that where detailed planning is required the appropriate planning domains need to be created. We consider that creating planning domains to be too complex for end user involvement and therefore we pre-code these.

Related Work. Interval-based reasoning, often based on Allen's temporal logic [2] (although for an alternative logic also see [14]), within 'smart homes' has been previously considered by Sciavicco [23] where a logical analysis is undertaken and is used to show that interval-based relations are "particularly adequate to express typical smart homes constraints". Augusto and Nugent [3] provide a language for expressing ECA (event-condition-action) rules (which are conceptually similar to our behavioural rules) that employ temporal relationships and apply these within a smart home environment using an active database. They specifically apply their formalism to emergency type situations and demonstrate that such analyses increase the possibility of complex event detection. Jakkula and Cook [10] also consider how temporal relations could be learned in a smart home environment, and they suggest that learning of such relations would be of much benefit, especially in relation to elderly persons. In our work, we are primarily concerned with robot behaviours within the home, therefore many of the decisions on which behaviours execute will be based on real-time considerations of sensor readings and their current or historical values. Our approach takes a pragmatic view of dealing with temporal relationships and provides a simple mechanism to apply such relationships in a practical way. Our future work also includes research into learning such relationships from occupant activity within the house.

Temporal Relationships. We constructed our sensor tables to reflect both the event driven nature of the system and to allow immediate decisions on sensory durations. We created two tables, the first holding a historical log of all sensor value changes, and a second table holding one row per sensor with the current value and the previous value (if different) of that sensor. Thus each sensor event, for example, a light switch being turned on, creates a time-stamped single row in the sensor log table which then triggers the update of the immediate state/time and previous state/time of that sensor on the sensor table.

By constructing the sensor table in this way fairly complex decisions based on the temporal rules can be constructed. Take for example a doorbell sensor. This type of sensor is 'on' only for a short period of time. Although we would normally, when constructing a behaviour using the doorbell, say "If the doorbell rings, then make the robot say 'someone at the door' ". However, due to the short period of sensory activity of the doorbell, we would need a more precise definition, for example, "If the doorbell rang within the last 'n' seconds, then make the robot say 'someone at the door' ". Given such considerations we defined three basic conditions:

1. *"is* the value of sensor X equal to Y *now?"*
2. *"has* the value of sensor X *been* equal to Y *for time period 'now - T'?"*
3. *"was* the value of sensor X equal to Z *at any time during time period 'now - T'?"*

where X is a sensor, Y is the current real-time value of sensor X, Z is the previous value of sensor X and T is a time unit (e.g. seconds, minutes, hours, days),

The first condition is simply a real-time reaction to a sensor value, for example, 'Is the microwave on?'. The second condition adds a duration to the current sensor state, e.g., 'Has the microwave been on for 30 minutes?'. The final condition considers the containment of the condition during some time period, for example, 'Was the microwave previously on at any time during the last 2 hours?'. Clock-based decisions can also be added. For example, 'is the current time greater or equal to C' and 'is the current time between C and D' (where C and D are clock times in hours, minutes and seconds). This allows for further complexity, for example, assume that the house occupant likes to sleep in the afternoon, but wants to be woken by the robot if they sleep longer than 1 hour. The following rule could be used:

"If the sofa has been occupied for 1 hour, at any time between 1pm and 5pm, make the robot say 'It's time to wake up' ".

Using the user GUI this would translate to the following behavioural template (note that the function $spBetweenTimeCheck$ is a SQL stored procedure which checks time intervals and returns a single row if the check is true).

```
SELECT * FROM Sensors WHERE sensorId = 15
        AND value = 0 and lastUpdate+INTERVAL 3600 SECOND <= NOW()
CALL spBetweenTimeCheck('13:00:00','17:00:00')

speak,0,it's time to wake up    (makes the robot say 'It's time to wake up')
```

The sensor table, by holding two timed events, can immediately yield duration information useful for real-time actions. The sensor log table, on the other hand, can then be used via our context analysis program, to carry out a deeper analysis of events (this is also discussed by Sciavicco [23] in the context of sleeping). For example, we may want to know if the user is having lunch. This might be expressed as a series of behavioural pre-conditions such as, dining room chair occupied, time is between 12am and 2pm, the fridge has been opened in the last 30 minutes etc. However, if the user vacated the chair temporarily, the 'having lunch' context may still be true, but using only real-time sensor information as pre-conditions would yield the opposite result. In this context an analysis of the sensor log, biased with appropriate behavioural parameters (for example, lunch typically takes 30 minutes) would avoid the 'noise' inherent in the activity. Furthermore, by considering 'having lunch' as simply a new sensor, all of the previous temporal rules can then be applied. Thus we could ask 'has the occupant had lunch today?'. These encoding facilities can therefore cope with a wide range of possibilities and capture information related to both current activity, past activity and used to encourage socially desirable and non-passive activities in the house occupant. This latter function is primarily set through the creation of predicate sensors from contextual rules.

5   Ongoing Experiments in the Robot House

The approach outlined above is, at time of writing, being tested and evaluated in a typical elderly person's apartment in Heerlen, Netherlands, by ZUYD

University (one of our project partners). This involves 11 elderly persons inter-acting with the robot in a 'fetch and carry' task, and with the robot instructed to check that the person has been drinking adequately over the period (to avoid de-hydration). This and the previous and following experiments are based on realistic scenarios derived from user requirements [12]. In the first of these sce-narios the user was reminded to take medicine at a particular time (medical re-ablement), asked to accompany the robot to the kitchen (a form of physical re-ablement), gave a reminder about medicine 10 minutes after the first reminder (warning reminder), warned that the fridge had been left open (safety warning), and suggested to the user that they watched TV together (social partner). In total around 30 behavioural components were created using the approach out-lined above. All operated successfully. This behaviour creation and scheduling system using the temporal rules outlined above also ran in real-time during an artistic event for over 20 persons held at the robot house in May 2013 [13].

6   Conclusion

In this paper we have described an approach where we integrate the ontology of a sensorised house, robots and house occupants with a behaviour execution mechanism embedded within the same ontology. We thus hold the semantic, procedural and episodic knowledge in one memory context (an SQL database). Behaviours and behavioural rules are held as tables and database statements (SQL statements) within the database, and operate directly within it. This allows us to both create behaviours relatively easily and apply complex temporal logic on physical sensors as well as on context or logically created abstract sensors. We hope that such an approach will be useful in demonstrating that complex systems, such as those described in this paper, can be implemented in a practical and pragmatic way using readily available technologies such as database servers.

Using such an approach has allowed us to explore one of the major goals of our project in studying how co-learning could operate with a robot in a domestic environment and allow the robot to act as a re-abling device for the user [22].

One of the many challenges in our ongoing work will be to extend these ideas by studying how the robot can learn behavioural rules directly from human actions and human behaviours. In order to achieve this goal an understanding of the temporal nature of human behaviours within the house will need to be understood and learned.

Acknowledgments. The work described in this paper was partially funded by the European project ACCOMPANY (Acceptable robotics COMPanions for AgeiNg Years). Grant agreement no.: 287624. The authors are grateful to colleagues in the ACCOMPANY consortium (The University of Hertfordshire, United Kingdom; Hogeschool Zuyd, The Netherlands; Fraunhofer, Germany; University of Amsterdam, The Netherlands; University of Sienna, Italy; Main-tien en Autonomie, Domicile des Personnes Agees, France; and University of Birmingham, United Kingdom; University of Twente, the Netherlands; Univer-sity of Warwick, United Kingdom).

References

1. ACCOMPANY: EU integrated Project ACCOMPANY Acceptable robotiCs COM-Panions for AgeiNg Years (2012), http://accompanyproject.eu/
2. Allen, J.F.: Maintaining knowledge about temporal intervals. Communications of the ACM 26(11), 832–843 (1983)
3. Augusto, J.C., Nugent, C.D.: The use of temporal reasoning and management of complex events in smart homes. In: Proc. of the 16th European Conference on Artificial Intelligence (ECAI 2004), pp. 778–782 (2004)
4. Duque, I., Dautenhahn, K., Koay, K.L., Willcock, I., Christianson, B.: Knowledge-driven user activity recognition for a smart house. development and validation of a generic and low-cost, resource-efficient system. In: The Sixth International Conference on Advances in Computer-Human Interactions (ACHI 2013), pp. 141–146 (2013)
5. Eurostats: Population projections. online database (2013), http://epp.eurostat.ec.europa.eu/statistics_explained
6. Freed, M.: Managing multiple tasks in complex dynamic environments. In: Proc. 15th National Conf. on Artificial Intelligence, pp. 921–927. AAAI Press (1998)
7. Ho, W.C., Dautenhahn, K., Burke, N., Saunders, J., Saez-Pons, J.: Episodic memory visualization in robot companions providing a memory prosthesis for elderly users. In: Proc. 12th European Conf. Advancement Assistive Technology in Europe (AAATE 2013) (2013)
8. Hu, N., Englebienne, G., Kröse, B.J.A.: Bayesian fusion of ceiling mounted camera and laser range finder on a mobile robot for people detection and localization. In: Salah, A.A., Ruiz-del-Solar, J., Meriçli, Ç., Oudeyer, P.-Y. (eds.) HBU 2012. LNCS, vol. 7559, pp. 41–51. Springer, Heidelberg (2012)
9. IIghami, O.: JSHOP2 Download, http://sourceforge.net/projects/shop/files/JSHOP2/ (last referenced February 5, 2013)
10. Jakkula, V., Cook, D.J.: Learning temporal relations in smart home data. In: Proc. 2nd Int. Conf. on Technology and Aging, Canada (2007)
11. Langley, P., Laird, J.E., Rogers, S.: Cognitive architectures: Research issues and challenges. Cognitive Systems Research 10(2), 141–160 (2009)
12. Lehmann, H., Syrdal, D., Dautenhahn, K., Gelderblom, G., Bedaf, S., Amirabdollahian, F.: What can a robot do for you? - evaluating the needs of the elderly in the UK. In: Proceedings of the 6th International Conference on Advances in Computer-Human Interactions, Nice, France (2013)
13. Lehmann, H., Walters, M.L., Dumitriu, A., May, A., Koay, K.L., Saez-Pons, J., Syrdal, D.S., Wood, L., Saunders, J., Burke, N., Duque-Garcia, I., Christianson, B., Dautenhahn, K.: Artists as HRI Pioneers: A Creative Approach to Developing Novel Interactions for Living with Robots. In: Herrmann, G., Pearson, M.J., Lenz, A., Bremner, P., Spiers, A., Leonards, U. (eds.) ICSR 2013. LNCS, vol. 8239, pp. 402–411. Springer, Heidelberg (2013)
14. Morchen, F.: A better tool than Allen's relations for expressing temporal knowledge in interval data. In: Proc. the 12th ACM SIGKDD Int. Conf. on Knowledge Discovery and Data Mining, Philadelphia, PA, USA (2006)
15. Nau, D., Cao, Y., Lotem, A., Muñoz-Avila, H.: SHOP: Simple Hierarchical Ordered Planner. In: Proc. IJCAI 1999, pp. 968–973 (1999)
16. Nilsson, N.J.: Teleo-reactive programs for agent control. Journal of Artificial Intelligence Research, 158 (1994)

17. Nilsson, N.J.: Teleo-reactive programs and the triple-tower architecture. Electronic Transactions on Artificial Intelligence 5, 99–110 (2001)
18. Przywara, B.: Projecting future health care expenditure at European level: drivers, methodology and main results. In: European Economy. European Commision, Economic and Financial Affairs (2010)
19. Quigley, M., Conley, K., Gerkey, B.P., Faust, J., Foote, T., Leibs, J., Wheeler, R., Ng, A.Y.: ROS: an open-source robot operating system. In: ICRA Workshop on Open Source Software (2009)
20. RACE: EU integrated Project RACE Robustness by Autonomous Competence Enhancement (2011), http://www.project-race.eu/
21. Reiser, U., Connette, C., Fischer, J., Kubacki, J., Bubeck, A., Weisshardt, F., Jacobs, T., Parlitz, C., Hagele, M., Verl, A.: Care-o-bot® creating a product vision for service robot applications by integrating design and technology. In: IEEE/RSJ International Conference on Intelligent Robots and Systems, IROS 2009, pp. 1992–1998. IEEE (2009)
22. Saunders, J., Burke, N., Koay, K.L., Dautenhahn, K.: A user friendly robot architecture for re-ablement and co-learning in a sensorised homes. In: Proc. 12th European Conf. Advancement Assistive Technology in Europe (AAATE 2013) (2013)
23. Sciavicco, G.: Using interval-based reasoning in smart homes. In: Proc. of the 4th International Conference on Ubiquitous Computing and Ambient Intelligence, pp. 307–314 (2010)
24. Welsh Social Services Improvement Agency: Demonstrating improvement through reablement (2006), http://www.ssiacymru.org.uk/reablement (2006) (last referenced November 23, 2012)

Empirical Methods for Evaluating Properties of Configuration Planning Algorithms

Lia Susana d.C. Silva-Lopez and Mathias Broxvall

Center for Applied Autonomous Sensor Systems, Örebro University, SE-70182 Sweden
{lia.silva,mathias.broxvall}@oru.se

Abstract. As the field of configuration planning grows, so does the need for objective comparisons of algorithms and results. As the community stands today, different approaches to formalise and solve the problem at hand exist, and little or no importance has been given to compare results of different research groups. In this paper we summarize the definitions used by a few different research groups, and we explain two empiric method for comparing planning algorithms, based on statistics. While the methods themselves do not solve all the problems of comparative studies, it is a first step towards numerically comparing performances of the different configuration planning methods proposed by the community.

1 Introduction

Currently the field of configuration planning is a growing community containing different ways of defining the problem, and approaches to solve it. An obstacle for a researcher intending to work in the field is the lack of objective, comparable evaluation that we can use to debate aboutthe different approaches. In strong computer science this is typically done with deductionistic approaches by proving properties such as complexities or the relative expressibility of the formalisms used. Due to the inherent complexity in planning, benchmarks [1] have been instead used in order to compare different planners. Where static benchmarks cannot be used, experiments more akin to empirical science are used to evaluate planners [5]. For the configuration planning community, no such benchmarks currently exist and due to the different ways of formalizing the problem at hand, it would be hard to reach an agreement on the best benchmarks to use. In this paper, we share sound experimental methodologies that can be used for evaluating quantitative aspects of configuration planning approaches, as an attempt to contribute to the state of the art on comparing configuration planning approaches.

2 Comparing Configuration Planning Approaches

Common points can be found between different flavours of configuration planning problems that we are examining in this section [6,7,2] and we assume the following. Firstly; sensors, actuators, programs, actions, percepts and other elements of the ecology are abstracted as elements to be connected with each other. Secondly, ways for relating most of the former elements exist in the representation. Thirdly, the process for generating configurations can be represented as a search problem.

M.J. O'Grady et al. (Eds.): AmI 2013 Workshops, CCIS 413, pp. 114–119, 2013.
© Springer International Publishing Switzerland 2013

ASyMTRe by Parker and Tang in [6] is and algorithm for configuring coalitions of single-task robots that uses schemas to represent collections of environmental sensors, percepts, motor and communication capabilities in robots. The configuration process in ASyMTRe involves greedily searching the space of potential solutions, and selecting the solution with the maximum local utility from each robots perspective, with the intention of maximising the sum of the utilities of all robots in the coalition. As for Lundh et al in [7], the capabilities of the members of an ecology are modelled as programs that can interact with the environment through sensing or actuating, and/or use information to produce additional information; such programs are called functionalities. Configurations are built by searching for ways to satisfy preconditions and inputs of functionalities as they were added into a configuration, with the help of task networks that held Information on how each action should decompose. Finally, Di Rocco in [2] proposes an approach in which configurations are represented with a pair of a set of activities and a set of temporal constraints over them. Configurations are obtained by five interacting solvers, and works in hand with an execution monitoring process.

We can compare the former approaches in terms of their properties and asymptotic complexities. However, when intending to compare them in terms of some metric, we see that such a thing is not possible since validation for these approaches was performed by means of scenarios, which are re-enactments of situations that are interesting for an application domain. Using scenarios for validating configuration planning approaches makes comparisons very difficult for two reasons: first, on each approach, a fairly different set of parameters is recorded, most likely to illustrate specific features of an approach; second, the exact same conditions for the scenario may not be available for other researchers, so a comparison is not always possible (no repeatability). To elucidate the former point, please compare section V of Parker and Tang [6], section 5 of Di Rocco et al [2], and section 6 of Lundh et al [7]. We can observe that there is a record of the execution time of the different ecology components in the scenarios, yet it is not possible to repeat them. It is also difficult to establish the influence of exogenous events on the measures. Finally, it is difficult to draw *unbiased* conclusions from only a small number of scenarios. There is a place for scenarios, as they often allows the researcher to observe a very specific aspect of an application domain, however it is not sufficient as an evaluation tool. Scenarios are best treated as complements to an empirical evaluation by means of experiments. In an experiment, the outcome of manipulating at least one independent variable is observed while other conditions remain controlled [9]. According to Hinkelmann [3], experiments can involve the observation of an assumed constant, of a varying property of a population, or of the response a group has to a procedure (treatment). Historically, experiments stem from the scientific method, and as such they are a repeatable way to test a hypothesis formulated from the important features of a research problem, and ultimately lead to conclusions.

3   Experimental Methodologies for Evaluation

As the configuration planning problem is a complex problem, the choice of using empirical methods for proving hypothesis to compare features of an approach is non-controversial. For the choice in *how* to prove these hypotheses, we propose to use sound statistical analysis of the behaviour of the algorithms over the infinite set $\mathscr{U}$ of all possible valid inputs. Since the computational tractability of the problem at hand prevents us from testing the algorithms using arbitrarily large input problems, we choose to prove only hypotheses that are valid for all problems up to a given size $|w|$ corresponding to the longest execution time that we are willing to let the algorithms run during practical use of the algorithms. Although the set of all possible problem instances of size up to $|w|$, for any non-trivial size $|w|$, is prohibitively large and cannot be exhaustively investigated we can prove properties of the algorithm using statistical analysis of randomly generated problem instances. This corresponds to measuring the mean and standard deviation of a stochastic variable whose value is the measured property for one problem instance taken from the space of all valid inputs using a uniform probability distribution.

To explain the methods, we will use a formalism based on some common points of the configuration planning approaches in section 2: sensors, actuators, programs and percepts are abstracted as elements to be connected with each other; we will assume some relation for connecting the former elements; and we assume that the process for generating configurations can be represented as a search problem. In this way, a configuration planning problem is represented as a set $\mathbf{w}$ of elements to be connected with each other, in which a goal and the initial conditions of the problem (as a set of effects) are included in $\mathbf{w}$. We have that each element in $\mathbf{w}$ can have between $\{0..k\}$ sensory and/or causal requirements, and can generate between $\{1..k\}$ information sources and causal effects. The goal of the problem is $f_g \in \mathbf{w}$, and the initial conditions are described by the causal effects $f_i \in \mathbf{w}$. f_i has no requirements. This single configuration planning problem $\mathbf{w}$ is a *scenario*. Before we can determine the size of the universe $\mathscr{U}$ of all valid inputs we need to determine the set of all possible elements from which valid inputs can be formulated. Since the set of all possible functionalities $\mathscr{F}$, where $\mathbf{w} \subset \mathscr{F}$, for an unbounded number of inputs and outputs is infinitely large we choose to look at the subset $\mathscr{F}_{m,k} \subset \mathscr{F}$ where m is the size of a dictionary determining compatible functionalities and where elements of the ecology a restricted to have between $\{0..k\}$ unique requirements and provide between $\{1..k\}$ unique sources taken from a dictionary of size $|m|$. The total size of $|\mathscr{F}_{m,k}|$ is given by $|\mathscr{F}_{m,k}| = \sum_{i=0}^{2k-1} \binom{|m|}{i}$. For convenience we will omit m,k and write only $|\mathscr{F}|$ when they are implicitly given. As we can see, $|\mathscr{F}|$ becomes intractably large even with a small dictionary. For instance, a dictionary with $m=18$ used to generate functionalities with $\{0..4\}$ requirements and $\{1..4\}$ sources, can generate 63004 unique functionalities. We write the universe of all possible scenarios using up to $|w|$ functionalities from $\mathscr{F}_{m,k}$ as $\mathscr{U}_{m,k,|w|} = \{ \mathbf{w}' \in \mathscr{P}(\mathscr{F}_{m,k}) : |w'| = |w| \}$. If we wanted to generate scenarios with $|w|=15$ unique functionality instances taken from a $\mathscr{F}_{18,4}$ we could generate up to $|\mathscr{U}_{18,4,15}| = \binom{|\mathscr{F}_{m,k}|}{|w|} = \binom{63004}{15}$ unique scenarios. For these numbers, the number of unique scenarios is in the order of octodecillions.

3.1   Method 1: Using Chernoff Bounds for Discrete Comparisons of Algorithms

As we can see in the previous section, comparing two independent configuration algorithms by exploring the space of all unique scenarios is infeasible as even small values of k,m and $|\mathbf{w}|$ would result in an intractable number of tests.

To make comparisons between configuration planning algorithms, we will conduct a series of $X_1, \ldots, X_N$ *independent* Bernoulli trials that test a given property for both algorithms using a boolean relation $\mathbb{R}$ (e.g. less-than relation). Examples of such properties would include the total execution time, number of nodes visited or if a solution was found. The outcome of each trial is zero or one, corresponding to if the relation is satisfied or not. With this formulation, it is possible to use tail inequalities to determine how many trials (n) are needed to determine a hypothesis H_a with an error of less than ε. To test the hypothesis, we use Chernoff bounds, since they provides tighter answers than Chebyshev bounds and the Markov inequality, given that we deal with independent Poisson trials, of which Bernoulli trails are a special case [4].

Define $\hat{p}$ by $\mathbf{Pr}[X_i = 1] = \hat{p}$, and $\mathbf{Pr}[X_i = 0] = 1 - \hat{p}$. We can now derive a *bound* for $\hat{p}$ based on Chernoff bounds. First, define $\hat{X} = \sum_{i=1}^{n} \hat{X}_i, X = \sum_{i=1}^{n} X_i$ where X_i is the outcome of the specific trials performed and $\hat{X}_i$ is the stochastic variable of the Bernoulli trials. We note that $\hat{X}$ has a binomial distribution [4]. Also, let $\hat{\mu} = \hat{X} = n\hat{p}$ and $\mu = X = np$. Next, consider the two variables $\varepsilon_{1,2}$ giving the error probability for our hypothesis to come, and the variable δ giving the tightness of the bounds – such that the following two equations hold.

$$n \geq \frac{4ln(\frac{1}{\varepsilon_1})}{(\delta)^2 p} \ , \ n \geq \frac{2ln(\frac{1}{\varepsilon_2})}{(\delta)^2 p} \tag{1}$$

Theorem 1. $\mathbf{Pr}[E(\hat{X}) > (1 + \delta^+)\mu] < \varepsilon_1$ *and* $\mathbf{Pr}[E(\hat{X}) < (1 - \delta^-)\mu] < \varepsilon_2$ *with the definitions of* $\hat{X}, \delta, \mu, \varepsilon_{1,2}$ *given above.*

Proof. Equations 1 holds for $\delta < 1$, and can be derived by rearranging equations 4.12 and 4.9 of Motwani [4].

Using the above theorem, and by replacing $\delta^+ = \sqrt{2}\delta^-$, we can now derive an expression for a bound on $\hat{p}$, valid for $\delta^2 < \frac{1}{2}$.

$$\hat{p} \in (\frac{1}{1 - \delta}\mu, \frac{1}{1 + \sqrt{2}\delta}\mu) \tag{2}$$

where $n = \frac{2ln(\frac{1}{\varepsilon})}{(\delta)^2 p}$. For determining the bounds on $\hat{p}$, we start by selecting a small value for p and perform as many trials as given in method 2. From the outcome of the trials, we compute the *actual* value of p. If this value is lower than the starting value of p we need to redo the trials with a larger number of runs[1]. Otherwise, we are ready to define our hypothesis H_a and corresponding null hypothesis H_0.

Hypothesis H_a: For any randomly selected scenario $w \in \mathcal{U}_{m,k,|w|}$ we have that $A(w) \ \mathbb{R} \ B(w)$ holds with the probability $\hat{p}$ given by Equation 2, where A,B are the two functions to sample the property of a w using the respective algorithm.

Hypothesis H_0: For any randomly selected scenario $w \in \mathcal{U}_{m,k,|w|}$ we have that $A(w) \ \mathbb{R} \ B(w)$ holds with the probability $\hat{p}$ *not* in the bounds given in Equation 2, where

---

[1] In this case, we cannot reuse any previous trials. Hence, it is important to pick the initial estimate of p small.

A,B are the two functions to sample the property of a w using the respective algorithm. Trivially, exactly one of H_a and H_0 must hold true. Using Theorem 1 we can reject the null hypothesis with $1 - \varepsilon$ certainty. Hence, hypothesis H_a holds with $1 - \varepsilon$ certainty.

This hypothesis formulation can be seen as a qualitative empirical proof of the behaviour of the algorithms, and is more appropriate for testing properties that can be established as true or false e.g. the planner being able to find a solution given certain conditions, or the planner returning a solution before a certain time is due. An alternative approach for determining quantitative differences of the algorithms is to estimate the mean of the property value within a given confidence interval, which we will look at in the next section.

3.2   Method 2: Using the Central Limit Theorem to Compute μ

This second experiment has the purpose of observing how treating a set of configuration planning approaches with a set of configuration planning problems, will vary the value of the mean and standard deviation of a parameter of the planner. A control group could be treating the set of problems with an algorithm that performs a random walk on the search space, or with published results of other configuration planning approaches.

The hypothesis formulation is slightly more flexible, and allows us to obtain and compare mean values and standard deviations of a stochastic variable $w \in \mathcal{U} : \mathbf{X}_A = A(w), \mathbf{X}_B = B(w)$ for the two approaches A, B. In addition to the impracticality of exploring such a space of problems, it is also very rare to know the actual distribution of the stochastic variables $\mathbf{X}$ beforehand, so choosing the most appropriate statistic for the distribution of the data is not feasible. However, we can obtain the mean $\hat{\mu}$ of the expected value of $\mathbf{X}$ with the mean μ of a *sampling distribution of sample means* S_m, and we can approximate the standard deviation $\hat{\sigma}$ of the expected value of $\mathbf{X}$ as a factor of the standard deviation σ of S_m (see [8]).

A sampling distribution of sample means is obtained by taking N independent samples of the same sample size n from $\mathcal{U}$, and calculating the means of each N. According to the central limit theorem, as $n \geq 30$ grows, the distribution of those sample means will approximate a normal distribution, with the same mean as the real population, and a standard deviation related to the standard deviation of the population and the inverse of the square root of n. To determine N, we use $N = 2 \left(\frac{\sigma erf^{-1}(c)}{M} \right)^2$. This equation [8] requires a margin of error M, a confidence level c, and a standard deviation σ of the population: the values of X that we are using to compare A and B are taken considering an error M and a confidence c. The method evaluates a Student t error function as *erf* (see [8]) with a confidence level c, which is an adequate error function since S_m follows a normal distribution. To determine c, a researcher may have a specific requirement, or perhaps use the *three-sigma rule* (also known as the 68-95-99 rule), which states that when a function follows a normal distribution, approximately 68%, 95% and 99% of the values are within 1, 2 and 3 standard deviations of the mean, respectively. The margin of error corresponds to half the width of a confidence interval. We can either use a-priori knowledge of the margin of error M and the standard deviation of the population σ, or we can express M as a small percentage of σ. When no a-priori knowledge is available for selecting these values, the latter method can ensure that no matter the sample size, the margin of error will remain as a small percentage of the standard deviation.

Now, we can perform N sets of $n \geq 30$ runs for each *category* of problems we want to discriminate upon e.g. different number of elements in the domain, and we record all information from these runs that we might want to look at a-posteriori. Then, we obtain the S_m of each observed variable and each category for each set of n runs, and obtain the mean and standard deviation of S_m as a descriptor for each variable in each category.

4 Summary

We have identified a problem in the configuration planning community, regarding comparability and repeatability of evaluations for new configuration planning approaches. We have analysed the size of the universe of all valid problem instances and have shown that although they are prohibitively large to analyse exhaustively, we can make scientific estimates of the behaviours of algorithms using statistical analysis. For this purpose we have presented and explained two methods, for which we can choose a hypothesis and a corresponding null hypothesis when analysing some given numerical property of a configuration planning algorithm. The first method, based on Chernoff bounds, allows us to make boolean comparisons between two algorithms and prove statements such as *"Algorithm A performs faster than algorithm B with a probability of atleast p for each scenario"* with a very low probability of error. The second algorithm, based on sampling sample means with a Gaussian distribution, allows us to prove statements such as *"The mean total time for executing any set of N scenarios for algorithm A is $\mu \pm \sigma$ seconds"* with a confidence level and a confidence interval.

References

1. Coles, A., Coles, A., Olaya, A.G., Jiménez, S., López, C.L., Sanner, S., Yoon, S.: A survey of the seventh international planning competition. AI Magazine 33(1), 83–88 (2012)
2. Di Rocco, M., Pecora, F., Sivakumar, P.K., Saffiotti, A.: Configuration planning with multiple dynamic goals. In: Proceedings of the AAAI Spring Symposium on Designing Intelligent Robots, Stanford, California (2013)
3. Hinkelmann, K.: Design and Analysis of Experiments, Special Designs and Applications, vol. 3 (2012), http://Wiley.com
4. Motwani, R.: Randomized algorithms. Cambridge University Press (1995)
5. Nebel, B., Koehler, J.: Plan reuse versus plan generation: a theoretical and empirical analysis. Artificial Intelligence 76(12), 427–454 (1995)
6. Parker, L.E., Tang, F.: Building multirobot coalitions through automated task solution synthesis. Proceedings of the IEEE 94(7), 1289–1305 (2006)
7. Lundh, R., Saffiotti, L.K., Autonomous, A.: Autonomous functional configuration of a network robot system. Robotics and Autonomous Systems. Elsevier (2008)
8. Rumsey, D.: Intermediate statistics for dummies. Wiley Publishing, Inc., Indianapolis (2007)
9. Winston, A.S., Blais, D.J.: What counts as an experiment?: A transdisciplinary analysis of textbooks, 1930-1970. The American Journal of Psychology, 599–616 (1996)

People-Centric Adaptive Social Ecology
between Intelligent Autonomous Humanoid Robot
and Virtual Human for Social Cooperation

S.M. Mizanoor Rahman

Dept. of Mechanical Engineering, Vrije Universiteit Brussel (VUB), Belgium
mizansm@hotmail.com

Abstract. The paper presents a simple people-centric adaptive ecology between a humanoid robot and a virtual human (social agents) to perform a real-world common complex social task. The social task was to assist the social agents each other in searching for a hidden object in a homely environment. In order to develop the ecology between the agents, we developed the agents with various similar functionalities, interaction modalities, sensing abilities, intelligence, autonomy etc., and integrated them through a common communication platform based on a novel control algorithm. In order to assess people's acceptance of the ecology between the social agents and to benchmark the ecology, we studied human's interactions with those agents and with some other allied agents for that task. We evaluated the attributes and performances of the social agents in their cooperations for the task, analyzed the attributes and performances and benchmarked them with the standards. The results showed that both of the social agents within the ecology could perform satisfactorily to accomplish the common social task though the performances varied slightly between the agents. We also found a trade-off between the attributes and the performances of the social agents. We then proposed to use the results to develop adaptive social ecologies with intelligent social agents of different realities to assist the humans in various real-world complex social tasks in smart spaces, or to get the real-world social tasks done in cooperation between the social agents.

Keywords: Adaptive social ecology, social robot, virtual human, system integration, human-computer interaction, human-robot interaction, smart spaces, benchmarking.

1   Introduction

1.1   The Virtual Humans and Social Robots (Social Agents)

The virtual humans are the software generated human-like animated characters. They can be developed with many social functions and attributes for their interactions with humans such as they can show human-like actions, motions, gestures, emotions, expressions, intelligence, autonomy etc., communicate and interact with the humans,

M.J. O'Grady et al. (Eds.): AmI 2013 Workshops, CCIS 413, pp. 120–135, 2013.
© Springer International Publishing Switzerland 2013

memorize the facts and retrieve them according to the dynamic context, and show reasoning and decision making abilities about what they perceive etc [1]-[2].

On the contrary, ideally, the social robots are the intelligent autonomous human-like robots, they may take inspirations from the humans, they are enriched with human-like communication and sensing abilities, they are capable of understanding human's affective states, emotions, expressions, intentions, actions, gestures etc., can interpret them based on contextual information and can act based on situations [3]-[4].

1.2   Performing Real-World Tasks by Virtual Humans and Social Robots

The virtual humans (VHs) are currently used to perform many tasks such as acting as the virtual tutor, student or trainee, patient, advertiser etc. They have increasing applications for anatomy education, psychotherapy, biomedical research etc [5]-[9]. However, the VHs still could not come beyond the virtual environments. We think that the applications of the VHs could be enhanced if they could perform the real-world social tasks for the humans or could cooperate with the humans to peform the social tasks. However, such applications are still not available. On the other hand, the social robots (SRs) are proposed for various social activities and interactions with the humans such as the therapies for social and cognitive development, autism etc [10]-[13]. However, their applications in performing social tasks in cooperation with the humans are still very limited. In most cases, either they do not look like the human [11], [13], or they may look like the human, but they may not act like the human [14]-[15], which may ultimately reduce their social acceptance.

1.3   Cooperations between SR and VH for Real-World Tasks in Social Ecology

The autonomous SRs and VHs have a lot in common in their objectives and performances though there is a difference that the SRs exist physically but the VHs are software-generated visual agents.We believe that SRs and VHs may separately cooperate with the humans and also with each other to perform the real-world tasks for the humans. However, such real-world social cooperations between VHs and SRs are usually not available. Of course, a few initiatives have been taken to stage the cooperations between VHs and SRs [16]-[17]. However, these initiatives are still in the concept design phases, and no real characters and cooperation methods have been proposed to realize the initiatives. On the other hand, social ecologies between the real-world social agents (e.g., networked multi-robots) have been slightly investigated [18], but the ecologies between social agents of heterogeneous realities such as the ecologies between the robots and the virtual humans for performing the real-world common complex tasks have never been investigated. We believe that such ecologies could enhance the individual performances, values and contributions of these agents.

1.4   Performances Evaluation and Benchmarking of the Social Agents

We think that there should have well-defined evaluation methods and standards for evaluating and benchmarking the performances of the social agents in their various social interactions with each other and with the humans within the ecologies, which may help improve their performances, social acceptance and social impacts. However, suitable evaluation and benchmarking techniques are still not available. Of course, a few evaluation and benchmarking methods of the social agents have been proposed, but the efforts are still limited in scope and applications [19]-[20].

1.5   Objective and the Paper Summary

Hence, the objective was to develop a simple adaptive ecology between a SR and a VH for social cooperations between them for a real-world common complex social task (searching for a hidden object). For this purpose, we aimed to develop a VH and a SR (social agents) with various similar functionalities, interaction modalities, intelligence, autonomy, sensing abilities etc. and integrate them through a common communication platform based on a novel control algorithm so that they can assist each other in the task. We aimed to study the human's interactions with these social agents and with some other allied agents for the task to benchmark the interactions between the social agents. We thus evaluate the attributes and performances of the agents in their interactions for the task in the ecology and benchmark them with the standards. We think that the results will help develop adaptive ecologies with intelligent social agents of different realities to assist the humans in various real-world social tasks, or to get the real-world social tasks done in cooperations between the artificial social agents of different realities.

2   People-Centric Adaptive Social Ecology

The central concept behind the agent ecology is that the complex tasks may not be performed properly by a single, very capable agent (e.g., a humanoid robot), instead the tasks are performed through the cooperation of many networked and bi-laterally communicating agents in a coordinated and goal oriented way. Building smart spaces in this way may reduce the application complexity and costs as well as enhance the individual values and contributions of the agents involved that may enable new services that may not be performed by any agent individually [18].Suitable integrating software platforms, intelligent controllers, actuating devices, communications, sensors etc. are necessary to build such ecolgy. The ecology should have cognitive and learning abilities and the ability to adapt with changes and uncertainties. It should be robust and efficient   and should gain users' acceptance and produce social impacts if it is   implemented in people-centric social environment [18].

3   Requirements for the Integration between Social Robot and Virtual Human in the Ecology

The effective integration of the SR with the VH for a specific real-world task needs to satisfy a set of requirements. The SRs need to have attributes for social interactions such as interactivity, intelligence, autonomy, perception, bilateral communication and interactions, social functions etc. [3]-[4], [10]-[15]. Similarly, the VHs should have intelligent decision technologies, autonomy, interaction modalities, personality, natural interactivity etc. [21]-[22].Kapadia *et al.* identified several key limitations in the existing representation, control, locomotion, multimodal perception and authoring of the autonomous VHs that must be addressed to generate successful interactions between the VH and the SR [23].Other requirements for creating interactive VHs for interactions with SRs are presented in [24]. Emotion, memory, recognition etc. for the social agents also seem to be important for their integration for multimodal social interactions for many cases [25]-[27].

The required interaction modes for the selected task might be vision, audition (speech), demonstration, recognition, gesture, locomotion etc. It means that, the social agents may need to see and recognize each other, the object and the environment, to speak and listen the counterpart for verbal instructions by the agents about the search path for the hidden object, to show gesture and understand/recognize the counterpart's gesture that may be used by the agents to demonstrate/understand the search path for the hidden object. They may also need to show movements to search for the object. They need to be enriched with the required technologies, control methods and algorithms, interfaces, sensors, communication platform etc.They should also be as human-like in appearances and performances as possible and their performances should be benchmarked to enhance their social acceptance.

4   Developing the Social Agents

4.1   The Virtual Human

We developed a realistic 3D virtual human (VH) with a woman face. We used the Smartbody (http://smartbody.ict.usc.edu/) for her control and animation. We created the model based on the joints and skeleton requirements of the Smartbody and then exported it to the Autodesk Maya 3D software (http://www.autodesk.com/).We estimated the anthropomorphic data (walking and running velocities, joint angles, whole body dimensions etc.) for the VH by being inspired by that for the human. We used Ogre for graphical rendering (http://www.ogre3d.org/).The software package included Application Programming Interfaces (APIs) for various functions such as expressions, gestures, actions, emotions etc. The VH was displayed in a screen as shown in Fig.1 (a). The VH was enriched with many social capabilities and attributes such as speech (from text to speech), locomotion (walk to a position), manipulation, gaze, nonverbal behaviours, facial expressions, emotions, actions, communications with the human, turn head, look at a position, point at something etc. The VH could perceive the environment through sensors (video, audio etc.). It could make decision based on some adaptive rules and stored information and react by moving, talking or showing internal emotions. The VH was interactive, intelligent and autonomous.

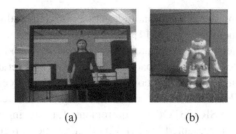

(a)   (b)

Fig. 1. The intelligent autonomous social agents, (a) the virtual human, (b) the social robot

4.2   The Social Robot

We used a NAO robot (http://www.aldebaran-robotics.com/en/) as shown in Fig.1 (b) as the social robot (SR). We developed various functions and attributes for the robot to make it intelligent, autonomous and social such as stand up, sit down, walk, shake hand, wave hand, grab and release object, look at a position, point at something, speech (text to speech) etc. Like the VH, it could perceive the environment through sensors such as video, audio etc. It could make decision based on some adaptive rules and stored information and react by moving, talking or showing internal emotions. Its software package included the APIs for the functions.

4.3   Developing Common Communication Platform for the Social Agents

Animation of each function of each character was commanded from a common command script (client) that was networked with the control server through the I2P (Integrated Interaction Platform) Thrift interface. The I2P was our in-house platform that we used to animate both the SR and the VH using the same command script (client) through specifying the character. However, each character had its own APIs for the functions called in the client script. The similar functions between the VH and the SR produced similar behaviours. Architecture of the common communication scheme for the social agents through the I2P is shown in Fig.2.

5   Experimental Setup

As Fig.3 shows, we arranged three rooms. We kept the computers in Room 1 to control the SR, VH and other hardwares. We kept 10 rectangular boxes of identical dimensions and appearance (black) in Room 2. We put five boxes randomly on a table in the left side of the room, and put the remaining five boxes randomly on two sofas in the right side. An object (a small doll) was hidden in any of the 10 boxes by the experimenter. One agent required assistance (called the assisted agent) from another agent (called the assistant agent) to search for the hidden object. Usually, the assisted agent stood at P1, and the assistant agent stood at P2 or appeared at the screen (e.g. the virtual human). Laptop 2 was used for Skype connection with Laptop 1 (in Room 3) if any human acted as the assistant agent but he/she did not appear physically, instead appeared in the screen through the Skype link. In addition, we put kinect cameras in Room 2, and also put other apparatus required for gesture recognition.

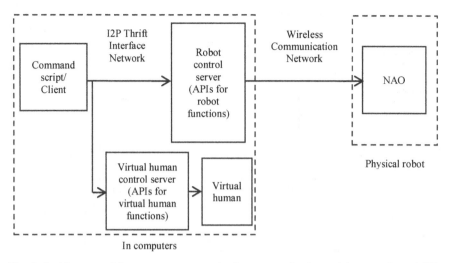

Physical robot

In computers

Fig. 2. Architecture of the common communication system for the social agents through I2P

6   Experiment Design

6.1   Experiment Protocols

We decided six experiment protocols to evaluate the cooperations between different social agents for searching for the hidden object as given in Table 1. In the protocols from 1 to 4, the human (assisted agent) received assistance from various assistant agents such as another human (protocol #1), another human appeared through Skype link (protocol #2), virtual human   (protocol #3), social robot   (protocol #4) etc. for searching for the hidden object. In protocols #5 & 6, the SR and the VH assisted each other for searching for the hidden object. We used the protocols from 1 to 4 to benchmark the interactions between the SR and the VH in protocols #5 & 6.

The VH possessed human-like functions, but it was screen-based and artificial. Consequently, it could not appear physically in front of the assisted agent. Similarly, the Skyped-human was also screen-based and it did not appear physically in front of the assisted agent, but it was natural. We recognized the Skyped-human as the physically non-appeared real human with the highest level of autonomy and intelligence. Hence, we assumed the Skyped-human as the standard for the VH. On the contrary, the SR was physically embodied, it existed like the human, it possessed human-like appearance, but it was artificial. The human is the physically embodied and physically existed natural agent with the highest level of autonomy and intelligence. Hence, we assumed the human as the standard for the SR. The SR and the VH were both artificial though they differed in the physical existence. We employed these protocols (#5 & 6) to examine the social interactions between the VH and the SR, which was our primary goal. These protocols could also help examine the effects of physical existence of the agents on their performances and social interactions.

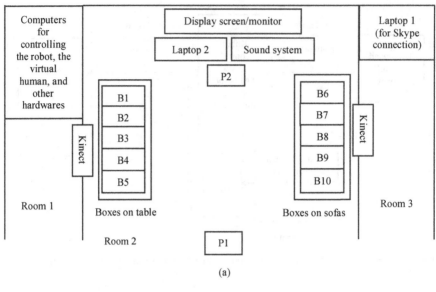

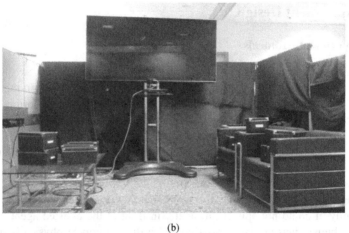

(b)

Fig. 3. (a) Layout diagram of the experimental setup, (b) inside of the room 2

Table 1. The social agents and their social interactions (as acronyms)

Protocol#	Assistant agent	Assisted agent	Interactions
1	Human (H)	Human (H)	H-H
2	Skyped human (SkypedH)	Human (H)	SkypedH-H
3	Virtual human (VH)	Human (H)	VH-H
4	Social robot (SR)	Human (H)	SR-H
5	Virtual human (VH)	Social robot (SR)	VH-SR
6	Social robot (SR)	Virtual human (VH)	SR-VH

6.2   Selection of the Subjects

We estimated the ideal requirements of 102 human subjects to take part in the experiments for different protocols (1 assistant human and 20 assisted humans for protocol#1, 1 assistant human appeared through Skype and 20 assisted humans for protocol#2, 20 assisted humans for each of the protocols #3 and #4, and 20 humans to evaluate the VH-SR and SR-VH interactions in protocols #5 & #6). The targeted subjects were mainly the students and staffs   (male and female) and they aged between 20 and 50 years. All the available subjects were right-handed and were physically and mentally healthy with sound eyes and ears. The subjects did not have prior experience with the SR and the VH. We individually instructed the subjects on how to conduct the experiment, but we did not arrange any formal training for them.

6.3   The Hypotheses

We adopted several hypotheses (research questions) to examine the cooperations between the agents as follows: (i) whether or not the performances of the assistant agents were satisfactory for the social task (for protocols#1-6), (ii) whether or not the performances of the assistant agents varied for the same assisted   agent (protocols #1-4) in the ecology, (iii) between the VH and the SR in protocols #3 and #4, whose performances were the better in assisting the human, (iv) whose performances were the better when the VH and the SR assisted each other (protocols#5 & 6), (v) whether or not the attributes of the agents could affect the performances of the agents, (vi) whether or not the adaptive social ecology between real and virtual agents was effective and justified   etc.

7   The Experiments

Protocol #1: The assistant agent (human) stood at P2   as in Fig.3 keeping the face towards P1.The experimenter needed to hide the object in any of the 10 boxes (say, it was hidden inside box B6). The assistant agent knew it. Then, the assisted agent stood at P1 keeping the face towards P2. Then, the assistant agent instructed (once only) the assisted agent on how to find the hidden object. The instructions included-

Speech: the assistant agent told "hello! I can assist you find the hidden object. The box containing the hidden object is lying on a sofa. It is not on top of another box. It may be closest to the screen".

Gesture, facial expressions, emotions and actions: the assistant agent turned towards the box where the object was hidden, looked at the box, pointed at the box with the hand, and made some facial expressions that matched the gesture and the actions.

Then, the assisted agent needed to determine the correct box based on the instructions of the assistant agent, then he/she moved to the box, pointed the box, touched it, grabbed it, told "the object is here" and then released it. The experimenter then opened the box and checked whether or not the object was found inside the box. The assisted agent then subjectively evaluated the attributes and performances of the assistant agent in his/her assistance for the assisted agent in searching for the hidden object. The evaluation was done based on a rating scale following a set of predefined criteria. The experimenter administered the evaluation. The evaluation criteria for the agent attributes were as follows: (i) anthropomorphism- how human-like the assistant agent was in appearance and performances, (ii) embodiments-how embodied the assistant agent was, (iii) gesture and action- whether or not there was any match between gesture and action of the assistant agent, (iv) stability-how competent the assistant agent was to avoid disturbances, noises etc. The performance criteria for the assistant agents were as follows: (i) cooperation- how cooperative the assistant agent was in assisting the assisted agent, (ii) clarity of instructions -how clearly the assisted agent understood the instructions of the assistant agent, (iii) effectiveness-how effective the instructions of the assistant agent were for the assisted agent in finding the object, (iv) cognitive load- how much cognitive load the assisted agent felt for finding the object (least cognitive load was to be the best), and (v) companionship- whether or not the assisted agent was motivated to establish a social companionship with the assistant agent based on the assistance. In the rating scale, (+1) indicates the worst and (+5) indicates the best evaluation for the assistant agent. The experimenter also objectively evaluated the peformances of the assistant agent based on two criteria as follows: (i) time-time taken by the assisted agent to find the correct box (we assumed that the performance of the assistant agent would be the best if the assisted agent could find the correct box within the least possible time), and (ii) accuracy- whether or not the assisted agent could find the correct box after all.

Then, the experimenter replaced the assisted agent by another subject keeping the assistant agent unchanged, and repeated the whole procedures as described above for the second subject (assisted agent). In this way, 20 subjects individually served as the assisted agent. Figure 4 (a) shows the experiment procedures for this protocol.

Protocol#2: A human standing at Room 3 appeared at the screen of Room 2 through the Skype and served as the assistant agent. Then, the same experiment procedures as employed for protocol#1 were employed as shown in Fig 4 (b).

Protocol#3: As Fig. 4 (c) shows, the VH appeared at the screen and acted as the assistant agent. Then, the same procedures as employed in protocol#1 were employed.

Protocol #4: The SR stood at P2 and acted as the assistant agent. Then, the same procedures as employed in protocol#1 were employed as shown in Fig. 4 (d).

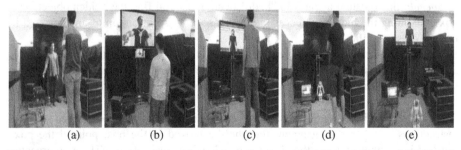

(a)   (b)   (c)   (d)   (e)

Fig. 4. The human receives assistance from (a) another human, (b) Skyped-human, (c) VH, and (d) SR for searching for the hidden object. In (e), the SR and the VH assists each other for searching for the object. The object was hidden inside any of the 10 black boxes as it is seen.

Protocol#5: Ten (10) relevant instruction methods for 10 locations of the 10 boxes were set (called) for the VH in the programming script (client). The VH could instruct the SR about the correct location of the box containing the hidden object if the object was hidden in any of the 10 boxes. However, the VH was to be taught the correct location of the box through the programming script. For example, in an experiment trial, the object was hidden in a box on the sofa that was also closest to the screen (box B6). We run the program and the VH instructed the SR to find the object based on the instruction methods set for that box as follows :

Speech: The same speech as implemented in protocol#1.

Gesture, emotions, expressions and actions: the VH showed emotions, facial expressions, gesture and actions matching her speech. For example, the VH turned towards the box containing the hidden object, smiled, looked at the box, moved towards the box (within the screen limit), pointed at it with the hand, told "the object is there" and then stopped working.

In the same programming script (client) as implemented for the VH, the required functions, expressions, gestures, emotions, speech, actions etc. for 10 different destinations (locations for 10 boxes) were set (called) for the SR. The SR could recognize the gesture of the VH and immediately determine the correct location of the box containing the hidden object based on the information it received from the VH through the gesture recognition, then turned towards the location and moved to that location, looked at the box, pointed at the box, took an attempt to grab the box (but, it could not grab due to its small fingers), then released the grab, then told "the object is inside this box" and then stopped working.Then, the experimenter opened the box and checked whether or not the hidden object was found there. The trial was repeated for 20 times and each of the 20 subjects evaluated the attributes and performances of the assistant agent based on the same criteria and methods as employed in protocol#1. The experimenter also recorded the time and accuracy data for each trial. Figure 4 (e) shows the experiment procedures for this protocol.

Protocol#6: the opposite of protocol#5 was staged when the SR assisted the VH in searching for the hidden object. The SR was taught the correct location of the hidden object through the programming script. The instruction methods for the SR were same as that for the VH.The VH could recognize the gesture of the SR and immediately determine the correct location of the box containing the hidden object, then turned towards the box and moved towards that location (up to the screen limit), looked at and pointed at the box, then told "the object is inside that box". Then, the experimenter opened the pointed box and checked whether or not the hidden object was found there. The trial was repeated for 20 times and the same evaluation procedures as employed in protocol#5 were employed.

8   Experiment Results and Analyses

Table 2 shows the mean evaluation scores with standard deviations for the performances of the assistant agents for interactions between different assistant and assisted agents. The table shows that the human, Skyped-human, SR and the VH secured the 1st, 2nd, 3rd and 4th position respectively for their performances when acting as the assistant agents for the assisted agents (human).The performances of the

Table 2. Mean (n=20) evaluation scores with standard deviations for the performances of the assistant agents for interactions between different assistant and assisted agents

Evaluation Criteria	Interactions between different assistant and assisted agents					
	H-H	SkypedH-H	VH-H	SR-H	VH-SR	SR-VH
Cooperation	5 (0)	4.7	3.9	4.2	3.8	4.1
		(0.1830)	(0.1062)	(0.1213)	(0.0762)	(0.1129)
Clarity	5 (0)	4.9	4.2	4.5	4.1	4.4
		(0.1162)	(0.1116)	(0.1215)	(0.0818)	(0.0781)
Effectiveness	5 (0)	4.8	4.1	4.3	4.0	4.2
		(0.1216)	(0.1167)	(0.1112)	(0.0998)	(0.1190)
Cognitive load	5 (0)	4.4	3.6	3.9	3.5	3.8
		(0.1164)	(0.1009)	(0.0897)	(0.0674)	(0.0962)
Companionship	5 (0)	4.6	3.7	4.1	3.6	4.0
		(0.1043)	(0.0921)	(0.1008)	(0.0459)	(0.0824)

assistant agents are satisfactory for the task that justifies the hypothesis (i). However, there are variations in the performances of the assistant agents for the same assisted agent that justifies the hypothesis (ii). The Skyped-human performed better than the VH. The reason may be that the VH was artificial, but the Skyped-human was the agent with natural origin. The results also show that the SR performed better than the VH probably due to the reason that the SR had physical existence, but the VH lacked it, which justifies the hypothesis (iii). Analyses of Variances (ANOVAs) for each criterion in each interaction showed that the variations in the evaluation scores due to the variation in the assisted agents (evaluators) were not statistically significant ($p>0.05$ at each case). The results also show that for VH-SR and SR-VH interactions where the VH and the SR assisted each other, the SR performed better than the VH that justifies the hypothesis (iv). It might happen probably due to the reason that the SR had physical existence, but the VH lacked it. Again, the performances of the SR and the VH as the assistant agents were evaluated for two conditions (protocols #3 & 5 for the VH, and protocols #4 & 6 for the SR). ANOVAs showed that the variations in performances for each of the two agents between these two conditions were not statistically significant ($p>0.05$ at each case), which indicates that the VH and the SR show similar performances in their assistance for natural (human) and artificial (VH or SR) assisted agents. It clearly justifies that the SR and the VH may be employed to assist each other in a remote or unmanned location or in any social location where human is not the performer but the beneficiary.

Table 3 shows the mean evaluation scores for the attributes of the agents. We see that the stability for the assistant agents except in protocol#1 is low. The reasons may be that the agents were slightly vulnerable to the external disturbances such as sound, noises etc. The SR might also be affected by floor properties and obstacles (if any). The results show that the assistant agents i.e. the human, Skyped-human, SR and VH secured the 1st, 2nd, 3rd and 4th position respectively in their attributes. The order for the agent attributes exactly matches that for the agent performancs (Table 2). In addition, the relationships for the attributes between (i) Skyped-human and VH, and (ii) VH and SR for different conditions were exactly same as that for the agent performances, which indicates that the agent attributes affect the agent performances [28]. The findings justify the hypothesis (v). It is true that the interactions between the SR and the VH were controlled by algorithms through programming script where there might have no influence of agent appearance or anthropomorphism. However, the performances of agents were evaluated by the humans who were influenced by the appearances of the SR and the VH.

Table 4 shows the mean times with standard deviations required by the assisted agents to find the correct box for interactions between various assistant and assisted agents. As the results show, the assistant agents in the interactions H-H, SR-VH, SkypedH-H, SR-H, VH-H and VH-SR secured the 1st, 2nd, 3rd, 4th, 5th and 6th position respectively for their performance for this time-based criterion. The order (except SR-VH) matches that of the performances and the attributes of the assistant agents in tables 2 and 3 respectively. In SR-VH interaction, the VH found the box based on the assistance of the SR. However, the interaction was controlled by software for a fixed speed of the VH (same speed as the assisted human in protocol#1 as we were inspired by the human while developing the VH). As a result, the time required by the VH was almost same as that required by the assisted human in protocol#1. Again, we see that there is no standard deviation in the mean time for the SR-VH interaction because there was no variation in the time required by the VH as it was controlled by the software for a fixed speed and the speed was not to be affected by disturbances. In VH-SR interaction, the input speed of the SR was the same as that of the assisted human of protocol#1, and the interaction was software-controlled. However, the SR took the time which was longer than that the assisted human took in protocol#1, and its time-based performance was ranked as the last. We also see that there is some small standard deviation for the VH-SR interaction. The reason may be that eventhough the SR was controlled by software for a fixed speed, it might be affected by disturbances (e.g. floor properties). It is also reflected in the lower stability of the SR (Table 3). The results show that, in general, the required time is related to the agent attributes, which justifies the hypothesis (v). ANOVAs show that the variations in time between the assisted agents were not significant ($p>0.05$ at each case).

Table 3. Mean ($n=20$) evaluation scores with standard deviations for the attributes of the assistant agents for interactions between different assistant and assisted agents

Attributes	Interactions between different assistant and assisted agents					
	H-H	SkypedH-H	VH-H	SR-H	VH-SR	SR-VH
Anthropomorphism	5 (0)	4.9 (0.1162)	4.6 (0.1043)	4.7 (0.1233)	4.6 (0.1043)	4.7 (0.1233)
Embodiments	5 (0)	4.8 (0.1216)	4.6 (0.1043)	4.8 (0.1216)	4.6 (0.1043)	4.8 (0.1216)
Gesture and action	5 (0)	4.9 (0.1162)	4.7 (0.1233)	4.8 (0.1216)	4.7 (0.1233)	4.8 (0.1216)
Stability	5 (0)	3.9 (0.1106)	3.6 (0.0878)	3.7 (0.0918)	3.6 (0.1030)	3.7 (0.0737)

Table 4. Mean ($n=20$) times with standard deviations required by the assisted agents to find the correct box

	Interactions between different assistant and assisted agents					
	H-H	SkypedH-H	VH-H	SR-H	VH-SR	SR-VH
Time (s)	17.12 (0.39)	21.09 (0.41)	25.63 (0.29)	23.71 (0.21)	26.57 (0.09)	17.12 (0)

Table 5. Accuracy (%) in finding the correct box by the assisted agents for various interactions between the assistant and the assisted agents

	Interactions between different assistant and assisted agents					
	H-H	SkypedH-H	VH-H	SR-H	VH-SR	SR-VH
Accuracy (%)	100	100	100	100	100	100

Accuracy of the assisted agents is shown in Table 5. The results show that all the assisted agents in all interactions could accurately find the correct box i.e., the accuracy or the success rate is 100%. This relationship also matches the relationships between the interactions in terms of performances, attributes and time in Tables 2, 3 and 4 respectively.

The results show that the VH in VH-H and VH-SR interactions was very close to the Skyped-human in SkypedH-H interaction, and the SR in the SR-H and SR-VH interactions was close to the human (assistant agent) in the H-H interaction in terms of the attributes. Similarly, the VH was able to achieve approximately 89% and 87% performances of the Skyped-human (standard for the VH) in the VH-H and VH-SR interactions respectively, and the SR was able to achieve approximately 90% and 88% performances of the human (standard for the SR) in the SR-H and SR-VH interactions respectively. However, as the assistant agent, the human's performance was better than the Skyped-human's performance, and hence the SR was still better than the VH in terms of performances.The results as a whole show that the adaptive social ecology between the real and virtual agents is effective, which justifies the hypothesis (vi).

9   Justification of the Adaptive Ecology with the Social Agents

The social robot and the virtual human were enriched with various attributes and skills and were integrated/networked through a common platform using appropriate sensing and communication channels for collaboration for the common goal (searching for the hidden object) in a homely smart human environment, which is the central theme of the social ecologies with the social agents [18]. Such social ecology reduces the application complexity and costs, enhances the individual values of the agents, devices and systems involved by enabling new services that cannot be performed by any of the agent, device and system itself [18].The especially developed social agents with various attributes, skills and capabilities, the in-house I2P integration platform, software packages, intelligent control algorithms and controller, sensors and communication devices and systems etc. have made the social ecology with real and virtual agents successful [18], [29]-[32].The ecology is adaptive, robust and efficient as the agents within the ecology possess intelligence to adapt with changes, decision making abilities, cognitive and learning abilities etc. Again, the ecology is people-centric and social as it has a common target to perform a common complex social task for the people in the homely environment.   The results also show that the ecology is able to cope with the key scientific and technical challenges such as goal priority, scalability, distribution, communication, heterogeneity, integration etc. [18].

10   Conclusions and Future Works

We implemented an adaptive people-centric   social ecology with a social robot and a virtual human to assist each other in a real-world social task based on a control algorithm through a common communication platform.We evaluated the interactions and cooperations between them and benchmarked the interactions and cooperations with some other allied interactions for the same task.The results showed that the performances of the interactions between the robot and the virtual human were satisfactory, which indicates that the integration betweeen the agents of heterogeneous realities were successful for the ecology.Their performances varied from each other and were affected by their attributes.The integration between robot and virtual human for real-world performances, methods for evaluation and benchmarking of social agents of different realities, implementation of communication for social agents of different realities through a common platform etc. that we proposed within the ecology are the most novel and have excellent prospects and applications. Thus, the findings will help develop adaptive social ecologies with intelligent social agents of heterogeneous realities (e.g., robots and virtual humans) to assist humans in real-world tasks, and to assist each other in smart social environment.

In future, we may employ human voice (only) and human video with voice as the assistant agents to further examine the effects of sound, vision and physical existence of the agents on agent performances.We will implement action and speech recognition to augment the decision making abilities of the social robot and the virtual human. We will improve the attributes, functions and capabilities of the virtual human and the social robot, apply advanced technologies and employ the social agents in the tasks with more complex social interactions in advanced social ecologies. We will also conduct extended studies to evaluate the social impacts of the social agents.

Acknowledgements. The author acknowledges the supports that he received from the Institute for Media Innovation, Nanyang Technological University, 50 Nanyang Drive, Singapore 637553, and from his past colleagues of the Institute.

References

[1] Swartout, W., Gratch, J., Hill, R.W., Hovy, E., Marsella, S., Rickel, J., Traum, D.: Toward virtual humans. AI Magazine 27(2), 96–108 (2006)

[2] Kotranza, A., Lok, B., Pugh, C., Lind, D.: Virtual humans that touch back: enhancing nonverbal communication with virtual humans through bidirectional touch. In: IEEE Virtual Reality Conference, pp. 175–178 (2009)

[3] Castellano, G., Peters, C.: Socially perceptive robots: challenges and concerns. Interaction Studies 11(2), 201–207 (2010)

[4] Leite, I., Martinho, C., Paiva, A.: Social robots for long-term interaction: a survey. International Journal of Social Robotics 5(2), 291–308 (2013)

[5] Hays, M., Campbell, J., Trimmer, M., Poore, J., Webb, A., Stark, C., King, T.: Can role-play with virtual humans teach interpersonal skills? In: Proc. of Interservice/Industry Training, Simulation and Education Conference (I/ITSEC), Paper No. 12318, Pages 12 (2012)

[6] SikLanyi, C., Geiszt, Z., Karolyi, P., Magyar, A.: Virtual reality in special needs early education. The International Journal of Virtual Reality 5(4), 55–68 (2006)

[7] Campbell, J., Hays, M., Core, M., Birch, M., Bosack, M., Clark, R.: Interpersonal and leadership skills: using virtual humans to teach new officers. In: Proc. of Interservice/Industry Training, Simulation, and Education Conference, Paper No. 11358 (2011)

[8] Saleh, N.: The value of virtual patients in medical education. Annals of Behavioral Science and Medical Education 16(2), 29–31 (2010)

[9] Lawford, P., Narracott, A., McCormack, K., Bisbal, J., Martin, C., Brook, B., Zachariou, M., Kohl, P., Fletcher, K., Diaz-Zucczrini, V.: Virtual physiological human: training challenges. Phil. Trans. R. Soc. A 368(1921), 2841–2851 (2010)

[10] Scassellati, B.: Using social robots to study abnormal social development. In: Proceedings of the Fifth International Workshop on Epigenetic Robotics: Modeling Cognitive Development in Robotic Systems, pp. 11–14 (2005)

[11] Dautenhahn, K., Werry, I.: Towards interactive robots in autism therapy-background, motivation and challenges. Pragmatics & Cognition 12(1), 1–35 (2004)

[12] Scassellati, B., Admoni, H., Mataric, M.: Robots for use in autism research. Annu. Rev. Biomed. Eng. 14, 275–294 (2012)

[13] Fischer, L., Alexander, E., Yan, X., Su, H., Harrington, K., Fischer, G.: An affordable compact humanoid robot for autism spectrum disorder interventions in children. In: Proc. of 33rd Annual Int. Conf. of the IEEE EMBS, Boston, USA, pp. 5319–5322 (2011)

[14] Nishio, S., Ishiguro, H., Hagita, N.: Geminoid: teleoperated android of an existing person. In: Filho, A. (ed.) Humanoid Robots: New Developments, ch. 20. InTech (2007)

[15] Kaneko, K., Kanehiro, F., Morisawa, M., Miura, K., Nakaoka, S., Kajita, S.: Cybernetic human hrp-4c. In: Proc. of IEEE-RAS Int. Conf. on Humanoid Robots, pp. 7–14 (2009)

[16] Dragone, M., Duffy, B., O'Hare, G.: Social interaction between robots, avatars & humans. In: Proc. of IEEE Int. Workshop on Robot and Human Interactive Communication, pp. 24–29 (2005)

[17] Forland, E., Russa, G.: Virtual humans vs. anthropomorphic robots for education: how can they work together? In: Proc. of ASEE/IEEE Frontiers in Education Conference, p. S3G (2005)

[18] Dragone, M., Rocco, M., Pecora, F., Saffiotti, A., Swords, D.: A software suite for the control and the monitoring of adaptive robotic ecologies (extended abstract). In: Proc. of the Workshop on Towards Fully Decentralized Multi-Robot Systems: Hardware, Software and Integration, IEEE Int. Conference on Robotics and Automation, Karlsruhe, Germany, May 6 -10 (2013)

[19] Madhavan, R., Pobil, A., Messina, E.: Performance evaluation and benchmarking of robotic and automation systems. IEEE Robotics and Automation Magazine, 120–122 (2010)

[20] Kipp, M., Kipp, K.H., Ndiaye, A., Gebhard, P.: Evaluating the tangible interface and virtual characters in the interactive COHIBIT exhibit. In: Gratch, J., Young, M., Aylett, R.S., Ballin, D., Olivier, P. (eds.) IVA 2006. LNCS (LNAI), vol. 4133, pp. 434–444. Springer, Heidelberg (2006)

[21] Kasap, Z., Thalmann, N.: Intelligent virtual humans with autonomy and personality: state-of-the-art. Intelligent Decision Technologies 1, 3–15 (2007)

[22] Kang, Y., Subagdja, B., Tan, A., Ong, Y., Miao, C.: Virtual characters in agent-augmented co-space. In: Proc. of the 11th Int. Conference on Autonomous Agents and Multiagent Systems (AAMAS 2012), Valencia, Spain, June 4-8 (2012)

[23] Kapadia, M., Shoulson, A., Boatright, C.D., Huang, P., Durupinar, F., Badler, N.I.: What's next? the new era of autonomous virtual humans. In: Kallmann, M., Bekris, K. (eds.) MIG 2012. LNCS, vol. 7660, pp. 170–181. Springer, Heidelberg (2012)

[24] Gratch, J., Rickel, J., Andre, E., Badler, N., Cassell, J., Petajan, E.: Creating interactive virtual humans: some assembly required. IEEE Intelligent Systems, 2–11 (2002)

[25] Kasap, Z., Moussa, M., Chaudhuri, P., Thalmann, N.: Making them remember-emotional virtual characters with memory. IEEE Computer Graphics and Applications 29(2), 20–29 (2009)

[26] Kasap, Z., Thalmann, N.: Building long-term relationships with virtual and robotic characters: the role of remembering. The Visual Computer 28(1), 87–97 (2012)

[27] Zhao, W., Xie, X., Yang, X.: Control virtual human with speech recognition and gesture recognition technology. Advances in Intelligent and Soft Computing 139, 441–446 (2012)

[28] Wainer, J., Feil-Seifer, D., Shell, D., Mataric, M.: The role of physical embodiment in human-robot interaction. In: Proc. of the 15th IEEE International Symposium on Robot and Human Interactive Communication, pp. 117–122 (2006)

[29] Bacciu, D., Chessa, S., Gallicchio, C., Lenzi, A., Micheli, A., Pelagatti, A.: A general purpose distributed learning model for robotic ecologies. In: Proc. of International IFAC Symposium on Robotic Control, September 5-7, vol. 10(1), pp. 435–440 (2012)

[30] Dragone, M., Swords, D., Abdalla, S., Broxvall, M., O'Hare, G.: A programming framework for multi agent coordination of robotic ecologies. In: AAMAS, Tenth International Workshop on Programming Multi- Agent Systems, ProMAS, Valencia, Spain, June 5 (2012)

[31] Rocco, M., Pecora, F., Kumar, P., Saffiotti, A.: Configuration planning with multiple dynamic goals. In: Proc. of AAAI Spring Symposium on Designing Intelligent Robots, California (March 2013)

[32] Saffiotti, A., Broxvall, M.: PEIS ecologies: ambient intelligence meets autonomous robotics. In: Proc. of the International Conference on Smart Objects and Ambient Intelligence (sOc-EUSAI), Grenoble, France, pp. 275–280 (2005)

A Portable and Self-presenting Robotic Ecology HRI Testbed

Anara Sandygulova and Mauro Dragone

University College Dublin
Belfield, Dublin 4, Ireland
anara.sandygulova@ucdconnect.ie,
mauro.dragone@ucd.ie

Abstract. Robotic ecologies are networks of heterogeneous devices (sensors, actuators, automated appliances and mobile robots) pervasively embedded in everyday environments, where they cooperate to the achievement of complex tasks. Their successful application opens important research questions for both their engineering and their interaction with human users. In this paper we illustrate a testbed built to support interaction studies between human users and robotic ecologies. The testbed consists of an interactive and autonomous robotic ecology that is able to engage with human users, react to their activities, and even introduce them to the main concepts behind robotic ecologies. We describe how such a testbed is built using a middleware purposefully designed for robotic ecologies, and we report our experiences in its application to a number of project demonstrations and human-robot interaction studies.

Keywords: Adaptive Robotics, Ubiquitous Robotics, Human-Robot Interaction, Testbed, Interactive Robotic Presentation.

1 Introduction

Robotic ecologies are an emerging paradigm, which crosses the borders between the fields of ubiquitous robotics, sensor networks, and ambient intelligence (AmI). Central to the robotic ecology concept is that complex tasks are not performed by a single, very capable robot (e.g. a humanoid robot butler), instead they are performed through the collaboration and cooperation of many networked robotic devices performing several steps in a coordinated and goal oriented fashion while also exchanging sensor data and other useful information in the process.

Robotic ecologies are expected to operate in dynamic and human-populated environments; their skills are the result of many interacting and heterogeneous components, both hardware and software. In addition, in order to help achieve broader adoption of the technology and attract the backing of investors, robotic ecologies must be purposefully designed for user acceptance. Human-Robot Interaction (HRI) studies for domestic or personal robot companions have raised the issues of personalization and social interaction as important considerations

M.J. O'Grady et al. (Eds.): AmI 2013 Workshops, CCIS 413, pp. 136–150, 2013.
© Springer International Publishing Switzerland 2013

for guiding the design of this type of robot application [1]. Studies on people's attitude to robots operating in smart environments have shown how the acceptability of robotic devices in those settings does not depend only on the practical benefits they can provide, but also on complex relationships between the cognitive, affective and emotional components of people's image of the robot [2].

In order to support our research into how robotic ecologies can be designed to be user-friendly and capable of effective and personalized interaction with their human users, we have built a self-presenting robotic ecology testbed. Our system is able to autonomously present itself to human users, and is designed to be easily transportable and re-configurable in order to adapt to different settings and requirements. The testbed has been used in a number of interactive demonstrations and HRI field studies, particularly to study personalization issues for robotic ecologies employed in public spaces, e.g. as receptionists or tour guides. Contrary to personal and companion robot scenarios, in this type of multi-party HRI application, robotic ecologies need to engage with a variety of previously unseen users, typically for short episodes of interaction.

While the details of those studies have been documented in other papers [21][23][24], here we give a detailed description of the testbed, and focus on the experiences that have allowed us to shape its current design and test its flexibility, autonomy, reliability and robustness in a variety of situations of increasing difficulty.

The remainder of the paper is organized in the following manner: Section 2 provides an overview of related work. Section 3 illustrates the components of our testbed and how they have been integrated. Section 4 reports our experiences using the integrated system. Finally, Section 5 summarizes the contributions of this paper and points to some of the directions to be explored in future research.

2   Related Work

Autonomous and interactive robots have been, or are being integrated with smart, sensorised home environments in a number of past and existing projects, most notably: CompanionAble[1], KSERA[2], Florence[3], Hermes[4] and ACCOMPANY[5]. In these projects, robots increase the user's acceptance of smart home and Ambient Assisted Living (AAL) technology, by offering added value with services such as cognitive stimulation, therapy management, social inclusion / connectedness, coaching, fall handling, and memory aid.

A number of testbeds have been developed to conduct HRI field studies outside home environments, for example in urban search and rescue scenarios [3],

---

[1] Integrated Cognitive Assistive & Domotic Companion Robotic Systems for Ability & Security, http://www.companionable.net

[2] Knowledgable SErvice Robots for Aging, http://ksera.ieis.tue.nl

[3] Multi Purpose Mobile Robot for Ambient Assisted Living, http://www.florence-project.eu

[4] Cognitive Care and Guidance for Active Ageing, http://www.fp7-hermes.eu

[5] Acceptable robotiCs COMPanions for AgeiNg Years, http://www.accompanyproject.eu

for child-robot interaction [4], and for applications in aid of mobility impaired individuals [5].

More in keeping with our work, an Actroid-SIT android system has been deployed in a shopping mall in Japan for an HRI experiment involving 1662 subjects. The gesture-centric android system [6] is able to adjust gestures and facial expressions based on a speaker's location in multi-party communication. Another example of a field experiment is the 6-day Fleet Week experiment that was conducted in New York with 202 subjects [7]. Groups of three people firstly trained a robot to memorise their soft biometrics information (complexity, height and clothes), then as the users changed their location, the robot was able to successfully identify them 90% of the time. Both systems successfully address multi-party HRI by exposing the systems to users in realistic conditions.

A number of initiatives explored humanoid robots in the role of presenters. In [8], a Multimodal Presentation Markup Language was designed for non-expert users to be able to program the presentation scenario for the robot. Specifically, the content of the presentation with images and videos, corresponding robot's behaviours, particularly basic emotions, pointing and gestures could be specified with simple commands. During the experimental comparison between the humanoid robot, HOAP-1, and a 2D animated character, the majority of the participants thought that the screen character was a better presenter. In a later study [9], which evaluated a humanoid ASIMO robot in a similar context, the audience appeared to receive a stronger impression of the presentation when carried out by the ASIMO rather than by the 2D animated agent.

Adaptability in presenting information is explored in [10] where a presenter robot serves as a knowledge medium for the user. A display installed on its arm plays tutorial videos of assembling/disassembling a bicycle. The system utilizes the positional information of the user, the objects and the robot in order to adapt to different users by a) finding a suitable position for the robot, b) playing an appropriate video, and c) adjusting the position of the display.

Another adaptive presentation system [11] comprises of a presentation by two 3D virtual reality agents and an eye-tracker, which provides a more personalized and 'attentive' experience of the presentation. Such intuitive and unobtrusive input modality is exploited in order to adapt the content of the presentation and the behaviors of the agents to the user's attention, visual interest and preference.

Compared to existing robotic ecology testbeds and robotic-driven presentation systems, our testbed is designed to leverage the heterogeneous abilities available in a robotic ecology, but also to be easily tailored to different requirements and settings. In addition, it has been equipped with specific features to facilitate the dynamic adaptation and personalization of its interaction style and the conduction of HRI studies with a large number of participants in a relatively short period of time.

3   System Design

Figure 1 illustrates all the devices currently integrated in the testbed to represent some of the typical elements in a robotic ecology, namely:

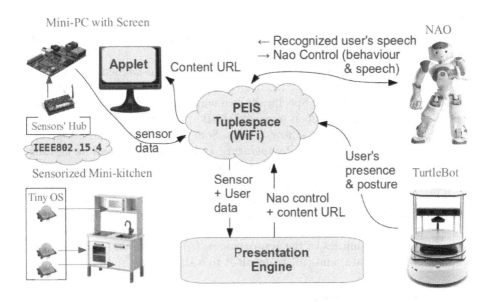

Fig. 1. Software and Hardware Components

- a toy mini-kitchen, equipped with a IEEE802.15.4[6] compliant Wireless Sensor Network (WSN);
- a Mini-PC, equipped with a monitor and a wireless network card;
- a Turtlebot[7] robot equipped with a Kinect 3D camera[8];
- a humanoid NAO robot[9].

In the following sections we briefly illustrate each of these elements, together with the software components sub-tending their operations and integration.

3.1 Middleware

Interoperability among robots, WSN and Mini-PC is ensured by using different clients (C/Java) to the PEIS middleware [13]. PEIS includes a decentralized mechanism for collaboration between software components running on separate devices. It offers a shared, tuplespace blackboard that allows for automatic discovery of new components/devices, and their high-level collaboration over subscription based connections. Specifically, Peis components can indirectly communicate through the exchange of tuples, key-value pairs, which are used to associate any piece of data, to a logical key.

---

[6] http://www.ieee802.org/15/pub/TG4.html
[7] http://www.turtlebot.com/
[8] http://www.xbox.com/en-US/kinect
[9] http://www.aldebaran-robotics.com/en/

3.2   Sensorised Mini-Kitchen

The mini-kitchen is a toy kitchen with an oven, a cupboard, a microwave, a sink and a cooker with simulated hobs, all in 72x35x50 cm.

In order to gather knowledge on the status of the mini-kitchen, we have installed a number of WSN *motes*, i.e. devices equipped with a micro-controller, a radio, and a sensor board. Specifically, we employ IEEE 802.15.4 compliant motes based on the original open-source "TelosB" platform [16]. Each mote can be equipped with a range of sensor boards. Some boards have sensors giving real-time information on the air temperature and humidity, as well as lighting conditions. Other boards are interfaced with magnetic switches, microphones and infrared passive sensors, which are used, respectively, to sense the opening/closing of drawers, the level of noise and the presence of humans moving in their proximity. Each mote runs a copy of a WSN communication software [17], based on the the Nesc/TinyOS 2.x platform, which can be exploited to (i) discover the capabilities of the sensor nodes, (ii) activate and configure the sampling of sensor data, and (iii) transmit it to a sink node.

3.3   Mini-PC and Sensor Hub and Perception Software

The mini-kitchen is equipped with a Raspberry Pi[10], a single-board computer running an optimized version of the Debian OS.

The Mini-PC is USB-connected to the sink node, and runs a Java-based server-side version of the WSN communication software [17], which is used to access the data read by the sensors installed on the mini-kitchen, and to publish it to the Peis tuplespace. The software publishes an index of sensors available in the WSN. In addition, it handles subscriptions to sensor data, which are fulfilled by (i) activating and configuring (through messages routed by the sink node) the sampling of sensor data, (ii) parsing the resulting data updates once they are received by the WSN sink node, and (iii) posting them as tuples in the Peis tuplespace.

3.4   Presentation Applet

The Mini-PC is furnished with a monitor to show presentation slides and other multimedia content, such as still pictures, html pages, slides and videos. To this end, we wrote a simple Web application consisting of a web-page with JavaScript functionalities, and a Java applet. The Java applet uses a Java Peis client to create a tuple, with the key "URL", whose value can be set by any component that wants to broadcast specific content on the monitor. Rather than actual media content, the value of the tuple represents the URL where the content is published, including locations in the local file system of the Mini-PC, or any resource available over the Internet. The Java applet subscribes to the URL tuple and every new URL request is relayed (using LiveConnect technology) to a JavaScript that takes care of retrieving the content and displaying it on the web-page.

---

[10] http://www.raspberrypi.org/

3.5   Turtlebot

The Turtlebot is a personal robot kit with open-source software based on the ROS software [19]. For the purpose of our demonstration, the Turtlebot is controlled by a netbook running ROS and the body tracking OpenNI framework [20]. This is used to process the 3D data gathered from the Microsoft's Kinect sensor mounted on the robot, in order to detect the presence of humans in front of the demonstration, and recognize their body posture. We employ the C Peis client to notify other components about the presence of users in front of the stand, supplemented with an estimation of the orientation of their gaze (deduced from their posture). Furthermore, the Turtlebot includes a number of pre-programmed behaviours and speech-synthesis functionalities, which can be used, respectively, to turn the robot to face the users, and to give them some basic information about the robot and its role in the robotic ecology.

3.6   Nao Humanoid Robot

The Nao is a programmable, 58cm tall humanoid robot acting as the main user interface toward the robotic ecology. It is equipped with a vast array of sensors, including cameras, microphones, sonars and tactile sensors, and with 25 degrees of freedom. In order to interface the Nao with our system, we wrote a interface combining the NAOqi C++ SDK with the C Peis client. The interface allows us to (i) publish information about objects and the user's speech recognized by the Nao, and (ii) activate, configure and deactivate the Nao's behaviours by simply setting the value of control tuples. To this end, the interface subscribes to changes to those tuples and forwards their value to the proxy classes, such as ALMotion, ALTextToSpeech, that are included in the NAOqi SDK to give direct access to the behavioural capabilities of the Nao.

3.7   Software for Users' Gender and Age Estimation

We have equipped our testbed with three open-source software tools from biometrics and computer vision research to gather information about the gender and the age of the person standing in front of the robotic ecology. Specifically, we use both the OpenBR[11] face-based gender estimation algorithm and a pitch detector algorithm to estimate the gender of the user based on the video and the audio captured by the Nao. In addition, we estimate the height of the user based on the coordinates of 20 skeleton points detected by the Microsoft Kinect sensor installed on the Turtlebot. The interested reader can find a complete description of these algorithms and the way they are used together for gender and age estimation in [24].

3.8   Presentation Engine

The last component of our system is a presentation engine that is able to execute a simple finite state machine where each state represents a possible situation

---

[11] http://openbiometrics.org/slides.pdf

or phase of the demonstration. Sensor and/or event updates originated by the other components in the robotic ecology are processed to build a picture of the situation and of the user, and are matched against a set of conditions describing the possible phase transitions in the presentation. Each time an event triggers a state transition and a new state is reached, our presentation engine sets the tuples required to control (i) the content that must be displayed on the monitor, (ii) the specific behaviours that must be activated in each of the robots, and (iii) the message that must be uttered to the users in front of the stand.

The presentation engine builds its confidence of certain events by integrating multiple sensor readings over time. For example, in order to detect the opening and closing of a drawer of the mini-kitchen, the engine monitors the readings of both a magnetic switch and a light sensor installed on the drawer.

The magnetic switch can only tell the engine when the drawer is properly closed but not when it is being handled by the user or when the user only partially opens/closes it. For this reason, the engine uses the light sensors installed inside each drawer and performs a simple online clustering algorithm to distinguish between situations when the light sensors perceive low levels of light (corresponding to the closed/semi-closed drawer) and the situations when they perceive high levels of light (corresponding to the open/semi-open drawer). In this manner, we do not need to specifically define high and low level thresholds for the level of light, but the system automatically adapts to the actual lighting conditions it finds when it is used.

4   Studies and Demonstration

We have used the architecture described in the previous section and complemented it with content, such as videos and presentation slides (converted to Html format in order to be used by the presentation Applet), to exercise our testbed in situations of increasing complexity. On each occasion, we placed both the robot(s) and the mini-kitchen on adjacent tables in order for them to engage more easily with the public.

4.1   Laboratory Study

Before deploying our system in fully autonomous settings, we have conducted a pilot study [21] in our laboratory to configure the behaviour and test the robustness of the testbed. The experiment was designed to promote and observe human-robot collaboration and to inform the design of social cues to be used by the Nao to efficiently engage with the humans. We adopted a simple collaborative cooking scenario, in which the Nao acted as a cooking assistant to a number of users who volunteered to participate in our study.

On this occasion, the system was manually reset before each user was introduced separately and instructed to approach the test-bed.

As soon as the system detected the user, the Nao welcomed the user and explained what food was to be prepared. We had a total of 16 users separated into two user groups: (i) A "Verbal Only" user group, with which the Nao used only verbal communication, and (ii) a "Face-to-Face" user group, with which the Nao used gaze and gestures to emphasise and facilitate the user's understanding of it's instructions (for instance by pointing to the drawer containing the salt, etc). Each trial lasted an average of 5 minutes and was fully autonomous and timed. The participants were asked to complete the Godspeed [22] questionnaire (with items measuring likeability, intelligence and safety) immediately after the experiment. As expected, the second group resulted in an increase to both the level of user engagement, and to the user's perceived intelligence of the robotic ecology.

The system behaved as specified by the presentation engine and we did not observe any technical problem during any of the short sessions. We adopted the Nao's gestures and gaze behaviours in all the subsequent tests.

4.2 University Open Day

The first outing of the testbed outside our laboratory was a half-day exhibition organized by our department to showcase a number of research projects.

Contrary to the more controlled laboratory settings described in the previous section, visitors and potential study participants on this occasion were wandering around the area clustered with many posters and other demonstration stands. We used this opportunity to test our system's ability to attract the attention and autonomously engage with an uninterrupted flow of users over a prolonged period of time.

As in our first pilot study, the robotic ecology was autonomous: it displayed a video on the screen in order to attract the attention of the visitors. As somebody approached the stand, the NAO greeted them and invited them to participate in an interactive presentation. First of all, the NAO talked over a few presentation slides to illustrate some introductory concepts about robotic ecologies. Secondly, it illustrated its own capabilities before presenting the other members of the ecology, by explaining the purpose of the sensorised kitchen, and by giving time to the visitor to engage with the Turtlebot. At each stage, visual content related to each of the topics illustrated by the Nao were projected on the monitor. Finally, the visitors were invited to interact with the mini-kitchen to open, close or use kitchen appliances. The ecology acknowledged each of these actions through the Nao and the monitor, in order to illustrate its ability to recognise the user's activities. If the visitors were detected leaving the stand, the Nao thanked them and waved goodbye while the monitor re-started displaying the project video.

Finally, after their interaction with the robotic ecology, users were approached and asked to complete a questionnaire evaluating their experience. When asked to indicate which member of the ecology they found most enjoyable, 45% of 30 participants preferred the smart kitchen, 5% liked the Turtlebot and the remaining 50% chose the Nao. These results, detailed in [23], contrasted with our past experiences when using the Nao on its own, which had the undesired effect of concentrating too much of the users' attention onto the robot and away from the actual content we wanted to present.

As in our first series of tests, we did not observe any technical problem with the operations of the test-bed.

4.3 Autonomous Exhibition

In order to further test the flexibility and the reliability of our testbed, we used it in conjunction with a showcase of research projects in which we were asked to give a project demonstration for an entire week. In order to meet this requirement, we used our middleware to prepare two configurations, respectively: (i) a configuration similar to the one we used at the University Open Day (but with different content), which we supervised on the first day of the showcase[12], and (ii) a fully-autonomous but partially simulated setup. For the latter, we replaced the actual Nao with its simulated counterpart. The simulated Nao was visualized on the monitor connected to the Mini-PC. This meant that, while in the original setup we ran the presentation engine inside the Nao's computer, in the autonomous setup we installed it on the Mini-PC, together with the Nao simulation software. Furthermore, since the simulated Nao does not have speech synthesis capabilities, we modified the visual content displayed on the screen to include subtitles.

Preparing and switching between the two configurations was straightforward, as the use of the Peis tuplespace meant that it did not matter from which computer we ran the presentation engine (the Nao or the Mini-PC) or which component we used to communicate with the user (the Nao's speech interface or the text included in the visual presentation).

Our autonomous but partially simulated setup performed satisfactorily throughout the week. However, we had to tackle a couple of problems. The first problem was due to a fault in the USB serial port of the Mini-PC. We solved the problem by adding an ad-hoc connection recovery step, which listed the available USB ports and pro-grammatically re-initialized the connection to the sink mote upon the detection of the first communication error. The second problem was that the Turtlebot's ROS component in charge of the skeleton tracking functionality would regularly become irresponsible if it was left operating for more than a one day-long shift. For this reason, we instructed the staff working at the exhibition centre on how to startup and shutdown the Turtlebot and the presentation engine at the beginning of each day.

4.4 Human-Robot Interaction in Public Spaces

We conclude the report of our experiences using our testbed with the description of a preliminary study we conducted to assess how effective it would be to adapt the robotic ecology's interaction style to suit each particular user. Specifically, we investigated the effects of the robot's perceived gender and age on levels of engagement and acceptance of the robot by children across different age and gender groups. The independent variables were variants of the robot voices: male, female, child, adult.

Method. The pilot study was conducted at a robotic summer camp with children aged between 8 and 15 years. The experiment was set up in a small room

---
[12] A video of the demo can be viewed at http://fp7rubicon.eu/index.php/ news/40/61/Successful-Project-Demonstration-in-Dublin

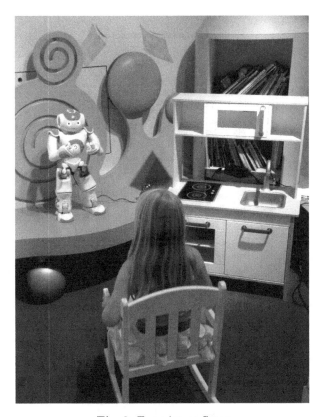

Fig. 2. Experiment Setup

(Figure 2). Participants were instructed to take a seat in front of the robotic system and follow the robot's instructions. After the session, each participant was given the Godspeed [22] questionnaire (with items measuring likeability) to fill. Rather than using the Turtlebot's sensors, the experimenter controlled the launch of each experiment session through a mobile phone application.

Results. The experiment involved 32 children aged between 8 and 15 years. Unfortunately, there was not a fair gender distribution with only 2 female participants. Therefore, we report the results of 30 male participants.

The questionnaire results showed internal consistency with Cronbach's alpha scores above 0.9 for all participants. A series of two-way ANOVA tests on perceived likeability were conducted in order to test for statistically significant differences between various combinations of the robots gender and age conditions. When comparing the average likeability score across age groups in relation to the robot's age, the results are significantly different: $F(1, 17) = 5.231$, $p = 0.10$ $(p < 0.5)$. Figure 3 represents the average likeability scores across the age groups of the participants. As can be seen from the chart, there are no results in response

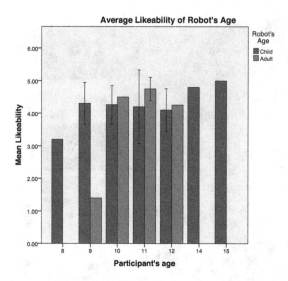

Fig. 3. Average Likeability of Robot's Age Across Age Groups for Boys

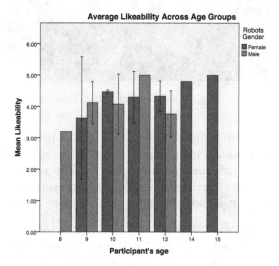

Fig. 4. Average Likeability of Robot's Gender Across Age Groups for Boys

to the adult voice of the robot for the 8 (1 participant), 14 (1 participant) and 15 (1 participant) age groups.

When comparing the average scores across age groups in relation to the robot's gender, the results are not statistically significant: $F(1, 17) = 0.659$, $p = 0.588$. Figure 4 details the results of the boys' likeability of the robot's voice for different age groups. The results of this pilot study suggest that boys statistically significantly disliked the robot with the voice of an adult at the age of 9.

These results are not conclusive, since we need a more controlled selection of a larger group of participants with similar gender and age distributions. However, they suggest that children relate differently to the robot's age and gender at different age groups. This is important to consider when designing robotic applications for children in order to increase a robot's perceived likeability, acceptance and engagement.

5   Conclusion and Future Work

We have described the design of a portable and self-presenting robotic ecology testbed, and illustrated our experiences in using it in a number of project presentations and HRI studies. The testbed has allowed us to engage with different types of users and explain the main concepts behind robotic ecologies by showing them a working example consisting of multiple robots, computers and sensors working together.

The system architecture illustrated in Section 3 lent us a lot of flexibility in the way we were able to design each presentation and user study, and deploy our system in different situations. The use of a centralized presentation engine simplifies the creation of synchronized behaviour among the various components in the ecology, while the peer-to-peer Peis tuplespace allows them to engage in loosely coupled, indirect collaboration. For instance, the system is able to function without the Turtlebot, as the presentation engine can be informed (although less accurately) about movements in front of the kitchen by monitoring the readings of a wireless passive infrared sensor belonging to the system's WSN, or it could simply be triggered with a phone-based Wizard-of-Oz interface. The information can be used by our presentation engine to decide that the ecology must enter a greeting state, but the presentation engine is unaffected if the Turtlebot is not present and the user is greeted only by the Nao.

One of the biggest limitations of its current implementation is that we need to prepare a new version of the presentation engine to suit the requirements of each of the outings of the robotic ecology. A developer can easily modify the scripts of existing presentations or create new ones by defining their states and transitions, using our C library. New robot behaviours can also be easily fitted into our system by leveraging our Peis/Nao interface. However, non-developers can only start and stop already defined scripts. In order to improve the usability of the system, e.g. by third parties, we plan to prepare an interpreted version of the presentation engine, following the example of [8].

The robustness of the testbed could also be improved. For instance, rather than relying on ad-hoc programming interventions each time a problem is found, the testbed should be equipped with generic error recovery mechanisms. For this reason, we are equipping our architecture with monitor components that will be able to detect when some of the devices in the ecology are not responding, and supervise their recovery.

The testbed has performed satisfactorily in the partially static settings in which it was tested, acting both in an autonomous (but pre-scripted) manner and in a Wizard-of-Oz modality. However, more work is necessary to address more complex scenarios, in which the robots may need to move around the presentation area, for instance, to get close to possible participants and invite them to interact with the system. We are currently extending our system to make it more autonomous and context-aware by using agent and plan-based control solutions and by leveraging existing functionalities, such as the Turtlebot's ability to localize itself, and the Nao's ability to use visual markers (that we place on the mini-kitchen and on the Turtlebot) to recognize the position of the other devices in the ecology.

Finally, our preliminary HRI studies suggest that alternative means of assessment need to be explored for future experiments with children. In order to supplement or replace the use of questionnaires, we could employ an interactive game structure to measure the time the child spends playing with the smart kitchen (i.e. opening and closing the appliances' doors). The number of doors the child opens and whether or not the child responds to the NAO by name can also be recorded by availing of our testbed. In order to evaluate the children's attitude toward the interaction experience, we plan to use the SHORE software [25], a high-speed, real-time tool for the recognition of facial expressions.

Acknowledgement. This work has been supported by the EU FP7 RUBICON project (contract n. 269914), in conjunction with funding from the Irish Research Council Embark Initiative and Science Foundation Ireland (SFI) under grant 07/CE/I1147. We thank the anonymous reviewers for their thorough review and highly appreciate the comments and suggestions, which significantly contributed to improving the quality of this paper.

References

1. Dautenhahn, K.: Robots we like to live with?! - a developmental perspective on a personalized, life-long robot companion. In: Proc. of the 13th IEEE International Workshop on Robot and Human Interactive Communication (ROMAN 2004), pp. 17–22 (2004)
2. Nugent, C., Augusto, J.C.: Human-robot user studies in eldercare: Lessons learned. In: Smart Homes And Beyond: Icost 2006, 4th International Conference on Smart Homes and Health Telematics, vol. 19, p. 31. IOS Press (2006)
3. Lewis, M., Sycara, K., Nourbakhsh, I.: Developing a testbed for studying human-robot interaction in urban search and rescue. In: Proc. of the 10th International Conference on Human Computer Interaction, pp. 22–27 (2003)
4. Goris, K., Saldien, J., Lefeber, D.: Probo, a testbed for human robot interaction. In: Proc. of the 4th ACM/IEEE International Conference on Human-Robot Interaction (HRI 2009), pp. 253–254. IEEE (2009)
5. Pineau, J., Atrash, A.: SmartWheeler: A Robotic Wheelchair Test-Bed for Investigating New Models of Human-Robot Interaction. In: AAAI Spring Symposium: Multidisciplinary Collaboration for Socially Assistive Robotics, pp. 59–64 (2007)
6. Kondo, Y., Takemura, K., Takamatsu, J., Ogasawara, T.: A Gesture-Centric Android System for Multi-Party Human-Robot Interaction. Journal of Human-Robot Interaction (1), 133–151 (2013)

7. Martinson, E., Lawson, W., Trafton, J.G.: Identifying people with soft-biometrics at Fleet Week. In: Proc. of the 8th ACM/IEEE International Conference on Human-Robot Interaction (HRI 2013), pp. 49–56. IEEE (2013)
8. Nozawa, Y., et al.: Humanoid robot presentation controlled by multimodal presentation markup language MPML. In: Proc. of the 13th IEEE International Workshop on Robot and Human Interactive Communication (ROMAN 2004). IEEE (2004)
9. Kushida, K., Nishimura, Y., Dohi, H., Ishizuka, M., Takeuchi, J., Tsujino, H.: Humanoid robot presentation through multimodal presentation markup language MPML-HR. In: AAMAS 2005 Workshop on Creating Bonds with Humanoids, pp. 23–29 (2005)
10. Nishida, T., Terada, K., Tajima, T., Hatakeyama, M., Ogasawara, Y.: Toward robots as embodied knowledge media. IEICE Transactions on Information and Systems 89(6), 1768–1780 (2006)
11. Hoekstra, A., Prendinger, H., Bee, N., Heylen, D., Ishizuka, M.: Presentation Agents That Adapt to Users' Visual Interest and Follow Their Preferences. In: The 5th International Conference on Computer Vision Systems (2007)
12. Amato, G., Broxvall, M., Chessa, S., Dragone, M., Gennaro, C., López, R., Maguire, L., Mcginnity, T.M., Micheli, A., Renteria, A., O'Hare, G.P., Pecora, F.: Robotic UBIquitous COgnitive network. In: Novais, P., Hallenborg, K., Tapia, D.I., Rodríguez, J.M.C. (eds.) Ambient Intelligence - Software and Applications. AISC, vol. 153, pp. 191–195. Springer, Heidelberg (2012)
13. Broxvall, M.: The peis kernel: A middleware for ubiquitous robotics. In: Proc. of the IROS 2007 Workshop on Ubiquitous Robotic Space Design and Applications, San Diego, California (2007)
14. Saffiotti, A., Broxvall, M.: PEIS Ecologies: Ambient intelligence meets autonomous robotics. In: Proc. of the International Conference on Smart Objects and Ambient Intelligence (sOc-EUSAI), Grenoble, France, pp. 275–280 (2005)
15. Saffiotti, A., Broxvall, M., Gritti, M., LeBlanc, K., Lundh, R., Rashid, J., Seo, B., Cho., Y.-J.: The PEIS-ecology project: vision and results. In: IEEE/RSJ International Conference on Intelligent Robots and Systems (IROS 2008), pp. 2329–2335. IEEE (2008)
16. Cunha, A., Koubaa, A., Severino, R., Alves, M.: Open-ZB: an open-source implementation of the IEEE 802.15.4/ZigBee protocol stack on TinyOS. In: IEEE Internatonal Conference on Mobile Adhoc and Sensor Systems (MASS 2007), pp. 1–12. IEEE (2007)
17. Amato, G., Broxvall, M., Chessa, S., Dragone, M., Gennaro, C., Vairo, C.: When Wireless Sensor Networks Meet Robots. In: Proc. of the 7th International Conference on Systems and Networks Communications (ICSNC 2012), Lisbon, Portugal, November 18-23, pp. 35–40 (2012)
18. Turtlebot.com, Home - TurtleBot (2013), http://www.turtlebot.com/ (accessed: September 20, 2013)
19. ROS (Robot Operating System) (2013), Documentation, http://www.ros.org/ (accessed: September 20, 2013)
20. OpenNI: Open-source SDK for 3D sensors (2013), OpenNI: The Standard Framework for 3D Sensing, http://www.openni.org/ (accessed: September 20, 2013)
21. Sandygulova, A., Swords, D., Abdel-Naby, S., O'Hare, G.M.P.: Face-to-Face Collaboration within Ubiquitous Robotics. In: Fifth Workshop on Gaze at the 8th ACM/IEEE International Conference on Human-Robot Interaction (HRI 2013), Tokyo, Japan, March 3-6 (2013)

22. Bartneck, C., Croft, E., Kulic, D.: Measuring the anthropomorphism, animacy, likeability, perceived intelligence and perceived safety of robots. In: Metrics for HRI Workshop, Technical Report, vol. 471, pp. 37–44 (2008)
23. Sandygulova, A., Swords, D., Abdel-Naby, S., O'Hare, G.M.P., Dragone, M.: A study of effective social cues within ubiquitous robotics. In: Proc. of the 8th ACM/IEEE International Conference on Human-Robot Interaction (HRI 2013), pp. 221–222 (2013)
24. Sandygulova, A., Swords, D., Abdalla, S., Dragone, M., O'Hare, G.M.P.: Ubiquitous human perception for real-time gender and age estimation. In: Proc. of the 10th International Conference on Ubiquitous Robots and Ambient Intelligence, URAI 2013 (2013)
25. Ruf, T., Ernst, A., Kblbeck, C.: Face detection with the sophisticated high-speed object recognition engine (SHORE). In: Microelectronic Systems, pp. 243–252. Springer, Heidelberg (2011)

A Comparative Study of the Effect of Sensor Noise on Activity Recognition Models

Robert Ross and John Kelleher

Applied Intelligence Research Center, School of Computing,
Dublin Institute of Technology, Ireland

Abstract. To provide a better understanding of the relative strengths of Machine Learning based Activity Recognition methods, in this paper we present a comparative analysis of the robustness of three popular methods with respect to sensor noise. Specifically we evaluate the robustness of Naive Bayes classifier, Support Vector Machine, and Random Forest based activity recognition models in three cases which span sensor errors from dead to poorly calibrated sensors. Test data is partially synthesized from a recently annotated activity recognition corpus which includes both interleaved activities and a range of both temporally long and short activities. Results demonstrate that the relative performance of Support Vector Machine classifiers over Naive Bayes classifiers reduces in noisy sensor conditions, but that overall the Random Forest classifier provides best activity recognition accuracy across all noise conditions synthesized in the corpus. Moreover, we find that activity recognition is equally robust across classification techniques with the relative performance of all models holding up under almost all sensor noise conditions considered.

Keywords: Activity Recognition, Sensor Noise, Support Vector Machines, Naive Bayes, Random Forests.

1 Introduction

Garbage In Garbage Out is as true of activity recognition as it is of any other part of computer science. However, while data driven predictive models for any domain will be negatively effected by noise in the input features, the structure of the activity recognition domain has a number of distinctive characteristics that complicate this problem. On one hand, in all but very limited situations, the activity recognition task is performed in environments with multiple agents and where activities can be inherently interleaved. A major consequence of this is that activity recognition is not simply a single class classification problem, but must instead accurately track multiple hypothesis in parallel. In such a case *noise* is not always simply noise and thus cannot always be filtered out. On the other hand, successful recognition for many activities is often dependent on observing a key characterizing action or event that captures the essence of that activity. Noise in these key features can have an extreme impact on predictive accuracy for individual activities [1].

M.J. O'Grady et al. (Eds.): AmI 2013 Workshops, CCIS 413, pp. 151–162, 2013.
© Springer International Publishing Switzerland 2013

Before we can design predictive models that are robust to noise in the specifics of the activity recognition domain, we must first understand how noise effects the performance of these models. Part of this task is to investigate whether different types of noise have different or similar impacts on a given activity recognition model. In the context of activity recognition, noise in the input features is primarily the result of sensors errors. A sensor could be mistakenly switched off, blocked or completely broken. Alternatively, a sensor could be miscalibrated resulting in either the sensor registering events that have not happened or in the sensor missing events when they do happen. Compounding these issues is the fact that often activities are interleaved and consequently not all of the events in an input stream relate to the same activity. Moreover, the noise from these different sources is often hard to differentiate within a particular stream of sensor data. For example, a broken sensor and a sensor that is miscalibrated and misses some events will both result in false negatives in the input feature. Conversely, assuming that activities are independent, the interleaving of events complicates the prediction of an activity in a similar way to a sensor that registers events that have not happened, in both cases input features will be marked as false positives for the target activity.

Clearly, noise of any type will have a negative impact on the accuracy on any particular recognition model; however, given that different model induction algorithms make different assumptions, in terms of their inductive bias, there is a possibility that different types of noise will effect the induced models in different ways. Some models may be more robust to a particular type of noise than another model resulting in a tipping point in the relative performance of the models as the amount of noise in the data increases. In light of the above, in this paper we present a study of the robustness of three different activity recognition models. We continue in Section 2 where we motivate our selection of the models used based on prior work in the area of Human Activity Recognition. Then in Section 3 we introduce the study dataset and describe all essential data pre-processing steps that were taken as well as the representation choices which we adopted. Following this, we present the results of our analysis in detail in Section 4. Following this we draw conclusions and outline proposed future work.

2   Model Selection

Machine learning based and probabilistic Activity Recognition determines to what extent evidence supports competing activity hypotheses. In recent years many different methods from statistical natural language processing and machine learning have been applied to the activity recognition problem (see for example [2] for a recent overview of techniques applied to situation recognition). While structured techniques such as statistical parsers or explicit sequence modeling techniques such as Hidden Markov Models [3–5] or Conditional Random Fields [6] do provide a theoretical firm basis for activity recognition, it has been widely shown that classifier based techniques often provide the best balance of performance while retaining effective computational tractability [6, 7]. Consequently, in this study we focused on the analysis of classifier based techniques.

Bayesian prediction models have a strong history in activity recognition. Early examples of probability based activity and plan recognition models application used Bayesian Networks (See e.g., [8] and [9]). Given the relative design costs and inference costs of applying non-trivial Bayes networks, their use in pure classification tasks has been widely superseded by the use of the more straightforward naive Bayes classifier. As is well known, the *naive* characterization of the Naive Bayes classifier is due to its the strong independence assumption that this classifier makes regarding input features. Particularly in the area of activity recognition an assumption of independence between sensors / features which characterize actions being performed in an environment may be too strong an assumption. Despite this, many, including for example Singla [5], have made use of a Naive Bayes classifier to identify activities in the case of interleaved data.

While the Naive Bayes classifier has arguably been the most widely applied classifier in the past 20 years, the class of maximum margin based classifiers and in particular the Support Vector Machine (SVM) have found ever increasing application. Essentially Support Vector Machines are discriminative classifiers built on the observation that the essential job for any classifier is to create suitable decision boundaries between different classes based on observed instances. Although SVMs require significant training in comparison to the Naive Bayes classifier; this drawback is outweighed both by the ability SVM's to deal with large numbers of features and also produce highly accurate models. Within the activity recognition domain the SVM is widely seen as one of the best performing yet computationally practical classification techniques, for example [10, 11] are examples of recent work that illustrates the application of SVMs models to activity recognition.

Whereas both the Naive Bayes classifier and the Support Vector Machine operate as individual classifiers, there exist a range of meta-classification or ensemble methods which work by aggregating the predictions of multiple (independent) models. There are two general approaches to creating such ensemble models: boosting and bagging. The essential difference between these two approaches is that during training boosting incrementally adapts how models are induced so that each new model added to the ensemble is biased to pay more attention to training instances that previous models mis-classified; by contrast, in bagging techniques each new model is induced using a randomly selected subset of features and examples. The motivation behind the use of ensemble methods is that the aggregated output of an array of weak prediction models may be more accurate over a datset than a single strong classifier. Indeed, within the Activity Recognition domain [12, 13] report a study where a LogitBoost ensemble outperformed a range of other classification models.

Given the above, in the study that follows we will investigate the relative performance of Naive Bayes classifiers, Support Vector Machines and ensemble methods. With respect to the ensemble method, given that our focus in on robustness to noise rather than pure model accuracy we chose to use a Random Forest model as our ensemble classifier. Random Forest is a bagging method and, we argue, that given bagging algorithms use randomly selected subsets of features during training (rather than the adaptive approach used by boosting) the Random Forest should be more robust to noise, such as missing input features.

3   Corpus Annotation and Preparation

We use the SCARE multimodal corpus as the base dataset for the study [14]. This dataset contains a collection of annotated videos and audio recordings of participant pairs performing joint tasks in a simulated environment . The environment itself is a 3D game like environment in which one individual, the instruction follower can navigate and perform activities, while the second participant, the instruction giver, directs the follower on how to conduct activities. Each Instruction Giver was informed of the five activities that were to be performed by each dyad, and was also given a schematic map of the virtual environment. The Instruction Giver was thus made aware of: (a) which objects were to be moved; (b) where these objects were to be moved from; and (c) where these objects were to be moved to. The Instruction Follower meanwhile could maneuver around in the virtual environment and manipulate that environment by moving objects, opening and closing containers, as well as picking up and placing down items. In the real environment, the Instruction Giver and Instruction Follower were placed in separate rooms and verbally communicated via headsets to jointly complete all five tasks. In total 15 dyad or session recordings are included in the corpus.

The SCARE corpus was selected as a testbed for a number of reasons. First, instruction givers and followers were not constrained in terms of the sequence in which activities were to be performed, and whether or not these activities could be performed in parallel. Thus there was wide variation in terms of the interleaving of activity completion in this tesbed. Second, the activities seen in the data are also varied in length with both very long and short activities present. Third, previous work by the authors [11] showed that the relative performance of Naive Bayes' and SVM activity recognition models was consistent across a range of datasets, including the SCARE corpus and two datasets from the CASAS Smart Home Project at Washington State University [15, 5]. As a result for this work we restricted the study to the SCARE corpus making the assumption that using a different dataset would not substantively alter the results.

Although the SCARE corpus includes a number of useful annotations such as time aligned speech transcriptions, Activity Recognition requires further annotation of the data. We therefore developed and applied an annotation scheme for activity recognition with the SCARE corpus. The annotation scheme included three distinct layers which labeled the data with respect to: (a) location of the instruction follower; (b) actions being performed by the instruction follower; and (c) activities or goals currently being pursued. Specifically, the *location* layer denoted which of 19 possible areas in the environment that the Instruction Follower was currently located in. The *action* layer on the other hand denoted what physical manipulation actions – if any – were currently being performed by the Instruction Follower. In total there were six action types where these types could in turn be parameterised. Examples of action types include *Pickup(Silencer)* and

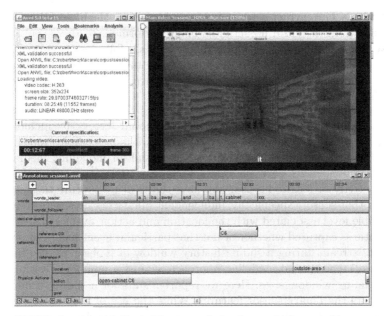

Fig. 1. ANVIL Annotation Tool. The top of the figure depicts a video recording of the Instruction Giver and Instruction Follower's view of the simulated 3D world. The bottom of the figure depicts the multi-tiered annotation tool interface.

Open-Cabinet(C1) where *Silencer* was an object in the environment and *C1* was a named container in that environment. The *activity* layer was a more course grained annotation layer that denoted what activities were currently being pursued by the participant pairing. In total 5 activities were pursued by each dyad, and these activities were frequently interleaved by participants. Thus the annotation scheme was defined to mark only the start and end of each activity; thus allowing for activities to be concurrently active. The annotation scheme was applied to each of the 15 SCARE session recordings. For annotation we made use of the ANVIL multimodal annotation tool [16] (See Figure 1).

3.1 Data Preparation

In the context of activity recognition, one critique that can be levelled at classifier models such as Naive Bayes', SVM and Random Forest is that they do not naturally handle the sequential nature of the information. In order to address this problem we developed a base-set of history-less features and augmented these with a suitable representation of event history. The base set of features of the SCARE dataset consisted of the following six features:

- **Step** - The number of observations since the beginning of this task.
- **Time** - The amount of time that has passed since the beginning of this task.
- **Place** - The current location of the instruction follower in the virtual environment.

– **Activity** - The current activity being performed by the instruction follower. Possibly none or null if no action is being performed.
– **LastPlace** - The last location of the instruction follower.
– **LastActivity** - The last action performed by the instruction follower - possibly none if no action has yet been performed by the instruction follower for this activity.

Although the baseline features capture a minimal history by including the *LastEvent* or *LastPlace* and *LastActivity* features, a more complex model which includes histories for individual features is essential for modelling medium and long range dependencies between events. For this model we made use of one feature per activity or location sensor and have that feature capture the activation history for that sensor. Specifically, independent binary features were created for each possible level associated with the location and action/event features. These binary features captured whether or not that particular event had been observed in the data stream during a sliding history window of n observations. In previous studies [11] we tested modeling approach against a number of variants and different sliding window sizes. Here we report results for a sliding window size of 100 events the binary sensor features. While the use of such binary features might seem an oversimplification where a more information rich occurrence count based set of features could instead be used, we have previously shown that the simple binary feature approach taken here considerably outperforms the more complex model across a range of data sets and models.

To illustrate the features made use of in this analysis consider the simplified data extract provided in Table 1. Here the first three sensor entries corresponding to an instance of the Activity *move-quad* are presented (for text compactness the following two acronyms are used: GR1 - Grey-Room-1, and OC_C3 - Open-Cabinet_C3). Along columns 3 through 8 we see the first 6 features of the data model, while from column 9 onwards each of the individual sensor features which make up the long rang history are captured. The first observed sensor value is an activation for Place at the Grey-Room_1. This activation occurs at step 0 and time 0 and since there were no previous LastEvent or LastPlace occurrences we record NA for these features. The sensor feature for the Grey-Room_1 also activates and will remain active for n rows (n=100 in the current work) past the following row. Similarly in row 2 we see an activation of the Open-Cabinet_C3 at a specific time and step and a subsequent activation of its corresponding sensor feature (column 10).

3.2 Introducing Noise

The baseline annotated dataset described above is used for training the Naive Bayes, Support Vector Machine, and Random Forest classifiers, but for testing we used modified data. Specifically to examine the effect of the noise on the resulting accuracy of the activity recognition models, we generated three collections of test

Table 1. Sample Data Extract. (GR1 - Grey-Room-1, and OC_C3 - Open-Cabinet_C3)).

Row	Goal	Place	Event	Step	Time	LastEvent	LastPlace	GR1	OC_C3	..
0	move-quad	GR1	NA	0	0	NA	NA	1	0	..
1	move-quad	GR1	NA	1	12.6	NA	GR1	1	0	..
2	move-quad	GR1	OC_C3	2	15.2	NA	GR1	1	1	..
..	..	..	..	..	..	..	..	..	..	..

data. Each collection of test data captured a potential source of error in the data as follows:

- **Collection A - Random Insertions:** Miscalibrated sensors may lead to false sensor positives in any activity recognition scenario. Proximity and inertia detectors may be influenced by environmental factors or other non-human agents in the environment. In the Random Insertion collection we took the baseline data set and inserted a proportion of random observations into the existing sensor event stream. We will report on a range of different insertion rates, i.e., between 1% and 32% extra random data in the data stream.

- **Collection B - Random Deletions:** Similarly miscalibrated sensors may lead to false sensor negatives where movements in the environment or interactions with objects fail to be recognized by the sensor system. In the Random Deletions collection we synthesized such a situation by removing between 1% and 45 % of the real data.

- **Collection B - Dead Sensors:** False sensor negatives may also be due to the overall failure of one or more sensors in the environment. We modeled this possibility separately through the Dead Sensors collection. Here all results for between 1% and 16% of the sensors were systematically removed from the baseline data set for testing.

It should be noted that for each of the above test-sets the removal or addition of data was performed with respect to the raw data prior to its transformation to the specific features outlined earlier in this section. Therefore the consequences of insertions or deletions are fully expanded out and have consequence to the long range history features for subsequent observations.

4 Results

In the following we report on the evaluation of the activity classification techniques considered for each of the three sensor noise data collections.

For each of the error types considered we tested against models within which all original features were present and where Feature Selection had been applied to reduce the feature set. For Feature Selection we made use of an entropy based information-gain feature selection process where the ranking of individual features was based on their correlation with the target class. Features were ranked and a certain proportion of the lowest ranked features were removed. Given the relatively low number of features in the SCARE corpus, we limited feature selection to remove only the 1/3 lowest weighting features.

Accuracy scores were calculated using k-fold classification within each data set. Namely, for a given dyad d we built a multiclass classifier based on data from all other dyads except the one being considered, i.e., {training data - d}, which we refer to as d'. Predicted target classes for d were calculated using the model built from d'. This was done for all d with classification accuracy values accrued from the testing of each d individually.

Moreover, given the random nature of inserting or deleting elements in the methods discussed below, all tests were run on three distinct sets of synthesized values. For example, in the case of Random Insertions we built three distinct insertion data sets $I1$, $I2$, and $I3$. While all three were based on the original annotated data set, the randomly inserted values for all three were selected separately. Our aim here was to build a smoothed result which was less tied to the removal or deletion of one specific reading or sensor. In the results presented below we show the result averaged over all three evaluations for each data set.

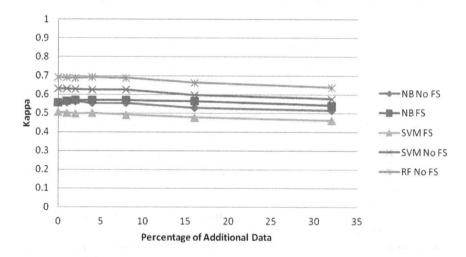

Fig. 2. Kappa Coefficient Scores for SCARE data with random noise insertions

Figure 2 summarizes the results for our Data Insertion evaluation for the Naive Bayes, Support Vector Machine and Random Forest classifiers across a range of data insertion volumes. Since the activity recognition problem is essentially a multi-class classification problem we report prediction accuracy in terms of Cohen's Kappa Coefficient. Cohen's kappa is a conservative measure of accuracy which takes into account the possibility of class agreement happening by chance. From the figure we can firstly note some of the general characteristics of the results. The Random Forest classifier significantly outperforms both the Support Vector Machine and Naive Bayes classifiers on the SCARE data set both in the presence of noisy data and in the original unaltered data, i.e., where Percentage of Altered Data = 0. Moreover we see that the application of Feature Selection results in positive gains for the Naive Bayes classifier over the case of using all features, whereas the opposite is the case for the Support Vector Machine classifier. We hypothesis that the interaction between Feature Selection and SVMs is caused by the fact that the Feature Selection process employed considered features in isolation whereas SVM models, unlike Naive Bayes classifiers, have the ability to consider interactions between input features. Consequently, the feature selection process may have removed features that in isolation were not information but in conjunction with other features were useful to the SVM models. Hence, the observed negative impact of Feature Selection on SVM model accuracy.

Considering the results specifically with respect to the insertion of noisy data, we see that all models generally held up well with respect to low volumes of noisy data insertion. To illustrate, the Random Forest classifier's performance deteriorated by only 0.6% between no inserted data and 8% extra inserted data. Following this point the rate of deterioration accelerated somewhat with a 4% reduction in the Kappa score between no inserted data and 16% inserted data. Looking at the relative performance we see that all models degraded in a broadly similar fashion with the exception that the Naive Bayes classifier with feature selection showed a marginally lower degradation than the Naive Bayes classifier based on a full set of features.

Turning to the case of poorly calibrated and broken sensors which may result in undetected events, let us first consider Figure 3. This figure shows the results for testing where a random proportion of the data has been removed. Similar to the results for the noise insertion study, we see that the Random Forest outperformed all other methods across a range of different test data volumes. Also, all the models are reasonably robust to low levels of noise with a relatively graceful degradation in performance as the noise level increased; for example, even at the point where 25% of the original sensor events had been removed the Random Forest's performance had decreased by only 7% as measured by Cohen's Kappa Coefficient.

Figure 4 meanwhile presents the case in which the results for entire individual sensors were omitted from the test data. This corresponds to the case of dead or broken sensors which fail to recognize any event occurrences. This differs from the case above in that whereas above events were removed randomly and from any sensor type, here events from some sensors are removed completely while other sensors retain all their readings. While these results are broadly similar to the case of randomly removed readings, it is worth noting the sharp drop at 2% of sensors removed which subsequently recovers. Since sensor selection for removal was random it is possible that very influential sensors can be removed. Even smoothed over three separate runs it is easy to see how dependent the activity recognition process can be even on the specific sensors operating correctly.

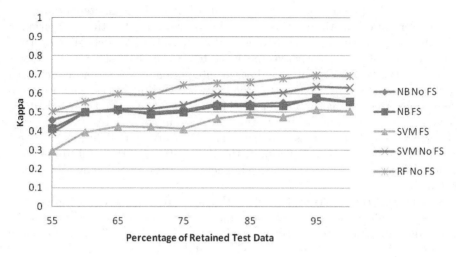

Fig. 3. Kappa Coefficient Scores for SCARE data with random deletions

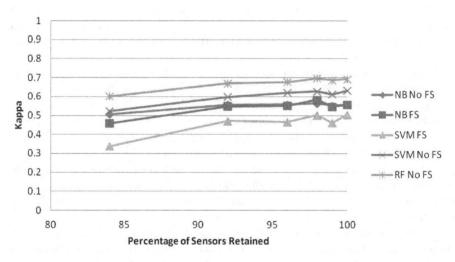

Fig. 4. Kappa Coefficient Scores for SCARE data with sensor removal

5   Conclusions

There can be no doubt that probabilistic and Machine Learning based classification techniques provide a sound theoretical and pragmatic solution to the
problem of activity recognition in uncertain and noisy environments. In this paper we have provided a brief study which both presented the relative merits
of popular Activity Recognition methods, and showed reassuringly that most
methods remain consistent in their relative performance across different types of
noise in the input data stream. We believe this is a highly useful finding in that

we can be assured that there is no need to consider different recognition models in different noise scenarios, and that developers can in general focus on selecting the method that provides the best balance between their accuracy requirements and training time constraints. In this context, the strong performance of the Random Forest models in this study provides some evidence the ensemble based methods may be an fruitful avenue for future research.

In analyzing the relative performance of methods on the activity recognition problem, it is worth noting that the sequential nature of activity data is arguably both a boon and a hindrance in the detection process. Since activity recognition is a sequential process, any noisy readings which are introduced are generally retained within sensor history models many steps after the false positive was initially detected. On the other hand, however, this may be balanced out by the fact that true positives also persist over time. Where the percentage of false positives is significantly outweighed by true positives the erroneous sensor readings can essentially be drowned out by the true history.

While performance degradation – particularly in the case of false positives – may not result in an extreme degradation of performance for low levels of errors, all reduction in performance is a challenge to be overcome in ensuring activity recognition performs acceptably in a real world interleaving and multi-agent environments. Given this, one avenue of future extension of work presented in this paper would be to conduct an initial pass of erroneous feature filtering based on anomaly detection. The difficulty here lies in detecting true noise in a real time basis where an unexpected sensor reading could be due to any number of reasons that are not necessarily due to defective sensors. Other avenues of future work include the extension of the studies presented here to other Activity Recognition corpora and indeed other sensor error models. At the very least we believe that an error model based on an empirical evaluation of error types in real world sensor deployments would be of great benefit to the study of Activity Recognition.

Acknowledgements. The authors wish to thank the Irish Research Council for Science Engineering and Technology (IRCSET) for their support through the IRCSET EMPOWER funding programme.

References

1. Geib, C.W., Steedman, M.: On natural language processing and plan recognition. In: International Joint Conference on Artificial Intelligence (2007)
2. Ye, J., Dobson, S., McKeever, S.: Situation identification techniques in pervasive computing: A review. Pervasive and Mobile Computing 8, 36–66 (2012)
3. Bui, H., Venkatesh, S., West, G.A.W.: Policy recognition in the abstract hidden markov model. Journal of Artificial Intelligence Research 17, 451–499 (2002)
4. Bui, H.: A general model for online probabilistic plan recognition. In: Proc. of the International Joint Conference on Artificial Intelligence (IJCAI), pp. 1309–1315 (2003)

5. Singla, G., Cook, D., Schmitter-Edgecombe, M.: Tracking activities in complex settings using smart environment technologies. International Journal of BioSciences, Psychiatry and Technology 1, 25–35 (2009)
6. Cook, D.: Learning setting-generalized activity models for smart spaces. IEEE Intelligent Systems 27, 32–38 (2012)
7. Singla, G., Cook, D.J., Schmitter-Edgecombe, M.: Recognizing independent and joint activities among multiple residents in smart environments. Journal of Ambient Intelligence and Humanized Computing 1, 57–63 (2010)
8. Charniak, E., Goldman, R.P.: A bayesian model of plan recognition. Artificial Intelligence 64, 53–79 (1993)
9. Pynadath, D.V., Wellman, M.P.: Accounting for context in plan recognition, with application to traffic monitoring. In: Besnard, P., Hanks, S. (eds.) Proceedings of the 11th Conference on Uncertainty in Artificial Intelligence (UAI 1995), pp. 472–481. Morgan Kaufmann Publishers, San Francisco (1995)
10. Krishnan, N., Cook, D.: Activity recognition on streaming sensor data. In: Pervasive and Mobile Computing (2012)
11. Ross, R., Kelleher, J.D.: Accuracy and timeliness in ml based activity recognition. In: Proceedings of AAAI Workshop on Plan, Activity, and Intent Recognition 2013 (PAIR 2013), Seattle, USA (2013)
12. Chen, C., Das, B., Cook, D.J.: A data mining framework for activity recognition in smart environments. In: Proceedings of the 2010 Sixth International Conference on Intelligent Environments, IE 2010, pp. 80–83. IEEE Computer Society, Washington, DC (2010)
13. Das, B., Cook, D.: Data mining challenges in automated prompting systems. In: Workshop on Interacting with Smart Objects (2011)
14. Stoia, L., Shockley, D.M., Byron, D.K., Fosler-Lussier, E.: Noun phrase generation for situated dialogs. In: Proceedings of the Fourth International Natural Language Generation Conference, pp. 81–88. Association for Computational Linguistics, Sydney (2006)
15. Cook, D., Schmitter-Edgecombe, M.: Assessing the quality of activities in a smart environment. Methods of Information in Medicine 48, 480–485 (2009)
16. Kipp, M.: ANVIL - A generic annotation tool for multimodal dialogue. In: Dalsgaard, P., Lindberg, B., Benner, H., Tan, Z.H. (eds.) INTERSPEECH, ISCA, pp. 1367–1370 (2001)

A Comparison of Evidence Fusion Rules for Situation Recognition in Sensor-Based Environments

Susan McKeever[1] and Juan Ye[2]

[1] School of Computing, Dublin Institute of Technology, Ireland
susan.mckeever@dit.ie
[2] School of Computer Science, University of St Andrews, UK

Abstract. Dempster-Shafer (DS) theory, and its associated Dempster rule of combination, has been widely used to determine belief based on uncertain evidence sources. Variations to the original Dempster rule of combination have appeared in the literature to support particular scenarios where unreliable results may result from the use of original DS theory. While theoretical explanations of the rule variations are explained, there is a lack of empirical comparisons of the DS theory and its variations against real data sets. In this work, we examine several variations to DS theory. Using two real-world sensor data sets, we compare the performance of DS theory and several of its variations in recognising situations. The empirical results shed insight on how to select these fusion rules based on the nature of sensor data, the relationship of this data over time to the higher level hypotheses and the choice of frame of discernment.

Keywords: Evidence theory, Dempster Shafer theory, situations, situation recognition, uncertainty, uncertain reasoning.

1 Introduction

Situations are human understandable representations of the environment that are of interest to a pervasive application. In the context of smart-homes, the term situation is often used interchangeably with activities, where the ambient system detects situation such as 'taking a shower' or 'preparing breakfast'. This task of situation recognition is a critical, continuous process in ambient environments, such as those monitoring the health of elderly patients in their homes.

Sensor data is inherently unreliable, noisy, prone to delay and imprecise. i.e. it suffers from uncertainty. For pervasive systems which rely on sensor data, the input such as a location tag reading is ambiguous [1], so inference from sensor data cannot be treated as fact, but simply evidence of fact. Users' actions can contribute to degradation of information quality, such as the failure of users to carry their locator tags [2]. Uncertainty of sensor information should be tracked and preserved to determine uncertainty at higher levels of context. Furthermore, the process of interpretation of sensed context is also subject to ambiguity and approximation. Some context concepts are fuzzy, so are subject to imprecision, such as the concepts of 'near' or 'warm'. Inference rules are not constant, such as a user 'sometimes' using a microwave when

M.J. O'Grady et al. (Eds.): AmI 2013 Workshops, CCIS 413, pp. 163–175, 2013.
© Springer International Publishing Switzerland 2013

engaged in 'preparing breakfast'. In our previous work [3], we have applied Demp-ster Shafer theory to quantify and accommodate this uncertainty in order to maximize our situation recognition results.

Dempster-Shafer theory is a theory of uncertain reasoning that is widely used in domains where information (evidence) is known to be imperfect and reasoning uncer-tain, such as medical diagnosis, quality control and process engineering. DS theory, and its associated Dempter rule of combination, has been widely used to determine belief based on uncertain evidence sources. In ambient environments, DS theory has been applied to situation recognition, based on sensors embedded in the environment [3-5]. The use of DS theory removes the reliance of training data required by learning approaches, such as Bayesian networks, Naive Bayes, Hidden Markhov models, and Decision Trees.

The field of evidence theory has widened beyond the original Dempster-Shafer theory, with variations to the theory proposed by other practitioners. Variations to the the original Dempster rule of combination from [6-9] have been proposed in order to support particular scenarios where unreliable results may result from the use of origi-nal DS theory. While theoretical explanations of the rule variations appear in the literature, there is a lack of *empirical* comparisons of DS theory and its variations against real data sets. In this work, we examine several variations to DS theory. Using two sensor data sets, we compare the performance of DS theory and these variations in recognising situations from the sensor data. By comparing the results, we empha-sise the nature of sensor data as a selection factor in the fusion rule, the impact of temporal spread of sensor data and the impact of multiple hypotheses in the frame of discernment.

The rest of the paper is organised as follows. Section 2 overviews the research in activity recognition and focus on the application of Dempster-Shafter theory in the area. Section 3 introduces the background of Dempster-Shafter theory and its alterna-tive fusion rules, which we evaluate and compare on two independent data sets (de-scribed in Section 4) in Section 5. The paper concludes in Section 6.

2   Related Work

The ability to recognise higher level situations or context is an ongoing area of re-search in the pervasive systems field.   Various machine learning approaches, have been applied to issue of uncertain sensor data environments. Naives Bayes classifiers have been used by Korpippa [10] and Tapia et al.[11]. Ranganathan et al.[12], Gu et al.[13] have applied Bayesian networks. Hidden Markov Models which considers the sequence of sensor data triggers have been applied by Clarkson et al.[14], Choujaa et al.[15] and van Kasteren [16].   The use of these approaches requires training data which can be problematic to collect and annotate in a sensored environment.

Dempster-Shafer theory has recently received greater attention in the domain of context-aware systems due to its lack of reliance on training data and its ability to cater for uncertainty in the reasoning process. The first use of the theory for context-aware systems was Wu's approach [17-18] to fuse sensor data into higher level contexts. Wu's main contribution is the definition of a dynamic discount factor for sensors that changes over time.

Hong et al. [19-20] apply Dempster-Shafer theory to define an evidence based activity (situation) model that uses sensor data for activity recognition in a smart home. Hong expands on Wu's work by using evidence propagation to bring evidence up through a hierarchy, so that *activities* can be recognised, as opposed to just abstracted contexts. Zhang et al. [5] use Dempster-Shafer theory for reasoning about activities. Their work focuses on resolving computation intensiveness of evidence fusion and addressing Zadeh's paradox [21], whereby conflicting evidence sources can give paradoxical results by granting majority belief to a minority opinion. In our previous work, we extended DS theory to allow for temporal knowledge to be incorporated into the evidential reasoning process [3].

DS theory has been extended by [6-8, 20] to allow for modifications to rules, in order to address particular limitations in the original DS rule of combination. In this paper, we examine variations to DS theory, and compare their performance for situation recognition on two sensor data sets. The purpose is to do an empirical comparison of DS theory and its variations, thus highlighting the subtleties of evidential rules when applied to real world sensor data. This will bolster existing theoretical work already done in this field with real examples.

3   Dempster Shafer Theory and Alternative Fusion Rules

3.1   Dempster Shafer theory

DS theory [9] is a theory of uncertain reasoning that is widely used in domains where information (evidence) is known to be imperfect and uncertain. In a DS theory reasoning scheme, the set of possible hypotheses are collectively called the *frame of discernment*. This frame Ω represents the set of choices $\{h_1, h_2, ...h_n\}$ available to the reasoning scheme, where sources (such as sensors) assign belief or evidence across the hypotheses in the frame. Hypotheses can be any subsets of the frame, ranging from singletons in the frame to combinations of elements in the frame. For example, a calendar sensor that monitors whether a user is scheduled to be in a meeting or not assigns belief across a frame of discernment that includes hypotheses {meeting, coffee break, busy at desk}. When the calendar indicates that the user does not have a meeting, belief is assigned by the calendar sensor to 'not meeting' situations i.e. the combination of {coffee break, busy at desk}. It assigns zero belief to {meeting}. Formally, 2^Ω denote the set of all subsets of   to which a source of evidence can apply its belief. The function $m : 2^\Omega \rightarrow [0; 1]$ is called a *mass function* that defines how belief is distributed across the frame, if the function satisfies the following conditions, for hypotheses A:

$$m(\Phi)=0 \qquad (1)$$

$$\sum_{A\in\theta} m(A) = 1 \qquad (2)$$

Based on these conditions, belief from an evidence source cannot be assigned to an empty or null hypothesis, and belief from the evidence source across the possible hypotheses (including combinations of hypotheses) must sum to 1, similar to probability theory. The least informative evidence (uncertainty) is the assignment of mass to a hypothesis containing all the elements $\{h_1, h_2, ...h_n\}$, because this evidence does not commit to any particular hypothesis. This uncertainty is denoted by the symbol θ

A crucial part of the process of assessing evidence is the ability to *fuse* evidence from multiple sources. In Dempster-Shafer theory, the combination of evidence from two different independent sources is accomplished by Dempster's combination rule:

$$m_{12}(A) = \frac{\sum_{X \cap Y = A} m_1 . m_1(X) . m_2(Y)}{1 - \sum_{X \cap Y = \emptyset} m_1(X) . m_2(Y)} \tag{3}$$

where $m_{12}(A)$ is the combined belief for a given hypothesis A, and X and Y represent all possible subsets of the frame. The numerator in equation (3) represents evidence for hypotheses whose intersection is the exact hypothesis of interest, A. i.e. the agreement across the two sources about the hypothesis A. This denominator, $1 - K$ is a normalisation factor, where K is a conflict factor representing all combined evidence that does not match the hypothesis of interest, A. The value of conflict, K, when combining evidence is indicative of the level of disagreement amongst the sources of their belief in hypothesis A. Dempster's rule can be considered as a strict AND operation of the evidence sources [22].

3.2   DS Evidence Fusion Issues

During our work on situation recognition [3, 23], we have noted three particular problems for when we apply Dempster's rule of combination to infer situations from sensor data:

1. Zadeh's Paradox: Zadeh's paradox is a well-documented problem with Dempster's rule of combination [21]. Zadeh highlighted the fact that when sources in high conflict are combined using Dempster-Shafer rule, the results can be completely counter intuitive.

2. Single Sensor Dominance: A second problem that has gained far less attention in the literature is the potential dominance of a single sensor. Murphy [8] described how a single disagreeing sensor can overrule multiple other agreeing sensors in the fusion process. A categorical belief function is where all belief is assigned to one hypothesis in a frame [24]. For example, if five sensors are used to determine the location of a user in the house, a single categorical sensor that assigns all of its belief to a contradictory option will negate the evidence from the other four sensors. We suggest that this is particularly problematic for binary sensors which are increasingly being used in smart home deployments. Binary sensors typically have small frames of discernment, with just three hypotheses: *{on, off, θ}*. Unless discounted, they will categorically assign all of their belief to the 'on' or 'off' states. A single malfunctioning binary sensor can in theory therefore overrule evidence from other correct binary sensors during the fusion process, unless its *off* state is assigned as evidence of uncertainty. A more intuitive result would be to allow the agreeing sensors to 'win' but to represent the disagreeing sensors' evidence as conflict.

3. Evidence Spread over Time: A third problem that we have observed [3] occurs when sensors' evidence of a higher-level state is spread over time. For example, the detection of a breakfast activity is the sequence of the triggering of a fridge sensor, then a kettle sensor, then the toaster sensor and so forth. At any point in time, only one of the sensors may be 'on', so fusion of all the sensor values at any point in time may result in the 'on' sensor evidence being lost. The fusion rule should capture that some evidence of the situation was observed even though it has been greatly contradicted by sensors that are off. It should not be wiped out by the overruling of the contradictory sensors, as will occur with Dempster's rule of combination.

3.3   Alternative Evidence Fusions Approaches

Dempster's rule of combination was the core fusion mechanism provided as part of the original Dempster-Shafer theory. The rule has been enhanced or changed by researchers in order to cater for specific applications of Dempster-Shafer theory because it is not suitable in all fusion scenarios, such as the work of Yager [6], Hong et al.[20], Dubois and Prade[7], Smets and Kennes [25] and Murphy [8]. To narrow down our focus, we examine the variations that address the particular fusion issues we have discussed in Section 3.2

Murphy's Combination Rule
Murphy's alternative rule of combination eliminates the dominance of a single sensor and allows contradictory evidence to be preserved to some degree. Evidence is averaged prior to combining it using Dempster's rule of combination. Formally, if there are n sources of evidence, we use equation (3) to combine the weighted averages of the masses $n - 1$ times. Evidence for each hypothesis, h, from n sources is summed, and averaged across all evidence sources. This eliminates the dominance of a single sensor by reducing its contribution according to the number of sources. Use of Murphy's combination rule will also eliminate Zadeh's paradox because the evidence is averaged prior to combination.

Averaging Rule
Shafer [9] combined belief functions by averaging all the evidence for each hypothesis (instead of the combination rule), as follows:

$$M(A) = \frac{1}{n}(M_1(A) + ... + M_n(A))$$ (4)

Averaging can be used to eliminate the influence of any strongly conflicting single belief [27], so would cater for both single sensor dominance and Zadeh's paradox. The use of averaging provides an accurate record of contributing beliefs because no belief is lost, but it lacks convergence. Both Dempster's and Murphy's rule allows evidence from sources that are in agreement to reinforce each other, and disagreeing evidence to be dropped. In contrast, averaging does not increase the measure of belief in the dominant subset but provides a less conclusive picture because conflict is not normalised out. However, it is simpler to compute with fewer calculations. We antici-pate that averaging will be useful to counteract the expected problem of conflicting sensors in binary sensors.

OR Combination Rule

Hong et al. [19] selected belief from two evidence sources by selecting the maximum belief. From our own work, we can see that this may apply well where a set of sepa-rate binary sensors are used for evidence of a situation. For example, the situation of 'preparing breakfast' may be detected by the kettle sensor firing *or* the toaster sensor. Mathematically, the highest mass associated with hypothesis A is selected from the evidence sources:

$$M(A) = \max(m_1(A)..m_n(A)) \tag{5}$$

This may be useful for task-driven situations where the sensors are triggering over a period of time. In theory, only a single piece of evidence needs to be triggered in or-der to detect the situation using the OR fusion scenario.

Temporal Knowledge in Fusion Rules

Temporal knowledge is a natural human way to reason about current activities or situations. For example, when assessing the current activity of a person at home, the time of day may determine whether they are preparing breakfast or dinner; the length of time they spent in the kitchen may help us decide whether they were preparing a meal or just getting a drink, and so on. Time durations of situations, sequential pat-terns in which situations occur and discernible patterns over time are examples of temporal knowledge that can improve our ability to recognise which situation(s) is occurring.

In [3], we set out an approach to incorporating time into situation recognition, us-ing evidence theory. To recap, we extended transitory evidence to increase the knowledge of our sensor datasets as follows.

We define transitory evidence [3] as evidence that does not last for the full duration of a situation. For example, during the situation of 'preparing breaking', the kettle sensor may fire briefly just one, even though the situation may be in progress over a number of minutes. During the inference process, when evidence for that situation is detected, the duration for that situation is triggered to start. Looking at the situation of 'preparing dinner' in figure Fig. 1, when any of the groceries cupboard, fridge, freezer, pans cupboard or plates cupboard sensors are fired, the reasoning system will 'start' the dinner activity. The lifetime of the triggered sensor evidence for that activ-ity will be extended to last for the remaining duration stored for that situation. As inference continues over time, the lifetime of any further evidence for the situation will be extended for the duration that is left of the situation (i.e. situation duration elapsed time). Once the full duration of the situation is reached, the evidence will expire. By extending the lifetime of the evidence, at any point in time, the evidence sources can be fused as if they are co-occurring.

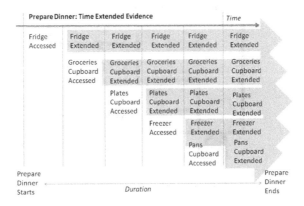

Fig. 1. Time extension of evidence for 'preparing dinner' situation

4   Sensor Datasets

In our work, we have used two annotated data sets containing data from sensors, allowing us to apply our various evidence approaches to situation recognition using the sensor data. Using the data sets, we will measure situation recognition success using Dempster's original rule of combination, Murphy's rule, Averaging rule and OR combination rule. In addition, we will do each of these using transitory and time extended evidence.

4.1   Van Kasteren DataSet

This data set originates from the intelligent autonomous systems group in University of Amsterdam [16]. The data is over a 28 day period using 14 digital sensors were installed in the house. The sensors are installed on the hall-toilet door, hall-bathroom door, hall-bedroom door, front door, microwave, fridge, freezer, washing machine and each of the cups/plates/pans cupboards. When a sensor is fired, it outputs a value 1 as its reading in the sensor output file.

Seven situations (termed 'activities') are annotated by the occupant of the house: 1) leave house; 2) use toilet; 3) take shower; 4) go to bed; 5) prepare breakfast; 6) prepare dinner; 7) get drink as shown in Fig. 2.

We timesliced the data to 1 minute timeslices, so that the sensor values are known at minute variations. The full data preparation, and domain knowledge attached to sensor readings is described in our previous work on temporal evidence theory in [3]. For the purposes of this work, it is worth emphasising that the sensor readings in Van Kasteren are from binary sensors, and generate transitory evidence – evidence which does not last for the full duration of the situation.

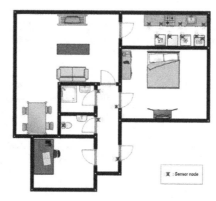

Fig. 2. Layout of sensors in van Kasteren house floor plan [109]

4.2   CASL Data Set

Our second data set, termed CASL, was generated in the Complex and Adaptive Systems (CASL) research laboratory of University College Dublin. We built our own infrastructure to capture the following data about a person in our research lab environment: their computer activity, their calendar entries, and their physical location in the building. Describing each sensor in turn:

- The *computer activity* sensor runs on the participant's desktop PC and monitors the rate of key presses and mouse clicks, along with the length of time since the last activity. The data from this sensor is used to indicate whether the user is 'active' or 'inactive' at their desktop. This data set is described and used in [2]. It is available to download at www.comp.dit.ie/smckeever/research.html
- The *calendar sensor* collects information about the user's scheduled Google calendar events, including meeting schedule state, start time and end time. The data from this sensor indicates whether the user has a meeting or not for the current time. The context values used are 'meeting' and 'no meeting'. The sensor mass function assigns its belief to 'meeting' if there is a meeting scheduled in the diary for the time in question, and assigns belief to 'no meeting' if the diary is empty.
- For *Location sensing,* we have a Ubisense system deployment on the third and fourth floor of our research lab. Ubisense is a tag-based 3-D location tracking system. It provides an X, Y and Z coordinate, based on the number of metres from an origin point – in our case the bottom corner of the third floor in CASL. Ubisense covers areas on the third and fourth floors in the CASL building, using 30 wall-mounted sensors. Ubisense tracks a location tag belonging to the user, providing co-ordinate readings for the location tag when the tag is moved. The participant gathered a data set over a 5-day period. For situation detection, as previously stated, we are interested in four particular locations: desk, cafe, meeting room and all other locations. Therefore, the context values are user desk, cafe, meeting room, other. The frame for the sensor mass functions contains the singleton elements: *{desk, cafe, meetingRoom, other}* and all possible combinations of the

singletons:{desk ∧ cafe; desk ∧ cafe ∧ meeting,...θ}: In practice, most of the combined elements are never used.

Six situations were annotated: (1) busy at computer, (2) busy reading at desk, (3) coffee break, (4) lunch break, (5) informal break, and (6) meeting. Each of these is detectable from the combination of the three sensor systems in our infrastructure. At any point in time, the participant can only be engaged in one of these situations, but is always engaged in one of the situations.

5   Empirical Comparison of Fusion Rules

The purpose of our experiment is to compare the situation recognition rates of various evidential fusion rules when used against our two data sets. We use the standard *f-Measure* metric, the weighted mean of *precision* and *recall* as our measure of comparison as also used in [3]. The full evidential reasoning for the van Kasteren dataset is described in [3] and for the CASL dataset in [23].

5.1   Results from Van Kasteren Data Set

Table 1. shows a comparison of situation recognition accuracies when each of the four rules is used with van Kasteren's data set. Dempster's rule is least accurate when transitory sensor evidence is used. We can anticipate this because Dempster's rule will allow a single sensor to overrule other sensors. Therefore, unless all sensors are fired at the same time in one time slice, the evidence from any firing sensors will be lost or allocated to uncertainty. When evidence from the sensors is extended for the duration of the situation, Dempster's rule improves greatly, as the problem of the single sensor dominance no longer exists.

Table 1. Recognition accuracies (f-measure) for four fusion rules on van Kastersen's data set

Fusion Rule:	OR	Averaging	Dempster	Murphy
Situation recognition with transitory evidence	**0.57**	0.54	0.48	0.55
Situation recognition with time extended evidence	0.66	0.65	0.60	**0.68**

Murphy's rule performs better than Dempster's in both cases. The agreeing sensors reinforce each other. In the case of transitory evidence, the categorical off sensors do not negate the evidence of the on sensors.

The averaging rule produces results that are almost as good as Murphy's rule. The averaging rule uses less computation but it does not provide any measure of conflict. At present, we do not use the conflict metric in our inference process so averaging may provide a faster alternative to evidence fusion, if the capture of a conflict measure is not an issue.

Interestingly, the 'OR' fusion rule performs best when used with transitory evidence. Only the 'OR' rule disregards co-occurrence of evidence, because it only relies on single pieces of evidence. The 'OR' approach also has issues distinguishing situations if they share sensors. For example, if a cup is used, and this is equally evidential of breakfast and drink, the system cannot distinguish which situation is occurring. When evidence is time-extended, all approaches, including the 'OR' fusion approach, benefit from longer durations of evidence, as previously discuss in [3].

5.2   Results from CASL Dataset

We run a similar analysis on the CASL data set, comparing results for fusion using averaging, Dempster's rule and Murphy's rule. We excluded the 'OR' combination rule because all evidence is co-occurring in the CASL situations so there is no theoretical benefit in using 'OR' fusion.

Looking at Table 2, in the CASL data set, Demptser's rule of combination performs slightly better than Murphy's rule. Unlike van Kastersen's data set, all evidence is continuous so the problem of single sensors being 'off' and overruling other firing sensors is not an issue. The averaging rule performs relatively poorly. In the CASL data set, evidence is frequently applied to combinations of situations (as opposed to the van Kasteren data set where evidence was applied to single situations). For example, if the computer activity sensor is 'inactive', this is indicative of any of the situations 'busy at desk', 'coffee break', 'lunch break', 'informal break' or 'meeting'. When averaging is used, the evidence is simply divided up amongst the elements prior to averaging. In Dempster's rule and Murphy's rule, agreeing evidence is merged so combined evidence converges more distinctly towards situations that have further evidence. As a result, the averaging rule results are more successful in van Kastersen's data set than in the CASL data set.

Table 2. Situation recognition (f-measure) for three fusion rules on the CASL data set

Fusion Rule	Averaging	Dempster	Murphy
Situation recognition	0.5	**0.62**	0.60

5.3   Discussion

The results confirm that the choice of evidential fusion rule has an impact on the success of inferring the correct situations on our data sets. From our analysis, we emphasise the following points for practitioners using evidence theory for analysing sensor data.

1. If the environment is generating sensors readings that are occurring over time, Dempster's rule of combination is useful for evidence that is *co-occurring*. In a monitored environment, multiple sensors may be used to detect a particular activity. If these sensors do not fire concurrently, Dempster's rule should be used with care. At any time, if most sensors associated with a situation are *off*, they will be evidential of the activity not occurring or uncertainty and may therefore give a misleading result.

2. In an environment where multiple sensors are used to detect a situation, and these sensors give short burst readings, consider the use of the OR fusion rule as a simple way to determine that if any sensor for a situation is on, the situation may be occurring.

3. The frame of discernment and allocation of evidence towards each element in the frame are a key consideration when choosing the evidence fusion in rule. We saw that for the CASL data set, a sensor may be evidential of more than one situation – in which case, the use of the averaging rule is weakened for reasons previously stated.

4. Finally, we note that *computational complexity* of the fusion rules is another consideration. For both Murphy's and Dempster Rule of Combination, evidence can be applied for any combination of hypotheses in a frame, so the number of permutations for n hypotheses in a frame can be as high as the power set, 2^n. But in reality, all combinations of hypotheses may never be used and there is no need to always build all the possible values of belief. There are many cases where the knowledge is very simple and where there are very few non-null masses - making the belief function computation lighter than its competitors. In addition, we noted that the simple averaging rule achieved comparable results with Murphy's decision rule on van Kastersen's data set. The averaging rule works well if applied to evidence that support single hypotheses only in a frame. Another way to reduce computational effort is to limit calculations to active parts of the environment. For example, using an example from Hong et al.'s [20] smart home, a motion sensor may detect motion in the kitchen. At that point in time, situation beliefs will only be calculated for kitchen-based situations.

6   Conclusions

In this work, we have compared a number of variations to the Dempster rule of combination, based on resolving specific issues encountered during previous work: Zaheh's paradox, single sensor dominance and transitory evidence. Our results for our first data set show that Murphy's rule produces the highest situation recognition rate when used with time extended evidence. When using binary trigger sensors, the simple OR rule produces the best results. In our second data set, where all sensors are continuously generating evidence, Murphy's rule is no longer needed to negate a single sensor dominating, and Dempster's rule performs best. Most importantly, to understand these results, a deep knowledge of the sensor data values and their use for inference over time is required in order to select the most suitable fusion rule. For example, Murphy's alternative fusion rule [8] negates the effect of a single dominant sensor overruling the evidence-based decision. While our work supports this observation, we note that this is applicable if all evidence is co-occurring. It is either less or not applicable if sensor readings for a situation are triggering over time and not occurring simultaneously The selection of suitable frames of discernments, either singletons or combined will also influence the outcomes.

References

1. Dobson, S., and Nixon, P.: Whole-Systems Programming of Adaptive Ambient Intelligence. In: Universal Access in HCI, Ambient Interaction, vol. 4555/2007, pp. 73-81, (2007)
2. McKeever S., Ye J., Coyle L., Dobson S.: A Context Quality Model to Support Transparent Reasoning with Uncertain Context, vol. 5786/2009, pp. 65-75,   Lecture Notes in Computer Science, (2009)
3. McKeever S., Ye J., Coyle L., Dobson S.: Activity recognition using temporal evidence theory, Journal of Ambient Intelligence and Smart Environments, vol. 2, (2010)
4. Wu H., Siegel M., Stiefelhagen R.: Sensor fusion using Dempster-Shafer theory: in Proceedings of IEEE Instrumentation and Measurement Technology Conference, vol. 1, pp. 7--12,(2002)
5. Zhang D., Guo M., Zhou J., Kang D., Cao J.: Context reasoning using extended evidence theory in pervasive computing environments, Future Gener. Comput. Syst., vol. 26, pp. 207--216, (2010)
6. Yager R.: On the Dempster-Shafer framework and new combination rules, Inf. Sci., vol. 41, pp. 93--137, (1987)
7. Dubois D. and Prade H.: Representation and combination of uncertainty with belief functions and possibility measures, Computational Intelligence., vol. 4, pp. 244-264, (1988)
8. Murphy C.: Combining belief functions when evidence conflicts, Decis. Support Syst., vol. 29, pp. 1--9, (2000)
9. Shafer G.: A mathematical theory of evidence.: Princeton University Press, (1976)
10. Korpipaa P., Mantyjarvi J., Kela J., Keranen H., and Malm EJ.: Managing context information in mobile devices, Pervasive Computing, IEEE, vol. 2, pp. 42-51, July-Sept. (2003)
11. Tapia E., Intille S., Larson K., Activity Recognition in the Home Using Simple and Ubiquitous Sensors, Springer Volume. 3001/2004, 2004, pp. 158-175 (2004)
12. Ranganathan A, Al-Muhtadi J, Campbell R.: Reasoning about uncertain contexts in pervasive computing environments, IEEE Magazine on Pervasive Computing, vol. 3, pp. 62-70, April-June, (2004)
13. Gu T., Pung H., Zhang D.: A Bayesian approach for dealing with uncertain contexts, Pervasive 2004, pp. 205—210, (2004)
14. Clarkson B., Pentland A., Mase K.: Recognizing User Context via Wearable Sensors, Wearable Computers, IEEE International Symposium, p. 69, (2000)
15. Choujaa D., Dulay N.: Activity Inference through Sequence Alignment,   LoCA 2009, pp. 19—36, (2009)
16. Van Kasteren T., Noulas A., Englebienne G., Krose B.: Accurate activity recognition in a home setting, Ubicomp 2008, pp. 1—9, (2008)
17. Wu H., Sensor fusion using dempster shafer theory, PhD Thesis (2003)
18. Wu H., Siegel M., Stiefelhagen R.: Sensor fusion using Dempster-Shafer theory, IEEE Instrumentation and Measurement, vol. 1, 2002, pp. 7—12, (2002)
19. Hong X., Nugent C., Wiu L., McClean S, Scotney B., Ma J, Mulvenna M.: Uncertain Information Management for ADL Monitoring in Smart Homes, Intelligent Patient Management, vol. 189/2009, pp. 315-332, (2009).
20. Hong X., Nugent C., Mulvenna M , Scotney B., McClean S,, Devlin B.: Evidential fusion of sensor data for activity recognition in smart homes, Pervasive and Mobile Computing, vol. 5, pp. 236-252, (2009).

21. Zadeh L.: A Simple View of the Dempster-Shafer Theory of Evidence and its Implication for the Rule of Combination, AI Magazine, vol. 7, pp. 85--90, (1986)
22. Sentz K., Ferson S.: Combination of Evidence in Dempster Shafer Theory, Sandia National Laboratories tech-report (2002)
23. McKeever S.: PhD Thesis: Recognising Situations using extended Dempster-Shafer Theory, phdthesis (2011)
24. Liu W.: Analyzing the degree of conflict among belief functions, Artif. Intell., vol. 170, pp. 909--924, (2006)
25. Smets P., Kennes R.: The Transfer Belief Model, Symbolic and Quantitative Approaches to Uncertainty, pp. 91-96, (1991)

In-Network Sensor Data Modelling Methods for Fault Detection

Lei Fang and Simon Dobson

School of Computer Science, University of St Andrews UK
lf28@st-andrews.ac.uk

Abstract. Wireless sensor networks are attracting increasing interest but suffer from severe challenges such as low data reliability. To improve the data reliability, many sensor fault detection techniques have been proposed. Behind these methods, mathematical models are usually employed to serve as comparing metric to find faulty data in the absence of ground truth. In this paper, we firstly discuss sensor data features and their relevance to fault detection. Criteria that should be met to become a competent data model for the purpose of fault detection is summarised. Some existing sensor data modelling methods for fault detection are presented and qualitatively compared.

1 Introduction

Wireless sensor networks (WSNs) typically consist of multiple battery powered sensor nodes, distributed over a large area, measuring and reporting real-world quantities through one or more powerful sink nodes. With the maturation of sensor network software, WSNs applications, which now range from scientific exploration [1], home and health control [2], [3], habitat monitoring [4] and environment monitoring [5] to infrastructure protection [6], have been attracting growing interests from both academia and industry. However, one problem that still prevents the further commercialising WSN technology is the low reliability of data gathered by sensors. It has been found that a substantial portion of the data gathered in real monitoring applications is actually faulty [7]. For example, 51% of the data collected in [1] was faulty; 3-60 % of data collected in the Great Duck Island experiment was incorrect [8]. Other data series [9],[10] collected by WSNs also have been found faulty.

Faulty data occurs when the data gathered and reported by the WSN application deviates from the true sample of the physical environment being measured [8]. Given the criticality of the applications envisioned for WSNs, the data collected by them should be accurate and reliable. To improve the data reliability, many solutions featuring different techniques have been put forward to calibrate sensor readings by filtering out faulty data in a on-line and in-network fashion.

Although server-side error filtering in which filters clean the received data at network sink is always an option, we believe on-line and especially in-network solutions have certain advantages over the traditional method. On-line solutions

M.J. O'Grady et al. (Eds.): AmI 2013 Workshops, CCIS 413, pp. 176–189, 2013.
© Springer International Publishing Switzerland 2013

can provide in-time alerts when things go wrong. Therefore, timely remedies can be given, like replacing the faulty sensors, to avoid the collected data set being completely useless. Moreover, in-network solutions are more scalable and flexible than their server side counterparts. For large scale sensor deployments, centralised solutions usually causes big overheads. And in-network solution is more flexible in that it can carry out casual sensor health inspection without sending all the data entries back to the sink. Furthermore, for some applications, in-network error filter may be the only feasible solution especially for those event driven deployments in which sensors do not send every data entry back to the sink [11]. Last but not least, the low yield of WSNs applications makes server side error filtering not practical. For example, the Redwood project [1] reported only 49 % of expected points are finally received at sink. The error filtering becomes challenging, if not impossible, with incomplete data set.

Most of the sensor fault detectors spot data faults by modelling historical sensor data as a norm and future data series are checked against the models to be classified as either normal readings or faulty data. This model-based solution is widely used because firstly it is a data centric method that usually does not require prior field expert knowledge and human intervention, which are not generally available or applicable for most WSNs applications. In other words, in the absence of ground truth, data model provides the metric for sensor data to be measured against their degree of being a fault. Secondly, the solution also fits the context of WSNs well due to its relative simplicity so that the whole operation can be carried out in a distributed, on-site and on-line manner, as sensor nodes with restricted processing power and memory space usually cannot cope with sophisticated machine learning methods. Thirdly, since mathematical models are usually employed, formal reasoning and inference can be naturally incorporated to the solution so that the solution is sound and accurate. For example, via a sound inference, not only faulty data can be detected but missing data or erroneous data can be reconstructed.

Numerous data modelling methods have been proposed for the task of fault detection. This paper provides a study on these different methods and qualitatively assess them in one metric. Section 3 introduces some sensor data features and their relationships with fault detection. Section 2 gives the definition of sensor data faults and as well as different types of sensor faults. Section 4 presents an evaluation metric for modelling method of sensor fault detection. Different modelling methods are then introduced and qualitatively compared in detail in Section 5. The paper concludes with future work and some research directions of data modelling methods.

2   Faulty Sensor Data

2.1   Data Faults and Data Outliers

Data-faults emerge when a node performs, or is forced to perform, a sensing task in an erroneous way resulting in faulty data which deviates from a true sample of the physical context to be measured. Data-faults in general are generated by either internal (i.e. system faults) or external factors. External source usually involves various kinds of malicious attacks, like unauthorised message spoof or node tampering [12], which lead to the received data altered therefore faulty. Intrusion detection or sensor network security [12], [13], [14], however, is another research topic which is beyond the scope of this paper. On the other side, internal sources include battery failure, weakening battery supply, connection failure, sensor hardware malfunctioning, calibration error, short-circuited connections and so on [15], [7]. Though different the sources, either external or internal, are, they all lead to faulty readings which do not agree with the ground truth of the interest.

One should also note the difference between data outlier and data-fault. Data-fault should be considered as a special kind of outlier. Outliers are data entries that deviate from expected normal patterns, which may either be caused by an unexpected genuine event, for example rainfalls, or other sources like malicious attacks or sensor failures. Sudden changes of the environment may cause turbulent sensor readings, which, however, usually is the main interest of a WSN application. For example, volcano eruption will give rise to radical sensor readings including temperature, humidity, and light; however, monitoring the eruption is the main purpose of the deployment. Therefore, separating real data faults caused by malfunctioning sensors from outliers is crucial for WSN applications as data fault detector may discard valuable information as data faults. But drawing a fine line between them is difficult especially for resource constrained sensors, which requires the data model adaptive and responsive to the changing underlying environment. The relationship between data-fault and outlier, and their corresponding causes are summarized in Fig. 1.

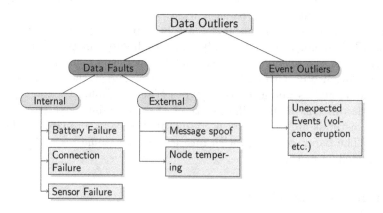

Fig. 1. The relationships between data-outlier and data-fault and their sources

2.2   Data Fault Types

By analysing the real world sensor data, sensor data faults can be categorised into four categories according to [7], [15]. The four types of faults: short, constant, noise and calibration have been constantly found in different WSNs deployments [1], [9], [10], [16], [17]. The definitions of the three types faults are listed below.

NOISE. Sensor readings exhibit an unexpectedly high amount of variation for a period of time. The noisy variance is beyond the expected variation of the underlying phenomenon. Usually high noise is due to a hardware failure or low batteries [15].

SHORT. A sharp momentary change in the measured value between normal consecutive readings. Hardware failures like fault in the analog-to-digital convert board may lead to short faults [7].

CONSTANT. Also known as "Stuck-at" fault. The readings remain constant for a period of time greater than expected. The reported constant value usually is out of the possible range of the expected normal readings and uncorrelated to the underlying physical phenomena [7].

CALIBRATION. Sensor readings may have offsets or incorrect gain, rendering reported data deviating from the true value. Drift faults occur when the offset or gain change with time.

3   Sensor Data Features

3.1   Multi-dimensionality

Sensor data gathered at the sink can be viewed as data stream indexed by time and their locations. For each deployed node, it usually has more than one type of sensor incorporated. The most commonly deployed classes of sensors include temperature, humidity, light, and chemical ones. Each data stream of the onboard sensor classes becomes a univariate time series. Therefore, the ensemble of the data streams becomes multivariate time series. Although different classes of sensor readings exhibit varying statistical features, they share similar fault types listed in Section 2.2; their relative frequencies present in different classes of sensor readings may vary though [15].

The multi-variate nature of sensor readings bring both benefits and difficulties with regard to fault detection for WSNs. The different classes of sensor readings tend to be correlated and such local correlations can be exploited to find outlier data entries in an energy efficient way as no data transmission is required. For example, the readings of humidity and barometric pressure sensors are related to the readings of the temperature sensors [18], as shown in Fig. 2. Capturing this correlation helps to improve the detection accuracy [19].

However, on the other side, higher dimensions bring higher computational complexity as well as modelling difficulty, whose impact on resource constrained sensors is apparent. Moreover, outlier detection may have to check multi-variate outliers as well. Because, as pointed out by Sun [20], occasionally, while each individual attribute reading appears normal, the ensemble of the attributes may display anomaly.

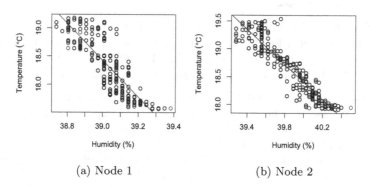

(a) Node 1   (b) Node 2

Fig. 2. Correlation between temperature and humidity sensors by real world sensor data [10]

3.2   Non-stationarity of Sensor Data

Stationarity is an important concept in statistical time series analysis [21]. Roughly speaking, a data series is stationary if its behaviour is self-similar therefore its statistical properties, like the first two moments mean and variance, does not vary according to time. Such an assumption is vital for all fault detection techniques as it provides the legitimacy to apply historic model learnt based on past data to future data series.

However, such an assumption is usually a "fair tale invented for the amusement of undergraduates" [22]. There is a clear loophole in this assumption: if the phenomena of interest were stationary, there would be no need to deploy sensors to monitor the ongoing changes whatsoever as the underlying process had been assumed to remain constant. The non-stationarity can be seen clearly from sensor data plots. As shown in Fig. 3a, the temperature readings change radically along the time stamps. In terms of data modelling for fault detection, dealing with the non-stationary sensor data is crucial as it may decide the detection accuracy of the technique: using a wrong historic model will lead to completely nonsense results.

3.3   Correlation of Sensor Data

Due to the fact that the underlying phenomenon usually is dominated by a smooth continuous process, sensor data tend to be correlated in both time and space, especially for those data collected from environmental monitoring applications [23].

Temporal Correlation. Temporal correlation means sensor readings sampled at closer time stamps tend to be similar. In other words, the readings observed at one time instant are related to the readings observed at the previous time instants [24]. Such an assumption is valid for most WSNs deployments because the underlying physical process usually evolves continuously and the sampling frequencies set for WSN applications are usually at sufficient granularity to capture the process smoothly.

Spatial Correlation. Spatial correlation implies that the readings from sensor nodes geographically close to each other are expected to be similar, i.e. correlated [24]. This assumption is usually held true because typical node-to-node spacings, usually in the range of 100-200 meters or less, are close enough to measure similar underlying evolving phenomena. Fig. 3a shows spatial correlation as the two data series collected at adjacent nodes exhibit the same pattern.

Capturing the spatio-temporal correlations can not only be used to filter out outlier readings from normal data but also can be used to further distinguish between faulty data and event outliers [18], [25], [19].

4   Evaluation Features of Modelling Methods

In general, a good fault detector should take both detection accuracy and complexity into account. First of all, to form an on-line solution, the cost of constructing and maintaining the model behind the detector should be within the storage and computational capabilities of regular sensor nodes. On the other hand, detection accuracy is the main metric to compare the performance of a fault detector. The faults reported by a detector can be categorised into the following four classes: data points correctly detected as faulty (true positive); data points correctly detected as non-faulty (true negatives); data points incorrectly detected as faulty (false positives); and data points incorrectly detected as non-faulty (false negatives). Good detection accuracy implies the method should be able to filter out the exactly amount of faulty data, i.e. achieve high true positive rate but keep false negative rate low.

Good data modelling methods should possess the following merits to form a accurate but cost effective fault detector.

Lightweight. As said before, a lightweight model is essential to produce an on-line and in-network solution. To be more specific, the model construction process should be lightweight enough to take place in local sensor nodes. Moreover, the learnt model should be lightweight enough to store locally as well.

Accurate Prediction Range. Each sensor data model, when applied to future data series, will produce a prediction range as the expected normal data limits; data entries outside this normal range is considered as faults. To achieve good detection accuracy, the range should be carefully selected so that it is neither too wide (lead to low true positive rate), nor too narrow (lead to high false positive rate).

Non-stationarity Resilient. As mentioned in Section 3.2, sensor data, by its nature, is non-stationary. Updating the stale model is an option to make the model commensurate with the stochastic phenomena being measured,

but it incurs extra computation or communication cost. Ideally speaking, a
constant data model, or a model with minimal updates, is the best option
for sensor fault detector.

Robust Learning. The learning data to construct the model at the first place
is unreliable as the rest; therefore, the data modelling method should be
robust to the errors present in the learning data. Otherwise, erroneous models
may be obtained, leading to detection accuracy degradation.

4.1   Model Data

Models can be constructed upon either raw sensor data or transformed data.
Most existing solutions use raw sensor data as learning series, like [7], [8], [26].
However, modelling on pre-processed data shows merits like making the model
resilient to non-stationary sensor data [19], [25].

The solutions presented in [19], [25] use synchronised difference between adjacent sensor readings as learning data. After the difference, the new data becomes
partially stationary or partially self-similar, i.e. the model learnt by historic data
remains true for most future data series. Fig. 3a shows temperature data series
from two correlated sensors. It is obvious that, comparing with the original data,
the absolute difference, shown in Fig. 3b, is more self-similar. It is shown that
the modified data stream becomes stationary in the sense it passes stationarity
statistical test and also the majority of future data series agrees upon the historic model learnt by the first 150 data entries [19]. One should, however, note
that models built on spatial data differences requires data sharing among local
neighbouring nodes at model construction phase, incurring extra data transmis-
sions. Also when it comes to operation phase, sensor data under test also needs
to be shipped among neighbouring nodes.

Bettencourt et al. also build statistical models on difference between each
node's own measurements at different times by making use of the temporal
correlation [25]; and similar results are found.

5   Data Modelling Methods

5.1   Regression Based Modelling

Statistical correlations among data attributes can be modelled by regression.
In sensor data context, simple linear models are commonly used. For example,
the spatial correlation between neighbouring temperature sensors, s_1 and s_2, is
modelled as:

$$X = \beta_0 + \beta_1 Y + u_i, \tag{1}$$

where temperature readings from s_1, X, is modelled as a linear combination
of its correspondent Y plus some random error u_i [27]. Similarly, linear model
between temperature and humidity can also be constructed.

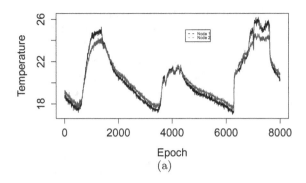

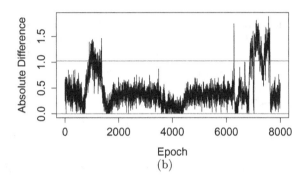

Fig. 3. Stationarity of Real World Sensor Data. The top shows the temperature series from two co-located and correlated sensors; The bottom shows the absolute difference between the two series. Over 87% of the future data agree upon the historic model.

Model parameters, β_0, β_1, may be learnt by the ordinary least-squares (OLS) estimation. The OLS estimators have closed-form solutions, as shown in (2).

$$\hat{\beta}_1 = \frac{\sum_{i=1}^{n}(X_i - \bar{X})(Y_i - \bar{Y})}{\sum_{i=1}^{n}(X_i - \bar{X})^2}$$

$$\hat{\beta}_0 = \bar{Y} - \hat{\beta}_1\bar{X} \tag{2}$$

Threshold for Fault Detection. According to the linear model, a prediction interval, which sets the boundary values for the value of interest, can be calculated formally at specific confidence interval:

$$X_{new} \in \hat{\beta}_0 + \hat{\beta}_1 Y_{new} \pm \varepsilon,$$

$$\varepsilon = t_{n-2,\alpha}\hat{\sigma}(1 + \frac{1}{n} + \frac{(Y_{new} - \bar{Y})^2}{S_Y})^{1/2} \tag{3}$$

where $\hat{\sigma}^2 = \frac{1}{n-1} \sum_{i=1}^{n} u_i^2$ is the residual sum of squares; and $t_{n-2,\alpha}$ is the significance test coefficient obtained from a t-table. When a new pair of observations, say (T_2, T_1), is sampled, the prediction interval can be calculated according to Eqn. 3. Any data entry which is outside of the interval is marked as a fault.

However, some works [27] use user specified error band, $\hat{\varepsilon}$ instead of the regressor-specific error ε. $\hat{\varepsilon}$ may be set as the maximum estimation error, i.e. $max\{u_i\}$, in learning data under the assumption the training data is error free.

Evaluation

Lightweight. The solution usually is **lightweight** enough to be carried out at local nodes, as the learning phase only involves the calculation of mean, variance and covariance [19], [28]; and the operational phase requires a storage of three floating numbers.

Accurate Prediction Range. The precision largely depends on the selection of error band ε, which involves some domain knowledge. One should also note regression-based solutions can be used to detect multi-variate outliers, as they naturally model the correlation relationship among the multi-dimensional attributes.

Non-stationarity Resilient. The model however is not resilient to the non-stationarity of sensor data. As pointed out in [19], the correlation model needs to be updated as the underlying correlation changes from time to time.

Robust Learning. Erroneous learning data's effect may be minimised by applying robust regression [19], [29].

5.2   Parametric Statistical Modelling

Parametric method is a statistical modelling method under the assumption that the modelling data has come from a specific type of probability distribution. It then models the data by estimating the distribution parameters. In WSNs applications, Gaussian model is the most commonly assumed distribution. Gaussian model is used because of its computational convenience and also its small model parameter size (a Gaussian distribution can be completely specified by its mean and variance [30]).

The model parameters are usually learnt through the maximum likelihood method [31]. The model parameters are selected based on their corresponding likelihoods towards the data. The maximum likelihood estimators for a Gaussian model are:

$$\hat{\mu} = \bar{x} = \frac{1}{n} \sum_{i=1}^{n} x_i$$

$$\hat{\sigma}^2 = \frac{1}{n} \sum_{i=1}^{n} (x_i - \bar{x})^2. \tag{4}$$

Threshold for Fault Detection. Based on the learnt Gaussian distribution, a new data entry, d_i, can be tested by comparing its p-value against some pre-specified significance level α. The p-value is simply the probability of observing a data as or more extreme than d_i, as shown in (5). Commonly used significance level is 0.05 or 0.01 [25].

$$p_i = min\{P(d \leq d_i), P(d \geq d_i)\} \tag{5}$$

Evaluation

Lightweight Parametric solutions with Gaussian assumption is **lightweight** enough to be carried out at local nodes, as the learning phase only involves the calculation of mean, variance; and the operational phase requires a storage of two floating numbers, i.e. mean and variance.

Accurate Prediction Range The precision largely depends on the selection of significance level and also the validity of the Gaussian assumption. For example, the Gaussian assumption is widely made for sensor data; however, its validity remains uncertain.

Non-stationarity Resilient Depends on the model data. If modified data is used, like difference between neighbouring sensors, the model usually is robust to the stochastic evolution [25]. However, if raw sensor data is used, the model needs frequent updates to adapt itself to the changing phenomena.

Robust Learning Robust estimators of model parameters, like median and median absolute deviation (MAD), may be used to counteract the effects of faulty learning data [32].

5.3 Non-parametric Statistical Modelling

One drawback of parametric modelling is its immature assumption of the data distribution. However, in reality, this priori knowledge is not always available and it may not be even possible to conjecture a good distribution for some data sets. For example, To solve this problem, non-parametric methods model the data without pre-fixing a distribution model and the model is determined from the input data. Histograms [25], [33] and Kernel density methods [34] are the two most widely used approaches in this category [18].

Histogram Modelling. The method usually involves two steps. First, a histogram, or a frequency table, is constructed based on the input learning data. Parameters like bin size and number of bins are needed to specify the model. During the following fault detection phase, a new data entry is examined against the histogram. The corresponding frequency of the data entry can be served as an indicator of being an outlier.

Kernel Method. This method uses kernel density estimators to approximate the underlying distribution of the data. In essence, the method treat an observed data as an indicator of high probability density in its surrounding region so that data entries close to an observed data are of higher probability densities. After the distribution of the data is approximated, the following fault detection process is done by checking its corresponding probability against the kernel function. A threshold is needed to classify data with low estimated probability as faults.

Evaluation

Lightweight. Comparing with parametric methods, non-parametric methods in general involves more calculation to estimate model parameters and occupies larger memory space to store the parameters. For example, the model learning cost for kernel estimation is up to quadratic, comparing with a linear complexity for a parametric method [31].

Accurate Prediction Range. The precision largely depends on the selection of parameters both for the model construction and fault threshold. Both [31] and [25] found detection results of histogram modelling largely rely on a good guess of model parameters like bin size and bin numbers. For kernel method, the threshold for outlier detection is also crucial [31].

Non-stationarity Resilient. Depends on the model data. If modified data like spatial or temporal data differences are used, the model usually is robust to the stochastic evolution [25]. Otherwise, the model needs to be updated frequently.

Robust Learning. Faults in learning data may produce noisy model which later will lead to poor fault detection accuracy. Fault pre-filter may be useful to clean learning data but may rendering in incomplete learning data.

6   Conclusion

In this paper, we firstly investigated sensor data features and their association with fault detection. Sensor data faults were examined with regard to their causes and different types. After the discussion of the desired attributes of a good data modelling method for sensor data fault detection, various existing modelling methods were presented and qualitatively examined against the four attributes. In future work, we plan to carry out a quantitative comparison study of the different modelling methods regarding both their model sizes and fault detection accuracies.

We find all the three categories of modelling methods provide a distance metric to classify data outliers from normal data in the absence of ground truth. However, during both the model construction and fault detection phases, the methods require certain level of user involvement, which largely determines the detection performance. For example, model parameter selection for non-parametric methods and fault threshold selection for all the methods. Selecting appropriate or even adaptive model parameters for different applications to different situations and in different contexts becomes imperative to further improve the detection accuracy. Other research challenges include the detector's ability to draw a fine line between data faults and event outliers; timely but on-demand update of stale model to commensurate the non-stationary sensor data.

Acknowledgements. Lei Fang is supported by a studentship from Scottish Informatics and Computer Science Alliance (SICSA).

References

1. Tolle, G., Polastre, J., Szewczyk, R., Culler, D., Turner, N., Tu, K., Burgess, S., Dawson, T., Buonadonna, P., Gay, D., et al.: A macroscope in the redwoods. In: Proceedings of the 3rd International Conference on Embedded Networked Sensor Systems, pp. 51–63 (2005)
2. Noury, N., Hervé, T., Rialle, V., Virone, G., Mercier, E., Morey, G., Moro, A., Porcheron, T.: Monitoring behavior in home using a smart fall sensor and position sensors. In: 1st Annual International, Conference on Microtechnologies in Medicine and Biology, pp. 607–610 (2000)
3. Herring, C., Kaplan, S.: Component-based software systems for smart environments. IEEE Personal Communications 7(5), 60–61 (2000)
4. Szewczyk, R., Mainwaring, A., Polastre, J., Anderson, J., Culler, D.: An analysis of a large scale habitat monitoring application. In: Proceedings of the 2nd International Conference on Embedded Networked Sensor Systems, pp. 214–226 (2004)
5. Ingelrest, F., Barrenetxea, G., Schaefer, G., Vetterli, M., Couach, O., Parlange, M.: SensorScope: Application-specific sensor network for environmental monitoring. ACM Transactions on Sensor Networks (TOSN) 6(2), 17 (2010)
6. Xu, N., Rangwala, S., Chintalapudi, K., Ganesan, D., Broad, A., Govindan, R., Estrin, D.: A wireless sensor network for structural monitoring. In: Proceedings of the 2nd International Conference on Embedded Networked Sensor Systems, pp. 13–24 (2004)
7. Sharma, A.B., Golubchik, L., Govindan, R.: Sensor faults: Detection methods and prevalence in real-world datasets. ACM Transactions on Sensor Networks 6(3), 23–33 (2010)
8. Kamal, A.R.M., Bleakley, C., Dobson, S.: Packet-level attestation (pla): A framework for in-network sensor data reliability. ACM Trans. Sen. Netw. 9(2), 19:1–19:28 (2013)
9. SensorScope: EPFL SensorScope Project (2008), http://sensorscope.epfl.ch
10. INTEL: Intel Berkeley Laboratory sensor data set (2004), http://db.csail.mit.edu/labdata/labdata.html
11. Buratti, C., Conti, A., Dardari, D., Verdone, R.: An overview on wireless sensor networks technology and evolution. Sensors 9(9), 6869–6896 (2009)
12. Pires Jr., W.R., de Paula Figueiredo, T., Wong, H., Loureiro, A.A.F.: Malicious node detection in wireless sensor networks. In: Proceedings of the 18th International Parallel and Distributed Processing Symposium, p. 24 (2004)
13. da Silva, A.P.R., Martins, M.H.T., Rocha, B.P.S., Loureiro, A.A.F., Ruiz, L.B., Wong, H.C.: Decentralized intrusion detection in wireless sensor networks. In: Proceedings of the 1st ACM International Workshop on Quality of Service & Security in Wireless and Mobile Networks, Q2SWinet 2005, pp. 16–23. ACM, New York (2005)
14. Bhuse, V., Gupta, A.: Anomaly intrusion detection in wireless sensor networks. Journal of High Speed Networks 15, 33–51 (2006)
15. Ni, K., Ramanathan, N., Chehade, M.N.H., Balzano, L., Nair, S., Zahedi, S., Kohler, E., Pottie, G., Hansen, M., Srivastava, M.: Sensor network data fault types. ACM Transactions on Sensor Networks 5(3) (June 2009)

16. Ramanathan, N., Balzano, L., Burt, M., Estrin, D., Harmon, T., Harvey, C., Jay, J., Kohler, E., Rothenberg, S., Srivastava, M.: Rapid deployment with confidence: Calibration and fault detection in environmental sensor networks. Technical report, Center for Embedded Networked Sensing, UCLA and Department of Civil and Environmental Engineering, MIT (2006)

17. Mainwaring, A., Culler, D., Polastre, J., Szewczyk, R., Anderson, J.: Wireless sensor networks for habitat monitoring. In: Proceedings of the 1st ACM International Workshop on Wireless Sensor Networks and Applications, WSNA 2002, pp. 88–97. ACM, New York (2002)

18. Zhang, Y., Meratnia, N., Havinga, P.: Outlier detection techniques for wireless sensor networks: A survey. IEEE Communications Surveys Tutorials 12(2), 159–170 (2010)

19. Fang, L., Dobson, S.A., Hughes, D.: An error-free data collection method exploiting hierarchical physical models of wireless sensor networks. In: Proceedings of the 10th ACM Symposium on Performance Evaluation of Wireless ad Hoc, Sensor, and Ubiquitous Networks, PE-WASUN 2013. ACM, New York (to appear, 2013)

20. Sun, P.: Outlier detection in high dimensional, spatial and sequential data sets. PhD thesis, Citeseer (2006)

21. Box, G., Jenkins, G.: Time series analysis: forecasting and control. Prentice Hall (1994)

22. Thomson, D.J.: Jackknifing multiple-window spectra. In: 1994 IEEE International Conference on Acoustics, Speech, and Signal Processing, ICASSP 1994, vol. 6, pp. VI/73–VI/76 (1994)

23. Elnahrawy, E., Nath, B.: Context-aware sensors. In: Karl, H., Wolisz, A., Willig, A. (eds.) EWSN 2004. LNCS, vol. 2920, pp. 77–93. Springer, Heidelberg (2004)

24. Jeffery, S.R., Alonso, G., Franklin, M.J., Hong, W., Widom, J.: Declarative support for sensor data cleaning. In: Fishkin, K.P., Schiele, B., Nixon, P., Quigley, A. (eds.) PERVASIVE 2006. LNCS, vol. 3968, pp. 83–100. Springer, Heidelberg (2006)

25. Bettencourt, L.M.A., Hagberg, A.A., Larkey, L.B.: Separating the wheat from the chaff: Practical anomaly detection schemes in ecological applications of distributed sensor networks. In: Aspnes, J., Scheideler, C., Arora, A., Madden, S. (eds.) DCOSS 2007. LNCS, vol. 4549, pp. 223–239. Springer, Heidelberg (2007)

26. Fang, L., Dobson, S.A.: Unifying sensor fault detection with energy conservation. In: Proceedings of the 7th International Workshop on Self-Organizing Systems. IWSOS 2013. Springer (to appear, 2013)

27. Sharma, A., Golubchik, L., Govindan, R.: On the prevalence of sensor faults in real-world deployments. In: 4th Annual IEEE Communications Society Conference on Sensor, Mesh and Ad Hoc Communications and Networks, SECON 2007, pp. 213–222 (2007)

28. Kamal, A.R.M., Bleakley, C.J., Dobson, S.: Congestion mitigation using in-network sensor datasummarization. In: Proceedings of the 9th ACM Symposium on Performance Evaluation of Wireless Ad Hoc, Sensor, and Ubiquitous Networks, PE-WASUN 2012, pp. 93–100. ACM, New York (2012)

29. Myers, R.H.: Classical and modern regression with applications, vol. 2. Duxbury Press, Belmont (1990)

30. Ross, S.M.: Introduction to probability models. Academic Press (2006)

31. Han, J., Kamber, M., Pei, J.: Data Mining: Concepts and Techniques, 3rd edn. Morgan Kaufmann Publishers Inc., San Francisco (2011)
32. Maronna, R.A., Martin, R.D., Yohai, V.J.: Robust statistics. J. Wiley (2006)
33. Sheng, B., Li, Q., Mao, W., Jin, W.: Outlier detection in sensor networks. In: Kranakis, E., Belding, E.M., Modiano, E. (eds.) MobiHoc, pp. 219–228. ACM (2007)
34. Subramaniam, S., Palpanas, T., Papadopoulos, D., Kalogeraki, V., Gunopulos, D.: Online outlier detection in sensor data using non-parametric models. In: Proceedings of the 32nd International Conference on Very Large Data Bases, VLDB 2006. VLDB Endowment, pp. 187–198 (2006)

Non-intrusive Identification
of Electrical Appliances

Aqeel H. Kazmi, Michael J. O'Grady, and Gregory M.P. O'Hare

CLARITY: Centre for Sensor Web Technologies,
University College Dublin, Dublin 4, Ireland
Aqeel.Kazmi@ucdconnect.ie,
{Michael.J.OGrady,Gregory.OHare}@ucd.ie

Abstract. The aim of reducing greenhouse gases and increasing energy
efficiency faces a number of challenges to date. A significant portion
of overall energy expenditure in residential and commercial sectors is
considered as wastage. Finding technological methods in order to reduce wastage has been the main focus of researchers in recent years.
Non-Intrusive Load Monitoring (NILM) is perceived as a cost-effective
approach to monitor appliance level energy consumption in a building.
However, this approach still faces a number of problems that need to be
addressed. In this study, we propose an approach by which uncertainty of
appliance's identification that have similar signatures, is addressed. Unlike other approaches, our approach uses occupant's behavioural information to aid appliance disaggregation algorithms. We also demonstrate
our technique through experimentation in a household.

Keywords: Energy conservation, Energy monitoring, Energy disaggregation, Non-intrusive load monitoring.

1 Introduction

Energy demand throughout the world has been rising during the past few years,
whereas available energy resources continue to decrease. It is also known that a
significant portion of overall energy consumption is actually wastage, that is, energy that does not fulfil a definite purpose [12]. This makes energy conservation
an important objective worldwide. Buildings account for more than 40% of total
energy usage [4] [3]. Researchers have identified an opportunity for significant
energy reductions in both residential and commercial buildings, by providing
detailed real-time information about energy usage [2]. In order to avail of this
opportunity, access to accurate information about appliance-level energy consumption is required. Existing appliance level energy monitoring techniques can
be categorised into two major types: single-point sensing and distributed sensing; these are also referred to as Non-Intrusive Load Monitoring (NILM) and
Intrusive Load Monitoring (ILM) respectively [14]. However, NILM is considered as the more cost-effective and scalable technique for acquiring energy usage
information at appliance level.

M.J. O'Grady et al. (Eds.): AmI 2013 Workshops, CCIS 413, pp. 190–195, 2013.
© Springer International Publishing Switzerland 2013

An advantage of the NILM method is that it uses a single metering device to measure energy load of a building when compared to distributed sensing, which itself uses multiple sensors installed throughout a monitored environment. However, the challenge of identifying low power consuming appliances is remains outstanding [5]. This problem can be addressed by installing a metering hardware with high data frequency sampling; for example, sampling range from 1 minute to 1 second can enable identification of up to 10 major appliances. Higher frequency hardware will allow additional appliances be identified [13]. However, the technical specifications of available smart meters are not adequate to support such sampling rates. Moreover, the limitation of distinguishing between similar power consuming appliances still remains. In this study, an innovative approach for identifying appliances with similar power signatures by using additional information about occupant behavioural patterns is presented.

2   Related Work

Existing NILM techniques can be categorised into two major types: steady state analysis and transient state analysis. Steady state technique uses power-based features (e.g. real or active power measured in watts and reactive or imaginary power measured in Volt-Amps-reactive (VAr)) for identifying or disaggregating appliance level energy usage. Hart, who invented NILM, used steady state analysis of energy load for disaggregations [7]. Ruzzelli et al. [11], presented Recognition of Electrical Appliances in Real-time (REAR) that used real power and reactive power to identify appliance level energy usage from total energy load. An accuracy of 95% was reported with top power consuming appliance. However, REAR was unable to identify multi-state appliances and those with similar power signatures. Marchiori et al. [8], introduced a NILM approach for circuit level monitoring. A smart meter on each circuit breaker box in a building was installed. Higher accuracy was achieved due to low occurrence of similar signatures. However, installing multiple sensors increases installation cost.

Transient state approach uses electrical noise, which is created on an electrical circuit for a short period of time when an appliance is turned on. Unlike steady state methods, appliances with similar power signatures can be distinguished using transient state analysis. Patel et al. [10], used a single plug-in sensor to detect electrical noise to classify appliances when switched on. However, a separate smart meter was required to measure energy usage, as the plug-in sensor was only reporting appliance state. Gupta et al. [6], used continuous electrical noise produced by Switched Mode Power Supplies (SMPS) enabled appliances. However, this approach targets only SMPS enabled appliances and requires expensive hardware. Moreover it is sensitive to the wiring structure of a monitored environment. Existing NILM techniques have limitations e.g. steady state methods have issues in classifying appliances with similar signatures, whereas transient state methods are expensive. ABLE, described in the next section, is an appliance classification technique that addresses the challenge of identifying appliances with similar load signatures. The approach uses occupant's behavioural patterns as additional parameters to resolve uncertainty in appliance identification.

3 ABLE

ABLE is a interactive energy feedback (and control) system that motivates residents to engage in positive behaviour change regarding their energy usage patterns as well as in reducing energy wastage. The aim of ABLE is to reduce energy wastage and to shift energy load from high-demand periods to off-peak times. ABLE's methodology for enabling energy usage monitoring is now considered.

3.1 Design and Implementation

ABLE uses NILM's low-cost steady state technique in order to obtain appliance level energy usage information from a single whole-building energy measurement. Energy usage data for the entire building is obtained using a smart meter. Machine learning algorithms are then used to identify appliance level energy usage from the acquired energy signal. Each step is now considered:

- *Energy Load Measurement:* A clip-on smart meter installed at the base-line entering a building measures total energy load and reports it in real-time. This measurement is received on a local workstation and is then uploaded to the ABLE server for further analysis.
- *Step Change Detection:* Energy usage information is analysed to detect step changes. A simple step-change detection algorithm that identifies sudden changes in energy usage data and separates those changes or patterns is harnessed. To improve step detection accuracy, the algorithm uses multiple threshold values to detect an event.
- *Appliance Classification:* At this stage, identified step changes are classified to appropriate appliance types. NILM's steady-state method, with supervised machine learning, requires a manual training process. Each appliance in a building is switched on and off to create an appliance signature database. These signatures are then labelled to build a training dataset. ABLE provides a simple GUI to accelerate the training process. For classification, ABLE uses Support Vector Machine (SVM) algorithms which takes a newly reported energy pattern and identifies appliance type by making reference to the training data set. To improve appliance classification accuracy, as in cases where patterns are similar, additional information about occupant's behaviour patterns must be utilised.
- *Occupant Behaviour Analysis:* In order to learn about occupant behaviour patterns, ABLE uses historical energy usage information. To further investigate activity patterns, a set of sensors, for example PIR, contact (door and so on), temperature, and acoustic, are deployed throughout the building for a shorter period of time, usually for a two week to four week period. Apart from occupant's activities, appliance state information is also inferred from the measurements of these sensors. For example, temperature and acoustic sensors placed close to a water heater tank can report activation and duration of appliance operation. ABLE's appliance classification technique uses behavioural information to distinguish between two appliances with similar power usage.

4   Experimentation

To validate ABLE, an experiment was conducted in a real household for over 8 months. The home was occupied by 4 adults and 1 child. To measure whole-house energy usage, we used Current Cost EnviR platform [1], a commercially available smart metering platform. The meter measures real power usage and has a data frequency rate of 6 seconds. We also deployed Current Cost's Individual Appliance Monitors (IAMs) at each socket within the home to acquire ground truth and thus validate findings. To track occupant behaviour, we used multiple low-cost TelosB motes equipped with PIR, temperature, acoustic, and magnetic sensors. These sensors were attached to living room and kitchen doors, walls, and to particular appliances having similar power consumption for a two week period, in order to validate inferred activities from historical energy data. Behavioural information is also utilised to identify various activity patterns, which were later investigated from a historical data perspective.

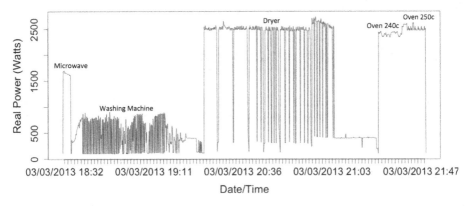

Fig. 1. A snapshot of energy usage load (above). X-axis shows date/time while y-axis represents real power (watts) consumption.

A snapshot of energy consumption is shown in Figure 1. The activity of 4 major appliances is noted between 03/03/2013 18:30 and 03/03/2013 22:00. Power usage of the microwave, washing machine, and cloth dryer are different, but the dryer (at high state) and oven (when turned to 250 degrees) have similar power usage. Due to having similar signatures, distinguishing between dryer and oven is complex. By providing additional information e.g. a step change of 2560 watts followed by washing machine activation is more likely to be the dryer (pattern verified by magnetic and PIR sensors attached with washing machine and dryer doors), classification accuracy is improved. Table 1 provides classification results of energy load shown in Figure 1. It is clearly seen that fine-tuned SVM classifier using radial kernel (with parameters e.g. gamma=2 and cost=16) could not classify oven's 250c state accurately. As this has been highlighted in the confusion matrix, 60 out of 61 (smart meter's) readings were classified as dryer

Table 1. Classification results: SVM alone vs additional information

(a) Confusion matrix: using SVM alone.

True Predicted	dryer	microwave	oven 240c	oven 250c	washing machine	Total
dryer	422	0	3	60	90	**575**
microwave	0	19	0	0	0	**19**
oven 240c	1	0	55	0	0	**56**
oven 250c	0	0	0	0	0	**0**
washing machine	9	2	1	1	239	**252**
Total	**432**	**21**	**59**	**61**	**329**	

(b) Confusion matrix: using additional information.

True Predicted	dryer	microwave	oven 240c	oven 250c	washing machine	Total
dryer	415	0	0	6	43	**464**
microwave	0	19	0	0	0	**19**
oven 240c	1	0	58	0	0	**59**
oven 250c	0	0	0	55	0	**55**
washing machine	16	2	1	0	286	**305**
Total	**432**	**21**	**59**	**61**	**329**	

(due to similar power signatures), whereas identification with the help of behavioural information 55 out of 61 instances were correctly classified as oven at 250 degrees.

5   Future Work

On-going research seeks to improve the classification rate, fusing historic energy data with real-world constraints will be considered. The investigation of unique use cases (patterns) from historical data and contextual sensors will be undertaken. It is intended to incorporate ABLE into an Ambient Intelligence configuration, possibly using an agile agent approach [9], and to proceed with a usability study to validate the approach in a number of dimensions.

Acknowledgments. This work is part funded by IRCSET Embark Postgraduate Research Scholarship in conjunction with Intel. In addition this work is supported by Science Foundation Ireland under grant 07/CE/11147.

References

1. Current Cost EnviR, http://www.currentcost.com/product-envir.html (last accessed October 10, 2013)
2. Darby, S.: The effectiveness of feedback on energy consumption. A Review for DEFRA of the Literature on Metering, Billing and direct Displays 486 (2006)

3. U.S. Energy Information Administration, `http://www.eia.gov` (last accessed October 10, 2013)
4. European Commission Statistical book on Environment and Energy, `http://ec.europa.eu` (last accessed September 14, 2011)
5. Froehlich, J., Larson, E., Gupta, S., Cohn, G., Reynolds, M., Patel, S.: Disaggregated end-use energy sensing for the smart grid. IEEE Pervasive Computing 10(1), 28–39 (2011)
6. Gupta, S., Reynolds, M.S., Patel, S.N.: Electrisense: single-point sensing using emi for electrical event detection and classification in the home. In: Proceedings of the 12th ACM International Conference on Ubiquitous Computing, pp. 139–148. ACM, New York (2010)
7. Hart, G.W.: Nonintrusive appliance load monitoring. Proceedings of the IEEE 80(12) (1992)
8. Marchiori, A., Hakkarinen, D., Han, Q., Earle, L.: Circuit-level load monitoring for household energy management. IEEE Pervasive Computing 10(1), 40–48 (2011)
9. O'Hare, G.M.P., O'Grady, M.J., Keegan, S., O'Kane, D., Tynan, R., Marsh, D.: Intelligent agile agents: Active enablers for ambient intelligence. In: ACM's Special Interest Group on Computer-Human Interaction (SIGCHI), Ambient Intelligence for Scientific Discovery (AISD) Workshop, Vienna (2004)
10. Patel, S.N., Robertson, T., Kientz, J.A., Reynolds, M.S., Abowd, G.D.: At the flick of a switch: Detecting and classifying unique electrical events on the residential power line. In: Krumm, J., Abowd, G.D., Seneviratne, A., Strang, T. (eds.) UbiComp 2007. LNCS, vol. 4717, pp. 271–288. Springer, Heidelberg (2007)
11. Ruzzelli, A., Nicolas, C., Schoofs, A., O'Hare, G.: Real-time recognition and profiling of appliances through a single electricity sensor. In: 7th Annual IEEE Communications Society Conference on Sensor Mesh and Ad Hoc Communications and Networks, pp. 1–9 (2010)
12. Williams, E., Matthews, H.: Scoping the potential of monitoring and control technologies to reduce energy use in homes. In: Proceedings of the IEEE International Symposium on Electronics the Environment, pp. 239–244 (2007)
13. Zeifman, M., Roth, K.: Nonintrusive appliance load monitoring: Review and outlook. IEEE Transactions on Consumer Electronics 57(1), 76–84 (2011)
14. Zoha, A., Gluhak, A., Imran, M.A., Rajasegarar, S.: Non-intrusive load monitoring approaches for disaggregated energy sensing: A survey. Sensors 12(12), 16838–16866 (2012), `http://www.mdpi.com/1424-8220/12/12/16838`

Personalized Remotely Monitored Healthcare in Low-Income Countries through Ambient Intelligence

Soenke Ziesche[1] and Sahar Motallebi[2]

[1] Singularity University
sziesche@gmx.net
[2] Tehran University of Medical Schools
Sahar_motallebi@yahoo.com

Abstract. Ambient intelligence is increasingly used for monitoring of health data, which contributes to personalized and preventive healthcare. While efforts regarding well-being in technology-enhanced spaces are currently very much limited to high-income countries, this article explores the cost effectiveness, emerging necessities and existing opportunities to invest to the transfer of this technology to low and middle-income countries as soon as possible. While this transfer is appropriate for the prevention as well as treatment of many diseases, this article focuses on the particularly relevant example of diabetes, which has also become one of the major health challenges in low and middle-income countries.

Keywords: personalized healthcare, preventive healthcare, low-income countries, diabetes.

1 Brief Overview of Healthcare and Ambient Intelligence

For quite a while already the opportunities for providing healthcare through surrounding intelligence have been studied [1], but the transfer of this technology from high-income to low-income countries has hardly been considered. Of particular interest are possibilities to track all kinds of data about a person's daily life, e.g. movements, food intake, moods, sleeping patterns. Devices in the house and/or on the body nowadays often do this without active interaction with the concerned person. Another important aspect is the proliferation of smart phones and cloud computing. Thereby, large amounts of tracked data can be stored and compared over time, showing the trends. It also provides opportunities to analyse the trends of a pool of data of certain populations and not only the targeted individuals. This in turns creates the baseline data for defining the attributes and characters of a targeted population, enables the experts to generate scientific observation and triggers alarms for unpleasant outcomes and possibly suggests solutions for improved quality of life. With scientific progress made towards the invention of simpler and more sensitive surrounding intelligence more types of data can be tracked and also more health-related data is detectable such as vital signs (heart rate, body temperature and blood pressure), as well as disease-specific indicators (blood glucose) [2][3]. This is a

M.J. O'Grady et al. (Eds.): AmI 2013 Workshops, CCIS 413, pp. 196–204, 2013.
© Springer International Publishing Switzerland 2013

significant change compared to some years back, where hardly any medical sensing technology, apart from a fever thermometer, was available outside the health facilities.

The focus of this article will be why and how this methodology can be transferred efficiently as well as very fruitfully to low-income countries without delay. All too often the time span before new developments in healthcare reach low-income countries is very long. Here it is argued that for personalized remotely monitored healthcare the situation is different since 1) smart phones as well as the knowledge how to operate them are already widely spread, 2) the necessary ambient intelligence devices can be transferred economically (in general and for diabetes in particular) and 3) health experts on the ground are not required, but will be substituted by computers or health experts at another location.

2   Personalized Health through Continuous Monitoring

The above-mentioned achievements provide two innovative advantages:

2.1   Personal Preventive Data

Clinically, a one-time irregularity is not necessarily a sign for a disease, but for clinicians the trends of health data (certain repetition of irregularities) are important to be observed and traced. The detected frequent irregularity of health data then enables the health experts to take/suggest necessary preventive and curative measures, of which the majority more or less has a component of behaviour change for a healthier life style such as hygiene promotion, healthy diet and adequate exercise. Undoubtedly without tracking the data quite often an illness remains undetected until it breaks out or progresses to severe stages with irreversible damages. Therefore, such preventive data can address and potentially eliminate conditions while they are still pre-clinical and controllable. Moreover, the longer the period of recording the personal health data is, the better it enables the experts to compare and detect the irregularities. This will also expedite the clinical diagnosis at earlier stage, resulting in decreased necessity for more invasive and costly healthcare intervention.

2.2   Remote Monitoring

All these data can be uploaded to a cloud and analysed, via a smart phone link, almost in real-time either by computers or by a health expert, who, however, could be located on a different continent. The most comfortable ones are devices, which do not require any or almost none interaction for tracking the data or at the time of transmission to the cloud. The purpose of monitoring is to detect irregularities and to provide advices for prevention. The remote monitoring is suitable in pre-clinical as well as in clinical contexts, where the goal is to monitor the healing process and to prevent complications or deteriorations.

3   Global Approach

Almost always, new technologies are initially limited to early adopters in developed (high-income) countries and reach the rest of the world only after notable delays. The technology of tracking of personal data in daily life activities has not been an exception to this pattern. However, the concept of personalized and preventive healthcare through ambient intelligence technology seems to be even more beneficial for low-income countries since access to adequate quality healthcare for the population is usually way below the standard and implementing preventive health intervention is often impaired and beyond the capacity of local authorities. As a result the health risks and hazards are often much higher and more diverse in low-income countries. Through economic lens the DALY[1] of low-income countries is higher as well.

With effective global initiatives for controlling communicable diseases epidemics the attributed mortalities and morbidities have decreased significantly through the past century. This concluded in higher life expectancy in most of the countries (unless affected by man-made disasters and conflicts). However the impatient desire of low-income countries to make rapid progress in their own development process has resulted in increased industrialization and urbanization often with insufficient infrastructure and preparation, which itself in turn imposes more health hazards on the population. All above said contributes to chances of enjoying longer lives, but with higher prevalence of non-communicable diseases compared to the past when communicable diseases were more common [4].

Yet, the same wave of industrialization and urbanization of today's life all over the globe also offers chances for instant adaptation of ambient intelligence technology in low-income countries. An indicator is that, unlike previous new technical inventions, smart phones have already spread to many of these places, surprisingly shortly after they were introduced to the market in high-income countries. Besides, competitive markets are of benefit for lower incomes as sensor technology is getting constantly cheaper and simpler. In addition, due to user-friendly interfaces and an omnipresent knowledge how to operate smart phone apps (at least among the young and middle-aged generation) not much training is required. This means that also in remote areas, wherever people have phone network, together with a smart phone and access to surrounding intelligence, tracking of personal data is possible including the upload to a cloud for storage and analysis. Therefore, as far as health-related data are concerned the same benefits apply: 1) the data can be analysed by a computer or a health expert far away from the person, who can track the data without ever meeting the targeted individual. 2) Then the data can be used for triggering preventive actions, not only to alert the subject and to advise on a remedy, but also, if necessary, to notify a nearby suitable health facility.

In order to apply such a global approach, the following steps are necessary: 1) Developing funding mechanisms and incentives to bring ambient intelligence to

---

[1] DALY, the disability-adjusted life year, is a measure of overall disease burden, expressed as the number of years lost due to ill health, disability or early death.

low-income countries (obviously some pilot places first), 2) Social mobilization and sensitization of communities on advantages of using the technology along with necessary behaviour change for a healthy lifestyle, if data indicate so, 3) Building institutional capacities to analyse data remotely and provide personalized health advice in plain and local language or voice messages for low literate population via smart phone, if data indicate so.

A critical part of preventive healthcare is a situation when data indicate the advent of an illness, which could be prevented by behavioural change. In Western countries this is usually based on appeals to the individual's rational choice, e.g. by text messages that explain what positive impacts specific behavioural change would have. Classical examples include a healthier diet, more exercise etc. However, there are on-going researches [5] in low and middle-income countries, to explore whether other methods would be more promising to achieve the desired behavioural change. Such methods are less focused on the individual, but more on the role of the community and social acceptance.

Another positive epiphenomenon of extending personalized remotely monitored healthcare to low-income countries is the significant enlargement of the data pool since according to statistics rules analyses are getting better the larger the pool is. But in addition to the amount of data, it is even more relevant that also the diversity increases: Currently this pool is primarily filled with data from populations of Western industrialized countries, with a focus on the prevalent diseases of these countries. Instead a global approach would provide a more diverse range of data, which could lead to whole new insights in comparison to the previously available data, but also in particular regarding diseases, which are endemic to these low and middle-income countries.

In addition to the technical feasibility and the usefulness it has to be looked into ways of funding the transfer of personalized remotely monitored healthcare to low-income countries, which is often the stumbling block why other new technologies remained for a long time limited to high-income countries. Several profitable models are possible:

For insurance companies, which are looking to expand to other countries, such data would be precious, since the database of the targeted population is quite essential in developing their own profit oriented policies and implementation strategies at the start of any investment. Also early detections of health danger signs of their potential clients can consequently help in reducing the economic burden of diseases, which they have to contribute into the expense. These are incentives for insurance companies to invest into such a transfer.

The market of low and middle-income countries is larger by population size and tax policies are quite often softer than in high-income countries, therefore it could be more attractive for the business world to make profit. Moreover, companies running a similar business in high-income countries can be also encouraged to invest in low-income countries as charity and to be exempted from taxes. The benefit of receiving a larger as well as more diversified data pool and their reputation are other added incentives for investors. Corporate social responsibility in the form of contributing to social good beyond the interests of the company is nowadays widely spread, but often such activities involve significant costs. However, for a company that is specialized already in personalized remotely monitored healthcare there would be only initial costs for the dissemination of the ambient intelligence system in the new country, for promotion to the communities and for the adaptation of the health advices to local languages and customs. On the other hand, the running costs, i.e. the computerized patient monitoring, are almost covered as such smart phone and cloud technology for analysis, diagnosis and provision of health advices are already in place for high-income countries.

4   Specific Example: Diabetes

Diabetes, widely reputed as disease of the rich, nowadays has become one of the major health challenges of low and especially middle-income countries. The 2012 Diabetes Atlas of the Internal Diabetes Federation (IDF) reported that 80% (291 million persons [6]) of diabetic people live in low and middle-income countries, whereas 75 million people have been reported to be from high-income countries. Of the total population of low-income countries 5.6% and of those in middle-income countries 10.1% are struggling with diabetes. In addition to the larger number of the affected population and its ratio to the total population the age distribution of affected people in low-income countries also imposes another burden on these already economically challenged societies. In contrary to high-income countries, where diabetes normally occurs above the 60 years of age, in low and middle-income countries, it strikes people at their productive ages of below 60 years. Consequently, the poorly managed diabetic cases are most likely to miss work, which leads to the loss of productivity [6].

The middle-income countries by far have the largest mortality rate associated to diabetes at about 3.5 million deaths annually. There is also greater mortality rate due to diabetes in low-income countries (1.22 per 1,000) compare to high-income ones (0.51 per 1,000). In 2011, the expenses of curative measures of diabetes put a burden of US$383.8 billion on the shoulders of high-income countries. Despite of higher prevalence, this amount stood only for US$1.1 billion in low-income countries [6]. Nevertheless, this huge disparity clearly reflects lack of adequate investment in developing countries, which directly resulted in higher associated mortality and morbidity rates.

The studies on social determinants of diabetes conclude that speeded urbanization in low and middle-income countries is a phenomenon associated with growing prevalence of obesity, caused by drastic changes of lifestyle; the minimized physical activity twined up with increased high calories diets and intakes. Therefore, it has been predicted that there would be an explosion in the prevalence of diabetes in low and middle-income countries in the next 20 years [6], while even in high income countries this worsening situation has not been combated by an increase of dedicated care providers for diabetes management [7].

It is proven that preventive interventions are undoubtedly more cost effective than curative interventions, being often non-invasive, cheaper and addressing bigger population. In this context, engaging the business communities into investing in early detection and control of diabetes by ambience intelligence technology for health indicators of diabetes could be an innovative way and win–win situation to bridge the gap and bring the simple and user friendly health monitoring devices to the daily life of consumers in developing countries, particularly as accessories of smart phones. This could also create a public–private partnership between different sectors of the society with the bonus of improved health and well-being of its population, by taking advantage of community's appetite and demand for fancy, handy and well marketed portable electronic gadgets such as smart phones.

Among chronic diseases, diabetes is on top of the list of those with treatment and control depending on behaviour change and daily adjustment of medication based on frequent para-clinical measurement and feedback from care providers [8]. One major step in good management of diabetes is glycemic control, which helps the early detection, timely adjusted curative care and prevention of severe irreversible damages [9][10]. It is proven that large portions of the daily life of diabetic patients are consumed by the management of self-measured data [11]. This motivates the drive to design intelligent devices for diabetic patients, which could not only store the blood glucose readings, but can also advise the patient about the next meal and insulin injection [12].

Scientists have worked to introduce a "Personal Health System (PHS)" with the aim to support the management of diabetes, i.e. the normalization of the blood – glucose level, by patients themselves; it has been also called Ambient Assisted Living (AAL). Several parameters should be monitored and interpreted by a personal health system. In this context monitoring means collecting, aggregating and communicating physical parameters, such as blood glucose, activity level and vital signs of the body, through an ambient system. Interpretation means that associated/connected intelligent agents use the parameters to derive important cause-effect relations about the patient's health status and then present them as active feedback to the patient through the device or an involved connected health expert [13]. The patients' information and care providers' feedbacks are presented on personal gadgets, which are connected to a portal based website [14].

Undoubtedly, internet has smoothened access to and exchange of information among individuals anytime and anywhere. It has subsequently resulted in a giant step in health education and promotion of population. Graham et al. in their survey of 512 patients presented that 60% of the cases felt that information provided by internet is as good as or even better than information they receive by health professionals [15]. On the other hand availability and affordability of mobile phones across socioeconomic, gender and age groups twined up with the unique abilities of real time processing and data communication have made them an ideal platform to create simple, effective and live diabetes management devices [16][17].

Kwon et al. and Kim et al. in their studies on the short term effect of over 3 to 12 months web-based and SMS interventions concluded that such applications improved the level of plasma glucose [7][18][19] and is an effective system for insulin dose adjustment for type two diabetes patients [20]. The associated reasons identified are continues monitoring and medical care through receiving medical advice based on the more recent and accurate data compared to those having traditional contact with their care providers [19][21]. This in turn had motivated the patients to eagerly control their glucose level. They also concluded that web-based services are as effective as face to face diabetes care and "are a viable strategy for bringing diabetes management services into patients' homes and improving their glycaemic control" [19].

In recent years, researchers have made massive progress by inventing simpler sensors for the detection of glucose of the human bodies' serum. The targeted sensors are partially passive and non-invasive sensors, to be used as regular glucose sensing devices [3]. For instance, a skin patch is available, which monitors the blood and wirelessly transmits glucose and potassium levels to a smart phone [22]. In the near future it is expected that other crucial biochemical factors and electrolytes will be incorporated into the patch. Now, at least two types of Bluetooth glucose meters are commercially available [23][24][25]. Another sensor detects glucose in saliva, tears, and urine [26]. A highly sensitive method is focusing on measurement of the interaction between the light and the glucose contained in the aqueous humour of the eye, between the lens and the cornea [27][28]. In another collective effort by researchers from the University of London, Imperial College London and University of Applied Sciences Western Switzerland, a more sophisticated personal health system was introduced as COMMODITY 12, which creates a technology-enhanced space (already available in the market) to monitor blood glucose (through a finger prick or arm patch), blood pressure [29], body weight (through a Wi-Fi enabled weight sensor at bathroom floor mat), respiratory (through a thoracic band tension sensor [30]) and cardiac rate (through a Wi-Fi enabled ECG device [31]), and activity (gait sensors along the walls or floors). Floor mats can additionally serve for the detection of diabetic foot ulcer [32]. Grandinetti et al. introduced a web-based software tool that is able to perform predictions on the glycaemia level for a specific period of time for diabetic patients using several parameters, which merges software engineering and operational research methods, creating a valid interactive support mechanism for diabetic patients and health care providers [33].

Although the above mentioned ambient intelligent system for diabetes control are costly several studies concluded that modern transmission of diabetic patients' data and clinicians feedback in the long run reduces significantly the cost and time needed for clinical visits, saving travel time and days off work [34][35].

The introduced personal health system has been designed, evaluated and validated by a multidisciplinary group consisting of patients, physicians and nurses to make it as user- friendly and accurate as possible. Yet, this system as well as others are currently only used in high-income countries, while a transfer to middle and low-income is not only technically feasible, but also much needed as described above. However some challenges are predicted and need to be addressed, such as the costs and affordability of devices in low income countries, adaptability of patients for using electronic gadgets, access to internet, architectural issues, security, privacy and confidentiality of patients' information [7].

5   Conclusion

Notable progress has been made towards architecture and functionality of technology-enhanced living environments. In the past, often new technologies prevail for a long time in high-income countries only. However, this article suggests that when it comes to personalized remotely monitored healthcare there are manageable steps left to create an ambient intelligent system in low-income countries, which is cost effective, marketable and affordable. An initial transfer of intelligent devices and global connectivity to low-income countries has already happened at this stage by availing intelligent personal devices and global connectivity. Such a transfer is highly desirable as health risks and hazards are often much higher and more diverse in low-income countries, while fewer health facilities are available; hence personalized remotely monitored healthcare would benefit the population significantly. The article explores the case of diabetes, which is also a major health challenge in low and middle-income societies, while available ambient intelligence devices can provide for early detection and control of diabetes as well as behaviour change towards this disease.

References

1. Riwa, G.: Ambient intelligence in health care. Cyber Psychology & Behaviour 6(3) (2003)
2. Swan, M.: Health 2050: The Realization of Personalized Medicine through Crowdsourcing, the Quantified Self, and the Participatory Biocitizen. J. Pers. Med. 2, 93–118 (2012)
3. Sarasohn-Kahn, J.: Making sense of sensors: How new Technology can change the patient care. California Healthcare Foundation (2013)
4. World health report (2013), http://www.who.int/whr/en/
5. Dupas, P.: Health Behavior in Developing Countries. Annual Review of Economics 3 (2011)
6. IDF Diabetes Atlas, Fifth Edition, http://www.idf.org/diabetesatlas/5e/diabetes-in-low-middle-and-high-income-countries
7. Azar, M., et al.: Web-based management of diabetes through glucose uploads: Has the time come for telemedicine? Diabetes Research and Clinical Practice 83, 9–17 (2009)
8. Graham, T.M., et al.: Web-based care management in patients with poorly controlled diabetes. Diabetes Care 28, 1624–1629 (2005)
9. Living with Diabetes, American Diabetes Association, http://www.diabetes.org
10. National Diabetes Fact Sheet, Centers for Disease Control and Prevention (2011), http://www.cdc.gov
11. Safford, M.M., Russell, L., Suh, D.-C., Roman, S., Pogach, L.: How much time does a patient with diabetes spend on self-care? Journal of the American Board of Family Medicine 18(4), 262–270 (2005)
12. Jara, A., et al.: Internet of thing-based personal device for Diabetes therapy management in Ambient Assisted Living (ALL). Personal and Ubiquitous Computing 15(4), 431–440 (2011)
13. Kafah, O., et al.: COMMODITY12: A smart e-health environment for Diabetes Management. Journal of Ambient Intelligence and Smart Environments 5, 479–502 (2013)
14. Fonda, S.J., et al.: Evolution of a web-based prototype Personal Health Application for diabetes self-management. Journal of Biomedical Informatics 43, S17–S21 (2010)
15. Diaz, J.A., Griffith, R.A., Ng, J.J., Reinert, S.E., Friedmann, P.D., Moulton, A.W.: Patients' use of the Internet for medical information. J. Gen. Intern. Med. 17, 180–185 (2002)

16. Quinn, C.C., Clough, S.S., Minor, J.M., Lender, D., Okafor, M.C., Gruber-Baldini, A.: WellDoc^{TM} Mobile diabetes management randomized control trial: Change in clinical and behavioral outcomes and patient and physician satisfaction. Diabetes Technol. Ther. 10(3), 160–168 (2008)

17. Quinn, C.C., et al.: Mobile diabetes intervention study: testing a personalized treatment/behaviorial communication intervention for blood glucose control. Contemporary Clinical Trials 30, 334–346 (2009)

18. Kwon, H.S., Cho, J.H., Kim, H.S., Song, B.R., Ko, S.H., Lee, J.M., Kim, S.R., Chang, S.A., Kim, H.S., Cha, B.Y., Lee, K.W., Son, H.Y., Lee, J.H., Lee, W.C., Yoon, K.H.: Establishment of blood glucose monitoring system using the internet. Diab. Care 27, 478–483 (2004)

19. Kim, S.I., Kim, H.S.: Effectiveness of mobile and internet interventions in patients with obese type 2 diabetes. International Journal of Medical Informatics 77, 399–404 (2008)

20. Kim, C.S., et al.: Insulin dose Titration System in Diabetes Patients Using a Short Messaging Services Automatically Produced by a Knowledge Matrix. Diabetes Technology and Theraputics 12(8) (2010)

21. Mougiakakou, S.G., et al.: SMARTDIAB: A communication and Information Technology Approach for the Intelligent Monitoring, Management and Follow up of Type1 Diabetes Patients. IEEE Transactions on Information Technology in Biomedicine 14(3) (2010)

22. Sano Intelligence Company, https://angel.co/sano-intelligence

23. Harris, L.T.: Designing mobile support for glycemic control in patient with diabetes. Journal of Biomedical Informatics 43, 537–540 (2010)

24. Entra Health Systems. MyGlucoHealth blood glucose meter, http://www.myglucometer.com/

25. BodyTel. Glucotel blood glucose meter, http://www.bodytel.com

26. Sensor detects glucose in saliva and tears for diabetes testing, http://www.purdue.edu/newsroom/releases/2012/Q3/sensor-detects-glucose-in-saliva-and-tears-for-diabetes-testing.html

27. Quantum Catch, http://www.quantumcatch.com/

28. Claussen, J.C., et al.: Nanostructuring Platinum Nanoparticles on Multilayered Graphene Petal Nanosheets for Electrochemical Biosensing. Advanced Functional Materials 22(16), 3399–3405 (2012)

29. Pressure Tel sensor, http://www.bodytel.com/en

30. Biopac Systems, http://www.biopac.com

31. BEAM® 3-channel ECG Loop/Event Recorder, http://www.iem.de/beam?_lang=1

32. Podimetrics, http://www.podimetrics.com

33. Grandinetti, L., Pisacane, O.: Web based prediction for diabetes treatment. Future Generation Computer System 27, 139–147 (2011)

34. Chase, H.P., Pearson, J.A., Wightman, C., Roberts, M.D., Oderberg, A.D., Garg, S.K.: Modem transmission of glucose values reduces the costs and need for clinic visits. Diabetes Care 26(5), 1475–1479 (2003)

35. Biermann, E., Dietrich, E., Standl, W., Telecare, E.: Telecare of diabetic patients with intensified insulin therapy. A randomized clinical trial. Studies in Health Technology and Informatics 77, 327–332 (2000)

A Visual Interface for Deal Making

Daniela Alina Plewe

University Scholars Programme, National University of Singapore, Singapore
danielaplewe@nus.edu.sg

Abstract. We assume that smart environments in combination with mobile devices will increasingly appear in contexts where interactions become transactions. Since most deal-making activities involve at least two parties and a process of negotiation, we propose a generic interface focusing on pre-negotiation, negotiation and contracting within *one* system. We present two prototypes based on the visual metaphor of a marketplace allowing for simple drag and drop actions. This combination of functionalities aims to bridge the gap between deal-making and its legal representation. Visualized interactive contracts introduced as a general convention may improve transparency of legal texts increasing the overall understanding and legal literacy of consumers and professionals alike. An intuitive visualization can differentiate between repetitive elements of standardized contracts, variables and amendments. The proposed platform is applicable to legal contractual contexts including b2b portals, ecommerce, online licensing agreements, financial instruments etc., and may help to transform social networks into transactional ones.

Keywords: Visualization, Visual Interfaces, Negotiation, Automated Conflict Resolution, Ambient Intelligence, Mobile Applications.

1   Motivation

In this paper we want to ask, how ambient intelligence practices [1][2][3][4][5] could inform transactional contexts, meaning any kind of situation, where interactions may lead to transactions. We believe that these contexts could - despite their obvious security challenges - benefit from the ideas subsumed under the tag *aesthetic intelligence* [6] [7].

In a first step we focus on what we consider a fundamental domain for any economic activity: that of negotiating and contracting. In the field of aesthetic intelligence interface design and visual forms of knowledge representation play a central role [5]. As elaborated under the concept of *strategic media* [8] we aim here at interfaces, which allow not only the representation of complex data/text but support activities within the same visual environment. In order to build a platform which generically supports all sorts of deal-making, ideally for any online community, we explore a visual approach and present two prototypes. Both are based on a visual metaphor of a market place.

Negotiation theory [9] suggests, there is a difference between the negotiators "designing the deal" and the actual legal representation of an agreement. This gap

M.J. O'Grady et al. (Eds.): AmI 2013 Workshops, CCIS 413, pp. 205–212, 2013.
© Springer International Publishing Switzerland 2013

between the intuitions of the deal-makers and legal documents is usually not bridged – often not in the domain of personal agreements interactions/transactions, but also rarely in commercial settings; even though, the legal expertise of the negotiators may be much higher than that of the laymen consumer. We aim to narrow and/or eliminate this gap through a strategic interface supporting the negotiation *and* the contract drafting phase within one visual language. Therefore the mental models of the deal maker and lawyers may converge within the same representation.

Deal design in David Lax' [9] sense involves more complex activities than mere negotiation. Deal-designers may need to consider and "bring to the table" completely new parties, take hidden and open motivations into account, design incentive structures, "increase the pie" and apply other rather complex strategies. All these heuristics may ultimately be represented via a visualized system, though we focus here in the first prototypes on a simplified pre-negotiation phase and the actual negotiation phase.

2   Advantages and Disadvantages of Visualized Negotiations and Contracts

Overcoming the gap between the negotiators "designing the deal" and the actual legal representation of an agreement seems an interesting goal for various reasons. Contracts may become much more transparent and signing parties could better understand what they are agreeing upon. This could be relevant not only for commercial and business contexts, but especially for consumers and laymen, who often sign agreements without having read those.

Visualised contracts [10] facilitate the reduction of complexity. Many consumer contracts are standardised; if a visualisation could effectively differentiate standard clauses from relevant and/or amended variables, the overall complexity could be reduced, therefore leading to an easier and more intuitive understanding. For consumers, this increase of transparency could result to in a stronger empowerment as market participants. Examples include online license agreements, financial products, such as insurances, rental and other simple contracts etc.

Another positive effect of visualizations is their potential for better deal making in general. If visualized negotiations and contracts could easily highlight standard procedures from new and unusual elements, we may focus on value creating strategies increasing the benefits for the parties involved. If negotiating and contracting would be less tedious yet representing the necessary legal details, then our overall deal making capabilities could significantly improve.

However, we can easily imagine contexts, where the lack of transparency is serving the interest of at least one party. Possible motivations may range from all sorts of deliberate omission of information and tactical manoeuvres to deliberate attempts for deceit. This could be the reason, why visual interfaces for negotiation are not a common application in the market. Nevertheless, we want to argue, that introducing a new convention for the representation of online negotiations and contracting drafts would lead to new conventions and along with these, as with any new technology, creative uses and abuses. The newly gained transparency could be counteracted by negatively motivated strategies – but yet, in an overall more efficient medium.

3   Visualization Approach: Market Place Metaphor

We introduce two prototypes for the front end; the first one applies a free style and ornamental visual language, the second one makes use of more familiar visual elements, such as window like text clusters etc. The here proposed interface may represent personalized, anticipatory and adaptive functionalities, such as automated negotiation and decision making [11].

Both display a simple negotiation scenario of two parties represented at the top ("others") and the bottom ("us") and a market place between them. Both parties have various layers below the market place which are not seen by the other side and support higher and lower level strategizing activities. Here (see second prototype), text elements may be clustered and organized linking high level preferences, mid-level goals and legal clauses. Text entities are represented either fully visually (and can be read via mouse over) or as expandable text elements. They are all completely editable thereby providing maximum flexibility. The first prototypes do not include anticipatory mechanisms, profiling practices or context awareness as we could expect them for ambient intelligent solutions. However, these could be implemented as further extensions.

Users may represent themselves via a hierarchy of personal values, preferences and even intentions [12] optionally made visible facilitating interest based negotiation, (see below). If wanted, they may break down higher level goals into lower level tasks and to-do lists via a simple tool allowing specifying hierarchical dependencies and clustering content according to contexts (comparable to brainstorming tools, such as mind maps). Similarly to the Balanced Scorecard [13] approach in the field of strategic management this form of representation enables the alignment of any activity towards higher level goals [14].

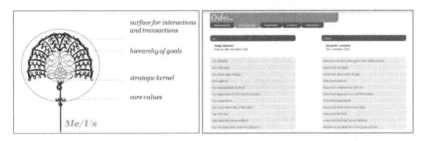

Fig. 1. Representation of the own party

In the second prototype the interface is organized vertically in order to allow for more elaborate textual inputs. The system may also represent the output of match making and intelligent algorithms for conflict resolution [11]. Market-participants with similar goals may learn about each other and explore opportunities for collaboration and synergies. Users with complimentary goods/services may also be connected via the system and can initiate their deal-making activities. The negotiation interface is scalable to the complexity of needs for individuals and organizations alike.

Any kind of negotiation between two users can be initiated through the interface.

The system facilitates the alternate dynamics of offer and counter-offer through highlighted buttons on the market place. Users may negotiate in real time or asynchronous, together within one space or remotely. Our approach is informed by the Harvard approach to negotiation as introduced by Lax and Sebenius [9] in continuation of Fisher, Ury and Patten [15] and integrates concepts from the Wharton School led by Richard Shell [16] as well. The interface facilitates the implementation of all their proposed strategies, since they result in different arrangements of the visual elements introduced here. For example, users may enter and structure information as "negotiable", "un-negotiable", "hidden and visible conditions", "target prices, "best alternatives to negotiated agreement" (BATNA) and other concepts [17].

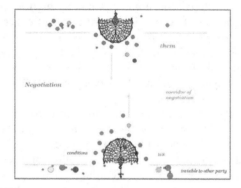

Fig. 2. Drag and drop interface for the asynchron negotiation between two parties

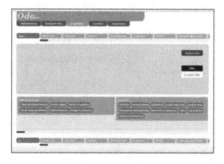

Fig. 3. Front-end implementation with preference layer, marketplace and offer and counter-offer buttons

After a negotiation phase and in case of an agreement the users may finalize the result in a visual contract. Every visual element of a contract refers to a section of a conventional contract, such as a clause. Since in various contexts contracts tend to be standardized the visualization of contracts as patterns can easily help to highlight the differing variables and amendments.

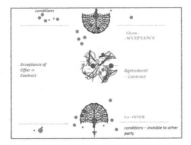

Fig. 4. If an agreement is reached it is captured as a visual contract

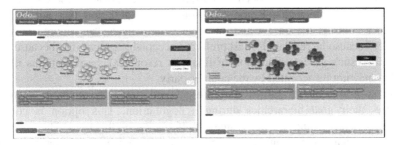

Fig. 5. Front-end implementation with visualized contract and preference layer, marketplace and offer and counter-offer buttons

Finally users may execute transactions through the platform. Here we will rely on existing transactional internet services such as PayPal. A clearing functionality is desirable as well; for example the freelancer portal Elance relies on its system Escrow which guarantees the timely clearing of transactions and reduces counterparty risk since funds have to be deposited in advance and are released according to the milestones reached.

The second prototype may operate with standard electronic payment services like a credit card or PayPal or could include a visual e payment module, to be developed.

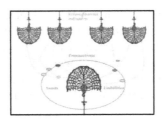

Fig. 6. Visualization of transactions between various parties

4   Research Challenges and Future Developments

Regarding the legal enforcement the system relies on current practices of cyber law, which requires basically defining all preliminaries of an international contract upfront. In relation to social networking sites and online market-places, such as Facebook, LinkedIn, Ebay, Search-a-Coder etc. social pressure and visibility reduce the risk of defaulting. For the context of financial services a clearing house is a prerequisite.

Informed by the field of interest based negotiation we may include algorithms facilitating win-win scenarios. Research [18] has shown that the display of goals may optimize the results of negotiations in certain situations. For example the bargaining and reframing protocol introduced by Pasquier [18] recommends the communication about underlying interests, if the first round of negotiation has not lead to an agreement. This is the case when an agent cannot make "any more concessions" (whether because he reached his last preferred acceptable proposal or because of other constraints, such as the exhaustion of financial resources), he repeats his last offer, which – may not be accepted by the counter-party.

The platform allows parties to represent and communicate - if wanted only partially- their goal hierarchies during a negotiation. This option is completely customizable according to the strategic preferences of the user: The spectrum of transparency may range from zero visibility to negation-specific disclosure of tasks to total visibility of a cluster of goals. By communicating higher level goals various opportunities for winwin situations may be discovered: e.g. if parties realize that they actually do not exactly compete for the same resources or that they may have complementary interests in other contexts than the currently negotiated one.

This is only one example, how a visualized negotiation platform can help to optimize the outcome of negotiations for all parties involved [19]. A platform may also serve as a research tool for the exploration of such strategies, automated via software agents or not [20][21].

5   Applications and Outlook

Due to its generic nature, this system can be customized to various media related processes of negotiation and contracting. Better online contracting practices may also facilitate the formation of new online value chains. Social networks could be easily transformed into transactional networks if wanted. If the system becomes a standard, then users may subscribe and form fast and easy agreements whenever they interact.

Using only the visual representations and the conventions around them may also help to communicate non-negotiable contracts, such as online license agreements, many financial and insurance products and e-commerce terms and conditions in the widest sense. For example, we could envision a visual market place for the design and trade of financial instruments, such as derivatives which are mostly used for risk management purposes. Derivatives such as options, futures and forwards are either standardized contracts or negotiable over the counter (OTCs) [19]. If they could be better designed, modified and customized they could also be more easily traded and therefore allow hedging and risk management strategies to be applied to arenas beyond financial service industries.

6   Implementation

The implementation of the first front end prototypes was based on client- and serverside software solutions. The client-side, an application run in a web browser, will be realized in Java Script enabling the strong focus on the GUI. PHP as a server scripting language will be used to implement the server-based database handling and content related interactions with the client-side. MySQL is used for the database implementation. The asynchronous communication between client and server relies on the web development technique AJAX (asynchronous JavaScript and XML).

Acknowledgements. The platform was developed in collaboration with Andreas Schlegel in charge of programming and the development of the front end. We are grateful for the discussions with Philippe Pasquier from Simon Frazer University, Vancouver for his input on Interest Based Negotiation and thank Horacio Falcao (Insead) and Nuno Delicado (Pluris7) for their valuable consulting on the Harvard negotiation approach. We also want to cordially thank the Harvard Law Lab at the Berkman Centre for Internet and Society for providing legal advice and the Centre for Future Banking at the MIT Media Lab.

References

1. Aarts, E., Marzano, S.: The New Everyday: Views on Ambient Intelligence. 010 Publishers, Rotterdam (2003)
2. Aarts, E., Harwig, R., Schuurmans, M.: Ambient Intelligence. In: The Invisible Future: The Seamless Integration of Technology Into Everyday Life, pp. 235–250. McGraw-Hill Companies, NY (2001)
3. Kasugai, K., Ziefle, M., Röcker, C., Russell, P.: Creating Spatio-Temporal Contiguities Between Real and Virtual Rooms in an Assistive Living Environment. In: Bonner, J., Smyth, M., O'Neill, S., Mival, O. (eds.) Proceedings of Create 2010 - Innovative Interactions, Elms Court, Loughborough, pp. 62–67 (2010)
4. Weber, W., Rabaey, J.M., Aarts, E. (eds.): Ambient Intelligence. Springer, New York (2005)
5. Röcker, C., Etter, R.: Social Radio – A Music-Based Approach to Emotional Awareness Mediation. In: Proceedings of the International Conferences on Intelligent User Interfaces (IUI 2007), pp. 286–289. ACM Press, New York (2007)
6. Kasugai, K., Röcker, C., Bongers, B., Plewe, D., Dimmer, C.: Aesthetic Intelligence: Designing Smart and Beautiful Architectural Spaces. In: Keyson, D.V., Maher, M.L., Streitz, N., Cheok, A., Augusto, J.C., Wichert, R., Englebienne, G., Aghajan, H., Kröse, B.J.A. (eds.) AmI 2011. LNCS, vol. 7040, pp. 360–361. Springer, Heidelberg (2011)

7. Röcker, C., Kasugai, K., Plewe, D.A., Kiriyama, T., Lugmayr, A.: Aesthetic Intelligence: The Role of Design in Ambient Intelligence. In: Paternò, F., de Ruyter, B., Markopoulos, P., Santoro, C., van Loenen, E., Luyten, K. (eds.) AmI 2012. LNCS, vol. 7683, pp. 445–446. Springer, Heidelberg (2012)

8. Plewe, D.: Towards Strategic Media, Ambient Intelligence. In: Wichert, R., Van Laerhoven, J. (eds.) AmI 2011. CCIS, vol. 277, pp. 19–24. Springer, Heidelberg (2012)

9. Lax, D.A., Sebenius, J.K.: 3D Negotiation: Powerful Tools to Change the Game in Your Most Important Deals. Harvard Business School Press, Cambridge (2006)

10. Haapio, H.: Contract Clarity through Visualization: Preliminary Observations and Experiments. In: Stuart, L., Ursyn, A., Wyeld, T. (eds.) 15th International Conference on Information Visualisation (IV), pp. 337–342. IEEE Press, New York (2011)

11. Kraus, S.: Automated Negotiation and Decision Making in Multiagent Environments. In: Luck, M., Mařík, V., Štěpánková, O., Trappl, R. (eds.) ACAI 2001 and EASSS 2001. LNCS (LNAI), vol. 2086, pp. 150–172. Springer, Heidelberg (2001)

12. Surie, D.: Egocentric Interaction for Ambient Intelligence, PhD. Thesis, Dept. of Computing Science, Umeå University, Sweden (2012)

13. Kaplan, R.S., Norton, D.P.: The Balanced Scorecard: Translating Strategy into Action. Harvard Business Press, Cambridge (1996)

14. Kaplan, R.S., Norton, D.P.: Strategy Maps: Converting Intangible Assets into Tangible Outcomes. Harvard Business Press, Cambridge (2005)

15. Fisher, R., Ury, W., Patton, B.: Getting to Yes: Negotiating Agreement without Giving. Penguin Books, New York (1981, 1991)

16. Shell, G.R.: Bargaining for Advantage. Penguin Books, New York (1999)

17. Nixon, P.: Mastering Business in Asia: Negotiation. Wiley and Sons Asia, Singapore (2005)

18. Pasquier, P., Hollands, R., Dignum, F., Rahwan, I., Sonenberg, L.: An Empirical Study of Interest-based Negotiation. In: Proceedings of the Ninth International Conference on Electronic Commerce (ICEC), Minneapolis. ACM International Conference Proceeding Series, vol. 258, pp. 339–348 (2008)

19. Plewe, D.A.: Transactional Art - Interaction as Transaction. In: Proceedings of the 16th ACM International Conference on Multimedia. International Conference Proceedings Series, pp. 977–980. ACM, New York (2008)

20. Luck, M., Mařík, V., Štěpánková, O., Trappl, R. (eds.): ACAI 2001 and EASSS 2001. LNCS (LNAI), vol. 2086, 437 pages. Springer, Heidelberg (2001)

21. Danfeng, Y., Shin, M., Tamassia, R., Winsborough, W.H.: Visualization of Automated Trust Negotiation. In: Proceedings of the Workshop on Visualization for Computer Security (VizSEC 2005) in Conjunction with Vis 2005 and InfoVis, pp. 65–74. IEEE Press, Minneapolis (2005)

22. Norman, D.: The Design of Everyday Things. Basic Books, New York (2002)

23. Weber, W., Rabaey, J.M., Aarts, E. (eds.): Ambient Intelligence. Springer, New York (2005)

Computer-Mediated Human-Architecture Interaction

Kai Kasugai and Carsten Röcker

Human-Computer Interaction Center, RWTH Aachen University, Germany
{kasugai,roecker}@comm.rwth-aachen.de
http://www.comm.rwth-aachen.de/

Abstract. One of the open questions in the concept of ambient intelligence regards user interfaces to these invisible computers. If at all, how do they show up – and how does ambient intelligence in general and the user interfaces in particular change architectural space. As computers become ubiquitous or ambient, they create spatial relations towards other devices and to the place that they are located in. This paper formulates chances and challenges for both architecture and HCI.

Keywords: Ambient Intelligence, Ubiquitous Computing, Smart Spaces, Aesthetics, Design, Architecture, HCI, Ambient Assisted Living.

1 Introduction

A few decades ago, computers in domestic environments were stationary objects bound to a fixed location. Monitor, keyboard and mouse where set on a desk, which was more often located in workrooms than living spaces. The location of the computer desk within the room does naturally follow basic architectural rules, however the layout of the rooms that those desks are placed in does little to react the presence of the desk.

Quite the contrary is the case with television sets. As television became a center in the family live around the middle of the twentieth century [1], the living rooms mirrored this change. Furniture was designed to perfectly house all the components of the home entertainment systems. Until today, the layout of a living room often clearly shows that the television screen is the center of activities and thus the center of this space.

But compared to the history of television, the history of (domestic) computing is a short one. While homes might actually be slowly changing to accommodate the personal computer [2], there is a rapid trend that is contradicting this movement. Not only does the design of personal computers become more important [3] and set or reflect trends of a certain life style, but the miniaturization of computers made it possible to liberate from the more or less fixed location on the desktop and to become mobile – ubiquitous computing [4] became reality.

M.J. O'Grady et al. (Eds.): AmI 2013 Workshops, CCIS 413, pp. 213–216, 2013.
© Springer International Publishing Switzerland 2013

2   HCI and Space

In first world countries, people often own and carry around multiple mobile personal computers such as notebooks, tablet PCs and smartphones. But the access to computing power is not limited to those mobile devices [5]. Computers have begun to being integrated into our everyday environment [6, 7].

With the trend of ambient intelligence arising [8], a computer is no longer disconnected from any spatial relationship. Even if the user directly interacts with the mobile device at hand, the devices themselves become a part of a spatial network. The location of the device (and at the same time the location of the user) becomes tremendously important, with an ever growing demand for precision.

2.1   Location

A few years ago, the location of a computer was mainly relevant for the system time. It was thus sufficient to set any country within the same timezone as the actual position. With the emergence of mobile phones, country boarders became more important as roaming contracts differ from country to country. Smartphones nowadays are often able to receive GPS signals and in combination with GSM localization which is possible with every mobile phone, the location of a smartphone is determinable with a precision down to around 10 meters. This enables to offer location based information on nearby points of interest as well as navigation and routing.

However, both GPS and localization via GSM becomes extremely unreliable or impossible when the devices move inside buildings. Also, the possible outdoor precision would not allow to distinct horizontally between rooms of a building, let alone the vertical distinction between floors.

The precise location is not only important for the device itself, but also necessary when integrating the device into a system of devices that relate to each other. The implicit situation and thus the way in that the user wants to interact with his environment differs depending on wether an interaction artifact is positioned on a table, held towards a screen, towards a lamp, placed on the floor, lying in bed or being carried around.

2.2   Urban Displays

Cinemas are not the sole domain for large displays anymore. As technology evolved, large screens gained presence in our every day urban landscape. While advertisement on large public displays is mainly dominant in large cities, urban screens nowadays regularly appear temporarily for public viewing of popular events.

On these occasions, the large screen for public viewing is the sole center of attention. The previous orientation of the place that was determined by adjacent buildings, landmarks or vegetation becomes obsolete. Basic planning rules regarding light, wind, circulation and emergency routes obviously have to be followed, but apart from that, the attraction of the displayed content should be strong enough to create a successful happening.

While content is not an issue at those temporary events, simply because the content is the main reason for the event itself, the situation may be completely different for permanent displays. Those might evoke different or even negative reactions from neighbors or passers-by if the location is not carefully chosen using methods of urban planning, similar to the planning and analysis necessary prior to the creation of a new building [9].

This may be one of the first examples of architecture and digital media intermingling, but we argue that in the future this connection will get stronger and more complex and that the role of computers in urban environments will exceed the displaying function.

2.3   Domestic Displays

However, when, speaking about concepts like ambient intelligence, one of the key questions is regarding the materialization of it [10–12]. Is ambient intelligence entirely invisible, or does it visually integrate into our environment? Following the developments in display technology, enabling to build larger, thinner and more affordable screens, large displays might soon reach our domestic space. When those are no longer literally screens that are somehow placed in our living rooms, but when they become wall sized, they will inevitably become an architectural element. As such, the configuration of the rooms with such a wall sized display will change, because at least one wall will obtain new, previously impossible and unthought of properties. Speaking of architectural properties, a large display is a light source, allows for communication with outside spaces and (if touch enabled) lets inhabitants control the environment [13].

New possibilities arise with the – ubiquitous or ambient – integration of displays into our environment, however there are also new challenges. Precise location of the user within the room becomes necessary to display the content on areas that are visible for the user. Furthermore, the distance of the user towards the display changes the perceptible level of detail and requires flexible user interfaces [14].

Wall sized displays need to be seamlessly integrated into the room [15, 16]. Functions and situations need to be envisioned and planned prior to the integration of the display, similar to the architectural planning of a house.

References

1. Spigel, L.: Make Room for TV: Television and the Family Ideal in Postwar America, 2nd edn. University of Chicago Press (1992)
2. Röcker, C., Feith, A.: Revisiting privacy in smart spaces: Social and architectural aspects of privacy in technology-enhanced environments. In: Proceedings of the International Symposium on Computing, Communication and Control (ISCCC 2009), Singapore, pp. 201–205 (2009)

3. Röcker, C.: Why traditional technology acceptance models won't work with future information technologies. In: Proceedings of the International Conference on Intelligent Systems (ICIS 2010), Tokyo, Japan (2010)
4. Weiser, M.: The computer for the 21st century. Scientific American Special Issue on Communications, Computers, and Networks 265(3), 94–104 (1991)
5. Röcker, C., Ziefle, M., Holzinger, A.: Social inclusion in AAL environments: Home automation and convenience services for elderly users. In: Proceedings of the International Conference on Artificial Intelligence (ICAI 2011), Las Vegas, NV, USA, vol. 1 (2011)
6. Aarts, E., Harwig, R., Schuurmans, M.: Ambient intelligence. In: Denning, P.J. (ed.) The invisible future - The Seamless Integration of Technology Into Everyday Life, pp. 235–250. McGraw-Hill, Inc., New York (2002)
7. Röcker, C.: Services and applications for smart office environments- a survey of state-of-the-art usage scenarios. In: Proceedings of the International Conference on Computer and Information Technology (ICCIT 2010), Cape Town, South Africa, pp. 385–401 (2010)
8. Ziefle, M., Röcker, C., Wilkowska, W., Kasugai, K., Klack, L., Möllering, C., Beul, S.: A multi-disciplinary approach to ambient assisted living. In: Ziefle, M., Röcker, C. (eds.) E-Health, Assistive Technologies and Applications for Assisted Living: Challenges and Solutions, pp. 76–93. IGI Global, Hershey (2011)
9. Moere, A.V., Wouters, N.: The role of context in media architecture. In: Proceedings of the 2012 International Symposium on Pervasive Displays, PerDis 2012, pp. 12:1–12:6. ACM, New York (2012)
10. Röcker, C., Kasugai, K., Plewe, D., Kiriyama, T., Lugmayr, A.: Aesthetic intelligence: The role of design in ambient intelligence. In: Paternò, F., de Ruyter, B., Markopoulos, P., Santoro, C., van Loenen, E., Luyten, K. (eds.) AmI 2012. LNCS, vol. 7683, pp. 445–446. Springer, Heidelberg (2012)
11. Röcker, C., Kasugai, K.: Interactive architecture in domestic spaces. In: Wichert, R., Van Laerhoven, K., Gelissen, J. (eds.) AmI 2011. CCIS, vol. 277, pp. 12–18. Springer, Heidelberg (2012)
12. Kasugai, K., Röcker, C., Plewe, D., Kiriyama, T., Oksman, V.: Aesthetic intelligence - concepts, technologies and applications. In: Keyson, D.V., Maher, M.L., Streitz, N., Cheok, A., Augusto, J.C., Wichert, R., Englebienne, G., Aghajan, H., Kröse, B.J.A. (eds.) AmI 2011. LNCS, vol. 7040, pp. 360–361. Springer, Heidelberg (2011)
13. Kasugai, K., Ziefle, M., Röcker, C., Russell, P.: Creating spatio-temporal contiguities between real and virtual rooms in an assistive living environment. In: Proceedings of CREATE 2010, Loughborough, UK. Electronic Workshops in Computing (eWic), pp. 62–67 (2010)
14. Heidrich, F., Ziefle, M., Röcker, C., Borchers, J.: Interacting with smart walls: a multi-dimensional analysis of input technologies for augmented environments. In: Proceedings of the 2nd Augmented Human International Conference, AH 2011, pp. 1:1–1:8. ACM, New York (2011)
15. Kasugai, K., Heidrich, F., Röcker, C., Russell, P., Ziefle, M.: Perspective views in video communication systems: an analysis of fundamental user requirements. In: Proceedings of the 2012 International Symposium on Pervasive Displays, PerDis 2012, pp. 13:1–13:6. ACM, New York (2012)
16. Heidrich, F., Kasugai, K., RÖcker, C., Russell, P., Ziefle, M.: RoomXT - advanced video communication for joint dining over a distance. In: Proceedings of the 6th International Conference on Pervasive Computing Technologies for Healthcare, PervasiveHealth, San Diego, CA, USA, pp. 211–214 (2012)

Applying Semantic Web Technologies to Context Modeling in Ambient Intelligence

Alexandru Sorici[1,2], Olivier Boissier[1], Gauthier Picard[1], and Antoine Zimmermann[1]

[1] Ecole Nationale Supérieure des Mines, FAYOL-EMSE, LSTI , F-42023 Saint-Etienne
{sorici,boissier,picard,antoine.zimmermann}@emse.fr
[2] University Politehnica of Bucharest, Department of Computer Science,
313 Splaiul Independentei, 060042 Bucharest, Romania

Abstract. Representation and reasoning about context information is a main area of research in Ambient Intelligence (AmI). Given the openness and decentralization of many AmI applications, we argue that usage of semantic web technologies for context modeling brings advantages in terms of standards, uniform representation and expressive reasoning. We present an approach for modeling of context information which builds and improves upon related lines of work (SOUPA, CML, annotated RDF). We provide a formalization of the model and an innovative realization using the latest proposals for semantic web standards like RDF and SPARQL. A commonly encountered ambient intelligence scenario showcases the approach.

Keywords: Ambient Intelligence, Context Modeling, Ontologies, Semantic Web.

1 Introduction

Ambient Intelligence is nowadays a well recognized area of research with work done in domains ranging from hardware (e.g. sensors, actuators) through middleware (e.g. information management, basic services) to innovative end applications and human computer interfaces. Ambient Intelligence applications are very often open and decentralized, involve a large number of heterogeneous devices and have to handle large amounts of information. Thus, the information management middleware and the notions of context representation and reasoning, as introduced by Dey [1], are very important. The past decade has seen many contributions in this particular field of research [3,5]. Due to the open and heterogeneous nature of ambient intelligence scenarios, recent works have recognized the need for interoperability and standards in terms of languages and approaches, thereby focusing on ontology models in support of context management. Amongst the proposed ontologies ever more [2,4] are seeing the need to offer explicit modeling of meta-properties of context information like accuracy or temporal validity. Few models however end up showing concrete ways of representation and reasoning for both context information and its meta-properties.

We therefore propose an extensive ontology model for representation of context, which extends and combines previous work [8,12] and handles the earlier presented aspects. Furthermore, we argue that the decentralized systems of ambient intelligence would benefit greatly from advances in semantic web technologies because they can

M.J. O'Grady et al. (Eds.): AmI 2013 Workshops, CCIS 413, pp. 217–229, 2013.
© Springer International Publishing Switzerland 2013

help with standardization and scalability. We therefore propose a new way of storing, querying and reasoning over context information and its meta-properties which uses the latest proposals of the semantic web community for standards like RDF and SPARQL.

In Section 2 we introduce supporting concepts and review previous work that inspired our own approach. We continue in Section 3 with a formal specification of our context representation and reasoning model and show how it maps to an ontology definition and use of semantic web technologies in Section 4. We provide an example scenario which highlights our approach in Section 5 before concluding in Section 6.

2   Background

This section reviews the research work which serves as background for our own proposal and shows how we build and extend upon it.

The field of context modeling has received a noticeable amount of contributions in the last decade [3,5] ranging from simple key-value models, through markup and graphical models [10,11] down to different ontology models [2,4,8]. As mentioned earlier, ontologies for context modeling are becoming a focus in many approaches and the authors in [9] note that the Standard Ontology for Ubiquitous and Pervasive Applications (SOUPA) [8] is one of the proposals that is often reused in other projects. Indeed, SOUPA is built in a modular way and reuses in its core many well established ontologies for modeling entities like persons (FOAF[1]), places (spatial ontologies in OpenCyc[2]), security or privacy policies (Rei policy ontology[3]) or even an agent's beliefs desires or intents (BDI). Though SOUPA was originally used in applications centered on user activity modeling, it is general enough such that it can be used as an upper-ontology for describing the entities involved in a wider variety of context management applications. Still, SOUPA does not provide a way to further characterize the type of properties defined between its core classes, nor does it offer direct support for annotations of these properties.

One approach which offers some answers to the above mentioned drawbacks is the Context Modeling Language (CML) model proposed by Henricksen [11]. CML builds upon the Object-Role Model (ORM) conceptual language for data modeling used in the Relational Database domain and extends it with constructs specific to the area of context representation. An important aspect of CML is that its basic representational unit is the *fact*, a relationship that holds between one or more entities. The model then provides a framework for classification of facts into categories denoting its type (static, sensed, profiled, derived, temporal), expression of uniqueness constraints and fact dependencies as well as annotation of facts with quality indicators (e.g. freshness, accuracy). CML also introduces a form of first-order predicate logic used to derive higher-level information called *situation* of entities based on the currently existing facts. One drawback of the model though is that it does not provide a base for the entities involved in the facts and its representation fails to easily capture potential subclassing hierarchies of entities or even facts themselves. Additionally, CML focused on custom relational database

---

[1] http://www.foaf-project.org
[2] http://www.cyc.com/opencyc
[3] http://rei.umbc.edu/

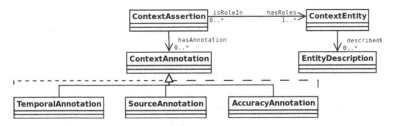

Fig. 1. The defining concepts of our proposed context model

techniques for model realization and it needed to provide its own implementation for the situation definition language. This could lead to difficuly in standardization of representation and scaleability. In contrast, our approach argues that semantic web technologies can mitigate these drawbacks. We propose a combination between an adapted version of SOUPA as the upper-ontology for modeling of application entities and an ontology model and RDF triple based realization that incorporates the strengths of CML. We also introduce an expressive derivation language that can be translated into equivalent SPARQL queries. We detail this proposal in Section 4.

Lastly, we noted earlier that an increasing number of works recognize the importance of modeling meta-properties like different measures of quality or provenance of context information. Yet, few of them focus on a systematic way of representing and reasoning about these annotations. On the other hand, work in the field of annotated RDF statements [6,7] provides formalization in terms of algebraic structures for the annotation language and the corresponding deductive system. Zimmermann et al. [6], for instance, define the semantics of a set of generic operators which are used to combine the annotations of statements during RDFS inferencing. They provide instantiations of these operators and the accompanying algebraic structures for the time, fuzzyness and provenance annotation domains. These works however do not concentrate on a concrete realization of their abstract annotation structures. As we detail further in Sections 3.3 and 4.3 our approach to context modeling adopts the more rigorous definition of annotation dommains proposed by work in annotated RDF while also explaining the mean for concrete implementation of the discussed meta-properties.

In summary, the context representation and reasoning model we detail in the following sections tries to combine the best of the 3 approaches presented above.

3   Context Representation

In this section we present a formalization of our context representation and reasoning models and then show (in section 4) their implementation using semantic web technologies.

3.1   Context Model Concepts

Let us first introduce the key concepts participating in the definition of the context model (cf. Figure 1). A *ContextAssertion* represents an informational fact, a basic truth unit used to describe the context situation of entities (e.g. a "person", a "place", an "object") "which are considered relevant for the interaction between a user and an application" (in the sense of Dey's definition of context [1]). Each assertion is therefore a relation involving one or more *ContextEntities*. As a short example consider the following relation of the form: *nearDevice(bob, lcdScreen)*. The *ContextAssertion* "nearDevice" involves two *ContextEntities*: *Person*("bob") and *Device* ("lcdScreen").

ContextAssertion (resp. *ContextEntity*) may be characterized by additional meta-properties through *ContextAnnotation* (resp. *EntityDescription*). Annotations of assertions can be their source (author of the statement), the timestamp of their generation, their validity (time intervals for which the assertion is considered to be true) or their accuracy. Since our model doesn't limit their number, other annotations can be imagined such as ownership (one or more entities which "hold control" of an assertion), access control (who is allowed to query or access the value of the assertion) or other.

EntityDescriptions are binary relations amongst *ContextEntities* and/or literals which don't need to be further annotated (as opposed to *ContextAssertions*). For instance, a context engineer can model *hasContactProfile(bob, bob_cp)* as a *ContextAssertion* where "bob_cp" is an instance of *ContactProfile* (a subtype of *ContextEntity*). Relations like *email(bob_cp, emailBob)* or *homepage(bob_cp, homepageBob)* are then modeled as additional descriptions of a *ContactProfile* instance (where in this case "emailBob" and "homepageBob" are literals).

3.2   ContextAssertion

Let us now give the formal definition of *ContextAssertion*. In the following, E denotes the set of *ContextEntities*, V the alphabet of variables, L the alphabet of literals and A_d the one of a *ContextAnnotation* domain d (which we discuss further in section 3.3). Further, let $\mathcal{F}$ be the set of all *ContextAssertions* and $\mathcal{A}$ be the set of all *ContextAnnotation* domains A_d.

A *ContextAssertion* F is then defined as an n-ary relation of the form $F(x_1, x_2, \ldots, x_n) : \{\lambda_1, \lambda_2, \ldots, \lambda_m\}$, where $x_i \in E \cup L \cup V, i = 1..n$ and $\lambda_j \in A_{d_j}, j = 1..m$. The function $role : \mathcal{F} \rightarrow 2^{E \cup L \cup V}$ returns the set of *ContextEntities*, literals or variables which play a *role* in an assertion, i.e. $role(F) = \{x_1, \ldots, x_n\}$.

Similarly, the function $ann : \mathcal{F} \rightarrow 2^{\mathcal{A} \cup V}$ returns all *ContextAnnotations* (instances or variables) which describe a *ContextAssertion* F, i.e. $ann(F) = \{\lambda_1, \ldots, \lambda_m\}$.

To each *ContextAssertion* we may also attach *key* and *uniqueness constraints* which are similar to the ones defined for the Relational Database domain and serve the same purpose of keeping the knowledge base consistent. It is important to note that we allow these constraints to be defined over a subset $K \subseteq role(F) \cup ann(F)$ of both context entities and annotations, meaning that annotations are important in determining the consistency of *ContextAssertions*.

3.3   ContextAnnotations

The definition of a *ContextAnnotation domain* A_d is inspired from work on annotated RDFS [6] and is defined to have the structure of an idempotent, commutative semi-ring $\langle A_d, \oplus, \otimes, \perp, \top \rangle$. Within this algebraic structure, the operators $\oplus$ and $\otimes$ can be considered similar to the meet and join operators of a bounded lattice. Following the observation in [6], we use $\oplus$ to combine information about the same statement, whereas $\otimes$ models the conjunction of two annotated statements. In what follows, we shortly present the form of the annotation domains for the common settings we discussed earlier in this section. We provide a more detailed working example of both annotated *ContextAssertions* and reasoning with those annotations in Section 5. The usually encountered annotation settings have the following domain definitions (partly adopted from [6]):

- source: A_{source} = set of URIs $\cup$ {*none, all*}, $\langle A_{source}, \vee, \wedge, none, all \rangle$
- timestamp: $A_{timestamp}$ = set of datetime strings down to ms precision, $\langle A_{timestamp}, max, min, -\infty, +\infty \rangle$
- time validity: $A_{validity}$ = the set of sets of pairwise disjoint time intervals, $\langle A_{validity}, \cup, \cap, \{\emptyset\}, \{[-\infty, +\infty]\} \rangle$
- accuracy: $A_{accuracy} = [0, 1]$, $\langle A_{accuracy}, max, min, 0, 1 \rangle$

3.4 ContextAssertion Derivation Rules

We now focus on the proposed reasoning model. It aims at combining several *Entity-Descriptions*, *ContextAssertions* and their annotations in order to obtain higher-level *ContextAssertions*. The reasoning is based on a deduction mechanism involving *Context Derivation Rules*. Each rule is made up of a head (the deduced *ContextAssertion*) and a body which expresses the conditions required for the rule head to be deduced.

The head of a derivation rule ρ is a *ContextAssertion* $F_{head}(x_1, \ldots, x_k) : \{\lambda_1, \ldots, \lambda_l\}$ where $x_i \in E \cup V \cup L$ and $\lambda_j \in A_{d_j} \cup V$. Notice that $role(F_{head})$ and $ann(F_{head})$ can include variables which will be bound during the reasoning process.

The body consists of so called *ConditionExpressions* (detailed further down in this section) and constrained forms of universal and existential quantification. The general form of a *Context Derivation Rule* is thus the following:

$$\rho : F_{head}(x_1, x_2, \ldots, x_k) : \{\lambda_1 \lambda_2, \ldots, \lambda_l\} \leftarrow body \qquad \text{where body may be:}$$

$$ConditionExpr$$

$$or \qquad \exists y_1, \ldots y_r \bullet F_c(z_1, \ldots, z_m) : \{\lambda_1, \ldots \lambda_p\} \bullet ConditionExpr \quad (EQC)$$

$$or \qquad \forall y_1, \ldots y_r \bullet F_c(z_1, \ldots, z_m) : \{\lambda_1, \ldots \lambda_p\} \bullet ConditionExpr \quad (UQC)$$

where $y_i \in V$, $Y_\rho = \{y_1, \ldots y_r\} \subseteq role(F_c) \cup ann(F_c)$ and $role(F_{head}) \cap role(F_c) \neq \emptyset$.

In the above rule, EQC (resp. UCQ) refers to existential (resp. universal) quantification constraint, meaning that the possible values of the variables y_i are those for which the constraining *ContextAssertion* F_c is true. In the existential case, at least one value assignment for each y_i has to also respect the conditions set in *ConditionExpr*. In the universal case, all possible value assignments have to do so. Additionally, Y_ρ and all the variables that appear in the rule head ($role(F_{head})$, $ann(F_{head})$) must also appear in *ConditionExpr*, which we discuss next.

A *ConditionExpression* contains a domain expression (*DomExpr*) and an annotation expression (*AnnExpr*) as follows:

$$ConditionExpr ::= DomExpr \wedge AnnExpr$$
$$DomExpr ::= ComExpr \mid DomExpr \wedge ComExpr$$
$$ComExpr ::= SimExpr \mid AggExpr$$
$$SimExpr ::= AssertionExpr \mid \neg AssertionExpr \mid TermExpr$$
$$AggExpr ::= aggregate(FuncExpr, FilterExpr, ResExpr)$$
$$AssertionExpr ::= F_{body}(x_1, \ldots, x_n) : \{\lambda_1, \ldots, \lambda_m\},\ x_i \in E \cup V \cup L,\ \lambda_j \in A_{d_j} \cup V$$

A *DomExpr* is a conjunction of positive or negated *ContextAssertions*, term expressions (*TermExpr*) and aggregations (*AggExpr*).

Term expressions contain terms $t \in E \cup L \cup V \cup A_{d_i}$ which are entities, literals, variables or annotations. Terms can be related by boolean operators ($>$, $<$, $\geqslant$, $\leqslant$, $=$, $\neq$), logical connectors ($\wedge$, $\vee$, $\neg$), *EntityDescription* relations and system or user-defined functions $func(t_1, \ldots, t_n)$. Functions in term expressions act like predicates which return a truth value when all their arguments are bound. If the arguments contain free variables, the function call binds them to values that make the function true.

An *AggExpr* contains three subexpressions: *FuncExpr*, *FilterExpr* and *ResExpr*. The *FuncExpr* is a list of one or more aggregation functions that take a single variable as their argument $[aggFunc_1(z_1), \ldots, aggFunc_k(z_k)]$. We employ the typical aggregation functions: $aggFunc \in \{count, sum, avg, min, max\}$. *FilterExpr* is the expression used to condition the values of the variables z_i over which we perform the aggregation. Its form is the same as that of the *SimExpr*. Therefore, all variables z_i must occur in *ContextAssertions* or *ContextAnnotations* contained in *FilterExpr*. Finally, *ResExpr* is a list of variables $[aggRes_1, \ldots, aggRes_k]$ which will store the result of the $k\ aggFunc_i(z_i)$ functions.

An *AnnExpr* is a conjunction of functions of the form $f_j(\lambda_{j1}, \ldots, \lambda_{jq})$ where each function f_j binds a free variable $\lambda_j^{head} \in ann(F_{head})$ (the annotations of the *ContextAssertion* in the rule head). All λ_{jk} and λ_j^{head} belong to the same annotation domain A_{d_j} and we additionally know that λ_{jk} belongs to the annotations of some *ContextAssertion* in *ConditionExpr*. The functions f_j are user-defined and can bind λ_j^{head} either to a constant (e.g. the default value for annotation domain A_{d_j}) or to a value computed using the $\oplus$ and $\otimes$ operators specific to each annotation domain.

4   Implementing the Model with Semantic Web Technologies

The formal model introduced in the previous section has been implemented using available semantic web technologies. In what follows we first present the ontology used to express the *ContextEntities* and the *ContextAssertions*. We then show how assertions and their annotations are inserted in an RDF quad store using the SPARQL query language[4] and the concept of Named Graphs. We then finish by detailing how and the way

---

[4] http://www.w3.org/TR/2013/REC-sparql11-query-20130321/

in which uniqueness constraints and context derivation rules are implemented using the SPARQL inferencing notation (SPIN).

4.1 Mapping ContextEntities and ContextAssertions to Ontology Models

In section 2 we discussed about SOUPA [8] as one of the most renowned and reused ontologies for representing context information [9]. Its modularity and reuse of existing vocabularies provides a good incentive to adopt it as the upper-ontology of our context modeling approach. We extend the original definition of SOUPA with a number of classes and properties which allow us to better express the particularities of our representation and reasoning models. These new concepts are part of an ontology we call ContextAssertion.

In the ContextAssertion ontology we define the generic class ContextEntity and use it as the new root for all classes existing in SOUPA. In section 3.1 we introduced the concepts of *ContextAssertion* and *EntityDescription* which are relations over *ContextEntities* and literals. In order to characterize the binary assertions and descriptions which already exist between classes of SOUPA, in the ContextAssertion ontology we define two OWL object properties (entityRelationAssertion, entityRelationDescription) and two datatype properties (entityDataAssertion, entityDataDescription) that help us "classify" SOUPA's object and datatype properties as either *ContextAssertion* with arity $n = 2$ (subproperties of *Assertion) or *EntityDescription* (subproperties of *Description).

Taking inspiration from work in [11], we further extend entityRelationAssertion and entityDataAssertion into static, sensed, profiled or derived properties, denoting the way in which those assertions are obtained within the system.

To express *ContextAssertions* with arities $n = 1$ or $n \geqslant 3$ we introduce two new classes of the ContextAssertion ontology: UnaryContextAssertion ($n = 1$) and NaryContextAssertion ($n \geqslant 3$).

For the unary case, a *ContextAssertion* like *occupied(bob)* entails the creation of the Occupied subclass of UnaryContextAssertion and the assertion of the statement :bob a :Occupied (in Turtle syntax). In the $n \geqslant 3$ case we make use of a mechanism which is similar to reification of RDF statements[5]. In the ContextAssertion ontology we define the assertionRole property relating an instance of a NaryContextAssertion to a ContextEntity or literal which plays a role in the assertion. In order to express a *ContextAssertion* like *personInMeetingAt(bob, teamMeeting, room123)*, we first create the PersonInMeetingAt subclass of NaryContextAssertion together with subproperties of assertionRole specifying its roles (personRole, meetingRole, locationRole). The assertion in our example is then expressed as the following group of statements: {:_a0 a :PersonInMeetingAt. :_a0 :personRole :bob. :_a0 :meetingRole :teamMeeting. :_a0 :locationRole :room123.}, where _a0 is an RDF blank node.

For instances of UnaryContextAssertion and NaryContextAssertion we also define an assertionType property which states if they are static, sensed, profiled or derived (like in the $n = 2$ case).

---

[5] http://www.w3.org/TR/rdf-mt/#Reif

4.2   Implementing ContextAssertions

Let us now discuss how we complete *ContextAssertions* expressed using the CONTEXT-ASSERTION and adapted SOUPA ontologies with the ability to become annotated statements. In doing so we make use of the concepts of quad stores and RDF named graphs[6,7]. RDF named graphs are a key concept of the Semantic Web. They allow a set of RDF statements (subject - predicate - object triples) called a graph to be identified by a URI. By naming the set of statements, additional meta-properties can then be asserted about the entire set.

We use this facility to our advantage with the purpose of expressing annotations of a *ContextAssertion*. We allow each individual RDF statement ($n = 1, 2$) or set of statements ($n \geqslant 3$) expressing a *ContextAssertion* to be wrapped within its own graph. Essentially, the graph URI becomes an identifier for the *ContextAssertion*. The *ContextAnnotations* are then expressed as RDF statements which have the graph URI (the identifier) as the subject.

Considering now an entire context model expressed in terms of the adapted SOUPA and CONTEXTASSERTION ontologies, our system performs the following steps for setting up and maintaining the named graph structure of the context assertions and their annotations. First, the RDF file containing the *ContextEntity* and *ContextAssertion* definitions is obtained and parsed. A SPARQL CREATE GRAPH <baseURL/#ContextEntityStore> statement is issued to create a named graph which will store all instances of ContextEntity subclasses as well as all *Entity-Descriptions* expressed with subproperties of entityRelationDescription or entityDataDescription. Next, for each type of *ContextAssertion* we use similar SPARQL statements to create a named graph with an identifier URI that follows a pattern (e.g. for an assertion called *nearDevice* we build the #nearDeviceStore relative URI). These named graphs will hold all *ContextAnnotations* made for instances of their respective type of assertions. Lastly, after building this supporting structure of named graphs, insertion of a new *ContextAssertion* requires the following actions: *(i)* issue a CREATE GRAPH request with a unique URI naming the graph that will wrap the new assertion and act as its identifier; *(ii)* use a SPARQL INSERT request to put the necessary RDF triples stating the assertion in the newly created named graph. *(iii)* issue SPARQL INSERT requests for *ContextAnnotations* in the named graph corresponding to the name of our assertion as seen above. The graph URI created at step (i) serves as the subject of the RDF triples expressing the annotations.

4.3   Implementing ContextAnnotations

We now describe our concrete representation for the annotation domains discussed throughout this article (source, timestamp, time validity and accuracy).

As described in Section 3.3, the vocabulary for the source annotation domain consists of the set of URIs identifying authors of *ContextAssertions*. In the CONTEXTASSERTION ontology we define the ContextAgent class, which describes the different type of actors

---

[6] http://en.wikipedia.org/wiki/Named_graph
[7] http://www.w3.org/TR/sparql11-query/#specifyingDataset

(agents) that we envision within the domain of discourse of an application (e.g. ContextSensingAgent, ContextUserAgent, etc). Thus, A_{source} is equal to the URIs identifying instances of the ContextAgent class.

For the timestamp annotation domain, the vocabulary $A_{timestamp}$ consists of the set of datetime strings. The RDF schema specification defines a rdfs:Datatype of xsd:datetime which suits our needs accordingly.

In the case of the time validity annotation domain, an element of the vocabulary $A_{validity}$ is a set of pairwise disjoint time intervals. We employ the "entry" sub-ontology of time in OWL[8] [13] to express a time interval using the ProperInterval class. In order to express a set of intervals we make use of the Ordered List Ontology[9] which describes a list in terms of Slot classes and next and previous properties. A time validity annotation is then an instance of the OrderedList class where each validity interval fills a slot.

Lastly, for the accuracy annotation domain the vocabulary consists of float values in the continuous interval [0, 1]. We can express them using the xsd:float datatype.

A named graph URI identifying a *ContextAssertion* is related to a particular *ContextAnnotation* instance by the assertedBy, hasTimestamp, validDuring and hasAccuracy properties defined in the CONTEXTASSERTION ontology for the source, timestamp, time validity and accuracy annotation domains respectively.

For each annotation domain, the respective $\oplus$ and $\otimes$ operators either already exist in the operational semantics of SPARQL ($\vee$, $\wedge$, *max*, *min*) or they are implemented as user-defined functions ($\cup$ and $\cap$ for the time validity domain).

4.4 Implementing ContextAssertion Uniqueness Constraints

Uniqueness constraints imposed on a *ContextAssertion* are enforced using SPIN constraints[10]. To explain, consider the example of a *personRoomLocation ContextAssertion*. A SPARQL ASK query saying that a person cannot be in two places of a room at the same time looks like the following:

```
ASK WHERE {
  GRAPH ?g1 {?P :personRoomLocation ?RoomLoc1} .
  GRAPH <:personRoomLocationStore> { ?g1 :validity ?v1 }.
  FILTER (
    EXISTS {
      GRAPH ?g2 {?P :personRoomLocation ?RoomLoc2}.
      GRAPH <:personRoomLocationStore> { ?g2 :validity ?v2 }.
      FILTER ( ?RoomLoc1 != ?RoomLoc2 && fn:overlaps(?v1, ?v2)).
    }
  )
}
```

The above query will return true when there is an overlap between the stated time validities of personRoomLocation assertions relating the same person *?P* to different locations inside the room (*?RoomLoc1, ?RoomLoc2*). The SPIN specification allows such queries to be attached to an OWL class definition using the spin:constraint property. In our system, for a given *ContextAssertion* (e.g. personRoomLocation) we attach

---

[8] http://www.isi.edu/~hobbs/damltime/time-entry.owl
[9] http://smiy.sourceforge.net/olo/spec/orderedlistontology.html#
[10] http://spinrdf.org/spin.html#spin-constraints

such a constraint to all ContextEntity classes which play a role in the assertion and are involved in the uniqueness constraint (e.g. the Person class in our example).

4.5 Implementing ContextAssertion Derivation Rules

To map the derivation rules which drive the reasoning process we again use SPIN which allows attaching different types of SPARQL queries to a subclass of rdfs:Class. Recall from Section 3.4 that the head of a derivation rule ρ is a *ContextAssertion* $F_{head}(x_1, \ldots, x_k) : \{\lambda_1, \ldots, \lambda_l\}$. We use the spin:rule[11] property to attach the corresponding body of ρ, expressed in SPARQL syntax, to a *ContextEntity* instance $x_i \in role(F_{head})$. At runtime, a SPIN compliant inference engine first searches all *ContextEntities* for attached *Derivation Rules*. It then inspects the rules to build a dictionary mapping all *ContextAssertions* to rule bodies where they appear. The engine can then execute those rule bodies every time the value of a mapped *ContextAssertion* changes. We now show how the *ConditionExpr* is expressed in terms of SPARQL requests:

- *AssertionExpr*: a *ContextAssertion* is expressed using RDF statements wrapped in named graphs as explained in Sections 4.1 and 4.2
- *AggExpr*: are expressed using SPARQL aggregates[12]
- *TermExpr*: *EntityDescriptions* are expressed as RDF statements encoding the binary description relations. Boolean operations, logical connectives and functions on terms are implemented using the equivalent SPARQL syntax and contained within SPARQL FILTER expressions.
- *AnnExpr*: the annotation assignment functions are user-defined. The value they compute is bound to the corresponding λ_j variable in the rule head ($ann(F_{head})$) using a SPARQL BIND statement.

Finally, let us consider the existentially and universally constrained quantifications. For the existential case support is already provided in SPARQL by the EXISTS filter expression (see Fig. 2). For the universal case the intuition behind the SPARQL query shown in Fig. 2 is the following: consider a substitution $\sigma = \{y_1/t_1, \ldots, y_r/t_r\}$ which binds each variable $y_i \in Y_\rho$ to a *ContextEntity* or literal. Let us then denote by $\Sigma_{F_c \downarrow Y_\rho}$ and $\Sigma_{DerivExpr \downarrow Y_\rho}$ the sets of all substitutions σ binding variables in Y_ρ for which the constraining assertion F_c and the assertions in *ConditionExpr* are true respectively. The interpretation of the universal constrained quantification rule then implies that $\Sigma_{F_c \downarrow Y_\rho} \subseteq \Sigma_{DerivExpr \downarrow Y_\rho} \Leftrightarrow \Sigma_{F_c \downarrow Y_\rho} \setminus \Sigma_{DerivExpr \downarrow Y_\rho} = \emptyset$. The SPARQL MINUS[13] filter expression used in Fig. 2 provides this exact semantics.

5   A Sample Use Case

To exemplify both our formal context model and its presented implementation with semantic web technologies we employ a fairly known ambient intelligence scenario: the ad-hoc meeting in a smart office. Alice, Bob and Charlie enter the smart office in room

---

[11] http://spinrdf.org/spin.html#spin-rules
[12] http://www.w3.org/TR/sparql11-query/#aggregates
[13] http://www.w3.org/TR/sparql11-query/#neg-minus

```
CREATE GRAPH <gURI>;                          CREATE GRAPH <gURI>;
INSERT{                                       INSERT{ assertion and its annotations }
  GRAPH <gURI> {new assertion}                WHERE {
  GRAPH <newAssertionStore> {annotations}       { SELECT (COUNT(*) AS ?count)
}                                                 WHERE {
WHERE {                                              {constraining assertion}
  { constraining assertion } .                      MINUS
  FILTER (                                           {ConditionExpr}
    EXISTS { ConditionExpr }                       }
  )                                             } . FILTER (?count = 0)
}                                             }
```

Fig. 2. SPARQL expressions for existentially (left) and universally (right) constrained quantifications

```
ContextEntity:{camera, microphone,
  roomLocation}                               :Device rdfs:subClassOf :ContextEntity
Literal:{noise level (in dB),                 :RoomLoc rdfs:subClassOf :ContextEntity
  skeleton position}                          :Kinect rdfs:subClassOf :Device
ContextAssertion: {                           :Mic rdfs:subClassOf :Device
  deviceRoomLoc(D,RL),                        :deviceRoomLoc rdfs:subPropertyOf :entityRelationAssertion
  sensesSkelInPos(Cam,S,P):{λvalid, λacc},    :SensesSkelInPos rdfs:subClassOf :NaryContextAssertion
  hasNoiseLevel(RL, NL):{λvalid, λacc},       :hasNoiseLevel rdfs:subPropertyOf :entityDataAssertion
  hostsAdhocMeeting(RL):{λvalid, λacc}        :HostsAdhocMeeting rdfs:subClassOf :UnaryContextAssertion
}
```

Fig. 3. Formalization of the ad-hoc meeting scenario

123 to have a meeting and discuss an important issue. The office walls are lined with Microsoft Kinect cameras and microphones near every desk. Sensed data from these devices is continuously processed by a computing agent which monitores the situations in the room. As the 3 friends sit down and start discussing, the Kinect camera near their desk observes 3 skeletons in the *sitting* position and the microphones in the vicinity inform of a signal level which is constantly over 60dB. Since this is going on for more than 5 minutes, the computing agent of room 123 recognizes it to be an *ad-hoc meeting situation* and relays this information to the user agents running on the smartphones of Alice, Bob and Charlie. Using customized rules these agents can decide to silence the ringtone or divert all calls to voice-mail as long as the meeting is in progression.

We focus on the *ContextAssertions* required to model this scenario and on the reasoning required to make the assertion that a desk in the smart office is host to an *ad-hoc meeting*. Figure 3 shows the formalization and representation within the SOUPA and CONTEXTASSERTION ontologies. In order to capture the described target situation

```
hostsAdhocMeeting(RL):{λsrc, λt, λvalid, λacc}:      ...
                                                     aggregate([avg(NL),avg(λaccN)],
  ∃K• deviceRoomLoc(K, RL) •                           hasNoiseLevel(RL, NL):{λtime, λaccN} ∧
  isA(K, camera) ∧                                     λtime ≥ now()-5 ∧ λtime < now(),
  makeInterval(now()-5,now(),λinterv) ∧                [AvgLevel, λAvgAccN]
  aggregate([count(S),avg(λaccS)],                   ) ∧ AvgLevel≥60 ∧ λAvgAccN ≥ 0.75 ∧
    sensesSkelInPos(K,S,sit):{λvalidS, λaccS}        assignAcc(λacc, λAvgAccS ⊗ λAvgAccN) ∧
    ∧includes(λvalidS, λinterv), [Ct,avgAccS]        assignSrc(λsrc, currentAgent) ∧
  ) ∧ Ct≥3 ∧ λavgAccS ≥0.75 ∧                        assignTimestamp(λt, now()) ∧
  ...                                                assignValid(λvalid, {[now()-5, now()]})
```

Fig. 4. Ad-hoc Meeting Context Derivation Rule

we need to model the *ContextEntities* (*Camera, Microphone, RoomLocation*) and the *ContextAssertions* that relate them (*deviceRoomLocation, hasNoiseLevel, sensesSkelIn-Position*). Notice that all 3 types of assertions ($n = 1, 2$ and $n \geqslant 3$) are present. Figures 4 and 5 present the *Context Derivation Rule* used to detect the ad-hoc meeting situation. We can observe again that all elements described throughout Sections 3 and 4 are present: *assertion expressions, aggregation expressions, term expressions* including predefined system functions (e.g. $fn : now()$ or $fn : includes()$ which determines interval inclusion), as well as examples of functions in *AnnExpr* like $fn : multiply()$ (implementing the semantics of *assignAcc* in Figure 4) which sets the value λ_{acc} for the assertion in the rule head. At the beginning of the SPARQL query we can also see the sequence of named graph creation and statement insertions discussed about in Section 4.2.

```
create graph <UUID>;                        graph <SensesSkelInPosStore> {
insert {                                        ?gCamera :validDuring ?validS;
  graph <UUID> {?RL a :HostAdhocMeeting}                 :hasAccuracy ?accS
  graph <HostAdHocMeetingStore> {           }.
  <UUID> :assertionType :Derived;           filter(fn:includes(?validS, ?interv))
         :assertedBy ?src;                   }.
         :hasTimestamp ?t;                  }.
         :validDuring ?valid;               filter(?Ct>=3 && ?AvgAccS>=0.75).
         :hasAccuracy ?acc.    }           {select (avg(?lvl) as ?AvgLvl)
} where {                                    (avg(?accN) as ?AvgAccN)
  ?K :deviceRoomLoc ?RL .                    where {
  bind (fn:makeInterval(fn:now()-5,            graph ?gNoise {?RL :hasNoiseLevel ?lvl}.
         fn:now())) as ?interv.               graph <hasNoiseLevelStore> {
  FILTER (                                       ?gNoise :hasTimestamp ?time;
  EXISTS { ?K a ctx:KinectCamera .                       :hasAccuracy ?accN
  {select (count(?S) as ?Ct)                   }.
    (avg(?accS) as ?AvgAccS)                   filter (?time>=fn:now()-5 && ?time<fn:now()).
    where {                                  }
      graph ?gCamera {                     }. filter(?AvgLvl>=60 && ?AvgAccN>=0.75).
        _n a :SensesSkelInPos;             }
           :cameraRole ?K;                ). bind (fn:multiply(?AvgAccS, ?AvgAccN) as ?acc).
           :skelRole ?S;                     bind (fn:currentAgent() as ?src).
           :posRole "sit"                    bind (fn:now() as ?t).
      }.                                     bind (?interv as ?valid)
  .......                               }
```

Fig. 5. SPARQL query mapping of Ad-hoc Meeting Context Derivation Rule

6   Conclusions and Future Work

In this article we presented a model for representation and reasoning over context information in ambient intelligence scenarios. We provided a formalization of the concepts involved in the model and have shown how they can be concretely implemented using an extended ontology (SOUPA + CONTEXTASSERTION) and the newest in semantic web technologies (usage of RDF Named Graphs and SPIN). Our proposed rule based reasoning model features a rich assertion derivation language capable of handling constrained quantification, aggregation and manipulation of context information annotations. It can therefore handle reasoning over complex situations involving things like averages over sequences of events and decisions over uncertain information. Additionally, the usage of ontologies and technologies of the semantic web offers our model advantages like interoperability, incremental knowledge build-up and decentralized control of information.

In future work we will test our model over different RDF quad stores and benchmark its performance in terms of resource consumption, reasoning throughput and delay. We plan to extend *ContextAnnotations* with domains we hinted towards (e.g. ownership, access control) and we will develop a query and subscription language which takes different policies (e.g. source of information, update frequency, access control) into account.

References

1. Dey, A.K.: Understanding and using context. Personal and ubiquitous computing 5(1), 4–7 (2001)
2. Strang, T., Linnhoff-Popien, C., Frank, K.: CoOL: A context ontology language to enable contextual interoperability. In: Stefani, J.-B., Demeure, I., Zhang, J. (eds.) DAIS 2003. LNCS, vol. 2893, pp. 236–247. Springer, Heidelberg (2003)
3. Strang, T., Linnhoff-Popien, C.: A context modeling survey. In: Workshop on Advanced Context Modelling, Reasoning and Management, UbiComp 2004-The Sixth International Conference on Ubiquitous Computing, Nottingham, England (2004)
4. Gu, T., Wang, X., Pung, H.: An ontology-based context model in intelligent environments. In: Proceedings of Communication Networks and Distributed Systems Modeling and Simulation Conference (2004)
5. Bettini, C., Brdiczka, O., Henricksen, K., Indulska, J., Nicklas, D., Ranganathan, A., Riboni, D.: A survey of context modelling and reasoning techniques. Pervasive and Mobile Computing 6, 161–180 (2010)
6. Zimmermann, A., Lopes, N., Polleres, A., Straccia, U.: A general framework for representing, reasoning and querying with annotated semantic web data. Web Semantics: Science, Services and Agents on the World Wide Web 11, 72–95 (2012)
7. Geerts, F., Karvounarakis, G., Christophides, V., Fundulaki, I.: Algebraic structures for capturing the provenance of SPARQL queries. In: Proceedings of the 16th International Conference on Database Theory, pp. 153–164 (2013)
8. Chen, H., Perich, F., Finin, T.: SOUPA: Standard ontology for ubiquitous and pervasive applications. In: Mobile and Ubiquitous Systems: Networking and Services (2004)
9. Krummenacher, R., Strang, T.: Ontology-based context modeling. In: Proceedings of Third Workshop on Context-Aware Proactive Systems (CAPS) (2007)
10. Indulska, J., Robinson, R., Rakotonirainy, A., Henricksen, K.: Experiences in using cc/pp in context-aware systems. In: Chen, M.-S., Chrysanthis, P.K., Sloman, M., Zaslavsky, A. (eds.) MDM 2003. LNCS, vol. 2574, pp. 247–261. Springer, Heidelberg (2003)
11. Henricksen, K.: A Framework for Context-Aware Pervasive Computing Applications. PhD Thesis, School of Information Technology and Electrical Engineering, University of Queensland (2003)
12. Henricksen, K., Livingstone, S., Indulska, J.: Towards a hybrid approach to context modelling, reasoning and interoperation. In: Proceedings of the First International Workshop on Advanced Context Modelling, Reasoning And Management, in Conjunction with UbiComp (2004)
13. Pan, F., Hobbs, J.R.: Time in OWL-S. In: Proceedings of AAAI 2004 Spring Symposium on Semantic Web Services (2004)

Proximates – A Social Context Engine

Håkan Jonsson and Pierre Nugues

Lund University, LTH, Box 118, SE-221 00, Lund, Sweden
{hakan,pierre.nugues}@cs.lth.se

Abstract. Several studies have shown the value of using proximity data to understand the social context of users. To simplify the use of social context in application development we have developed Proximates, a social context engine for mobile phones. It scans nearby Bluetooth peers to determine what devices are in proximity. We map Bluetooth MAC ids to user identities on existing social networks which then allows Proximates to infer the social context of the user. The main contribution of Proximates is its use of link attributes retrieved from Facebook for granular relationship classification. We also show that Proximates can bridge the gap between physical and digital social interactions, by showing that it can be used to measure how much time a user spends in physical proximity with his Facebook friends. In this paper we present the architecture and initial experimental results on deployment usability aspects of users of an example application. We also discuss using location for proximity detection versus direct sensing using Bluetooth.

Keywords: Mobile Phone Sensing, Proximity, Social Context, Social Sensing.

1 Introduction

The purpose of middleware for social context is to simplify development of applications that use social context. By social context we mean individuals and groups in proximity of a user and the relation of the user to the individual and group, for example family, co-workers, friends, sometimes referred to as pervasive social context [17]. Modeling a user's social context is not trivial. It requires knowledge about privacy, mobile sensing, power efficient data collection, data cleaning and analysis, clustering, etc. A mobile software component that addresses all this complexity is vital to save development effort and cost. The developer will then be able to focus on the task of using social context rather than extracting it.

There has been several studies investigating the relations between online social networks such as Facebook and social networks spanned by physical proximity or co-location retrieved from mobile phones. An early major research project into using proximity data for understanding a user's social context was the Reality Mining project [9]. This project studied social changes in organizations adopting proximity based applications, but also suggested consumer oriented applications, e.g. Social Serendipity [8], but did not include integration with an online social network. The SocioPatterns [1] project combined proximity sensing using directional RFID with online social networks, including Facebook. Later [16], this is used for link prediction in the proximity

M.J. O'Grady et al. (Eds.): AmI 2013 Workshops, CCIS 413, pp. 230–239, 2013.
© Springer International Publishing Switzerland 2013

network. Cranshaw et al. [7] model the social context of locations a user visits to do link prediction in the Facebook network. To this end they use location trails collected from GPS and Wifi networks on mobile phones. However, as shown by several studies [2, 6, 14] spatio-temporal granularity makes all the difference in modelling human social interactions, and location sensing rather than proximity sensing is not granular enough for our purposes. The Lausanne Data Collection Campaign has given rise to several important studies in this area, such as [5, 10, 13] but does not include Facebook data. WhozThat [3] use both sensed proximity and social network ids to bridge the gap between physical and online social network identities. However, the simplicity of the protocol raised some serious privacy issues as noted by the author, and it was not deployed in field trials with smartphone users. SocialFusion [4] address the privacy issues of WhozThat by proposing alternatives to K-anonymity for anonymization.

Middleware to address the complexities of developing pervasive social networking applications has been the topic of several studies as well. In a survey of mobile social network middlewares [12], requirements on such middleware is defined, which we use in the description of Proximate's architecture. Mokhtar et al. [15] suggest using Bluetooth for proximity detection. They discuss different potential deployment strategies of their architecture, and results are based on simulations using Reality Mining data and a social network derived from text message interactions.

In this paper we build upon the concept developed in Serendipity, to use the Bluetooth radio transmitter as a carrier of identity. In Serendipity a separate digital social network was created. In our project Proximates, we use Facebook and phone number as the digital identity of users and bridge it to the physical identities emitted by the users' devices. This allows us to analyze the relation between Facebook friendship and physical proximity, e.g. how much time a user spends with Facebook friends. We believe that Proximates can be used across many applications and used to build a corpus of social context data that can be shared across researchers. To satisfy users need of privacy as stated in the Obvious Data Usage Principle, we need to build value in proximity data. Proximates does this by supporting the bridging of physical and digital identities with low latency. We will use Proximates to study users perceptions of privacy regarding this bridging, architectures that satisfy scaling of research applications to large numbers of users, and spatio-temporal aspects of social dynamics.

In the first section(System Architecture) we present the architecture of Proximates (Figure 1) and how it bridges the gap between physical proximity space and online social networks. In section Applications and Results we present some early experimental results from a user study and example applications that was built on Proximates for the study.

2   The Proximates Social Context Engine

The purpose of Proximates is to simplify development of mobile phone applications that use social context. By social context we mean individuals and groups in proximity of a user and the relation of the user to the individual and group, for example family, co-workers, friends. By social context classification we mean the inference of the relationship class of such an individual or group. Which user identities and social networks

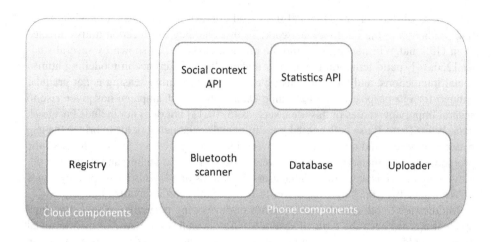

Fig. 1. Architecture of Proximates

to use is application specific, but can be shared across applications if desired. In its current deployment, Proximates use Facebook ids and phone numbers to identify users across applications.

2.1   System Architecture

Proximates consists of six components: a Bluetooth scanner, a database, two APIs, an uploader and a device registry.

Bluetooth Scanner and Social Context API Components. The Bluetooth scanner is a service that runs in the background on a mobile device. Periodically it performs a Bluetooth scan for nearby Bluetooth peers with the phone device class, and stores the result in the database. The data includes MAC ids, signal strength, and device class.

The social context API is a background service that carries out mining on the stored data in the database and triggers on events from the Bluetooth scanner. It performs smoothing of Bluetooth scans over time and group them for easy access and Bluetooth MAC ids are mapped to user ids. An API to application developers that allows applications to get notifications when a contact or group of contacts is in proximity, or when a user's social context change. The social context of a user is a ranked list of relationship labels, where the top label is the most common relation of the peers in proximity to the user, over a scan period. For example, if there are five peers in a scan where three are known to the user and two of them are classified as Family and three of them are classified as Colleagues according to the user's Facebook friend list, then the top ranked relation will be Colleagues, the second Family and the third Unknown.

To know the relation between a user and its friends, Facebook friend lists are used. When an application is notified of the proximity of a person, it can retrieve the classification of the relation to that person.

We use the labelled data to train classifiers of social context for users who don't use friend lists. The training of classifiers is ongoing work and results will be presented in future papers.

Registry Component. The purpose of the registry is to map Bluetooth MAC ids to any public ids of its owner. The public owner ids can be any application specific ids or general public ids, such as phone numbers or Facebook ids. It is up to the application that registers the device and its owner to determine which user ids to register and whether they should be hashed or not. Hashing makes it hard to make a lookup from a Bluetooth MAC id to a useful user id unless the user id is already known.

The registry is a web service and exposes a simple JSON REST API. The registry API performs all the operations on a single resource: the device. There are methods for adding, update, deleting devices, as well as retrieving a single device or a list of devices providing user ids and MAC ids as query parameters.

Applications are encouraged to cache results from device queries in order to minimize data traffic, server load, and power consumption. For known contacts, for example phonebook contacts, the Bluetooth MAC ids can be cached for a long time since they are not likely to change often. Some applications will not know the id they are looking for in advance and will need to lookup any new peers that are in proximity. These results should also be cached since transient peers often appear in at least some scans.

Database, Statistics API and Uploader. The database stores collected sensor data and events. The statistics API allows the application developer to query historical information, for example retrieve the most frequently occurring people, groups of people or social contexts of the user, over a specific time frame. The uploader pushes the stored data to a server. The uploader is an optional component that is deployed if Proximates is used for research applications, for example in computational social science, where extensive data logging is needed for analysis.

2.2 Requirements

As a middleware intended for real world deployment, Proximates needs to fulfill several requirements that are common to middleware for mobile social networking and pervasive social context. In the survey of mobile social middleware [12], the aspects below are analyzed, and we use them here as reference requirements. We also use the two social context modeling requirements [18] defined by Tran et al.

Simplification of Development Process. Modelling social context requires knowledge about privacy, mobile sensing, power efficient data collection, data cleaning and analysis, stream processing, clustering, etc.The social context API for detecting proximity of people, groups and social context is a very simple and high-level API.

Energy Efficiency. Power consumption is a major concern for opportunistic sensing applications. Recent availability of dedicated sensor processing subsystems in smartphone chipsets is improving the situation by allowing continuous sensing with low power consumption. However, application sensing of network data from Bluetooth, 3G and Wifi still needs to be done in the application CPU.

Proximates uses Bluetooth to detect proximity. By using Bluetooth, proximity is sensed directly rather than indirectly through a translation to location coordinates and distance calculation. Bluetooth consumes less battery than GPS and Wifi, and only needs to be sampled periodically. Using Bluetooth rather than GPS or Wifi avoids both translation to location coordinates in the case of Wifi, and more importantly removes the need for frequent uploading of location data for all users for which we want to detect proximity.

The power consumption of scanning can be traded off with latency. If an application needs to be notified of a nearby person with low latency, power consumption increases. The latency in Proximates is configurable through setting of the scan rate. The default rate of 2 minutes makes the power consumption very low and in general not noticeable to the end user.

Privacy. By using hashed identifiers for people, for example Facebook IDs and phone numbers, Proximate applications require their users to already know the identities of the people they want to detect proximity of. This means they already need to be friends on Facebook or to already have their phone numbers. This is a more secure approach than the one used in WhozThat which transmits Facebook IDs in clear text. It is up to the application to determine whether to used hashed IDs or not, depending on requirements. For applications that do not need the access to the registry to be open, for example in the case where the ID is entirely application specific, strict access control to the registry component can be enforced rather than providing shared access across applications.

However, the attitudes of users regarding mapping their phones' Bluetooth MAC ids to personal identities, such as Facebook identities, is unknown. As far as we know, no such studies has been done. Several studies on privacy aspects of location sharing has been done, but we cannot assume they apply directly to proximity. We believe that sharing of your social network identity connected to your Bluetooth MAC id is less sensitive than sharing location data, since within Bluetooth range it is hard to hide your identity anyhow. At least in the non-public case, where only people who know you can detect you when in proximity. This remains to be verified by user studies.

Scalability and Distributed Architecture. The architecture of Proximates is very simple compared to most mobile social networking platforms since it focuses on a specific problem, uses proximity sensing, and delegates management of social networks to the original social network services rather than aggregates. Using direct proximity sensing rather than via location makes it possible to do the sensing directly on the device. This eliminates scalability problems associated with pairwise distance computations. The registry is a centralized component, but it is not subject to heavy loads since registrations seldom change which allows for long caching in clients.

Heterogeneity and Dynamicity of Mobile Environments. Performing the proximity detection directly on the device removes the need for continuous network coverage and data connection, making Proximates insensitive to networks signal strength fluctuations. Regarding heterogenous evironment, this is ignored by selecting Android 4.0.4 or later as the target environment.

Social Context Modelling. Tran et al. defined requirements [18] for social context modeling. We show how Proximates fulfill these and elaborate on them:

> Social context needs to explicitly capture constructed relationships and inter-action constraints between actors. This set of constructed relationships and constraints needs to be managed, and modeled subjectively from an actor's perspective. The architecture of context-aware systems needs to externalize the management of social context from the implementation of actors.

Proximates explicitly models relationships through the integrated social networks, de-fined by the application. Currently integrated networks are Facebook and phone con-tacts. The user manages his Facebook relations using the Facebook service and his phone contacts through the phone book application, and are thus externalized. Inter-action constraints are not specifically captured, but are left to the application since these are application specific. The relationships are modeled subjectively since Face-book friend lists is managed by the user and only visible to him.

> The architecture also needs to support the adaptability of social context, and needs to be easily deployable.

The complexity and cost of integrating and deploying a social context engine in com-mercial applications must be low. Many companies are yet to understand the potential benefits of context aware applications. This means that a small and simple compo-nent that solves a specific problem in existing infrastructure is preferable to a complex system that solves a wide range of problems. Additional context information should be added through integration of additional simple components that integrate well. It should also utilize existing infrastructure and services, e.g. Facebook for management of a user's social graph. Furthermore, the social context model must be simple and usable across several applications. Proximates fulfill these requirements through its simplicity and integration with existing services.

Additional Requirements. In addition to the requirements used in [12] we have further requirements on Proximates.

- Low latency for proximity detection is a requirement for some applications, for ex-ample reminder applications triggered by proximity to a person. This requirement makes it impossible to use location for proximity detection.
- Robustness, i.e. not needing to rely on GPS satellite visibility, availability of nearby wifi access points and a network data connection, also makes us choose direct prox-imity sensing.
- Finally, accuracy of location based methods is at best 10 meters indoors which is not enough to detect actual social interactions. Using Bluetooth, 10 meters is the maximum distance. Also, as shown by Cattuto et al. [2, 6] spatio-temporal granu-larity makes all the difference in modeling human social interactions, and location sensing rather than proximity sensing is not granular enough for our purposes.

3   Applications and Results

3.1   SmartTodos

Proximates was used to develop SmartTodos, a contextual reminder application, that for allows a user to add a reminder that will trigger when he is in close proximity of a specific contact or Facebook friend, in addition to reminders based on time and location triggers. It was distributed to about a 100 users who installed it and who could also send invites to others. We sampled seven users out of this population to make a usability study. The users in the sample were advanced smartphone users with university degrees.

Task completion time and requests for help was measured for seven different tasks as shown in figure 2. Task 1 is the task of setting up Proximates, while the other tasks are related to SmartTodos as such, for example the creation of location alarms. It is clear from the study that setting up Proximates is a hard task. It includes the following manual steps for the users: Signing into Facebook and accepting requested permissions, entering phone number, accepting enabling of Bluetooth and location services if not enabled, and setting Bluetooth visibility timeout to infinity. The most complicated step is the last one. This step should not be needed at all, but exists due to a bug in Android. Entering of phone number is often needed since most operators do not provide the information on SIM cards. Preloading of Proximates, an option only available to phone OEMs, can remove some of these obstacles, but it is clear that it is important to reduce the complexity of these tasks in Proximates.

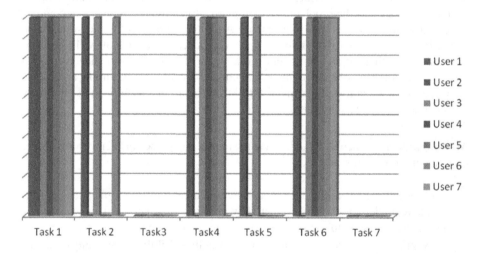

Fig. 2. Requests for help

3.2   Data Collection

In the SmartTodos trial we deployed the application with the upload component. Proximates collected proximity and Facebook data and uploaded them to a server where they were stored for analysis. Bluetooth scans were performed every minute, and only

Bluetooth with device class "phone" were stored for analysis. In the period July 2012 to March 2013, 2,466,036 Bluetooth scans containing 84,793 peers were collected by 135 devices. 161 users were registered with Facebook id in the registry, and they had 29,979 friends in total. 99 users had no user defined friend lists while the median number of friend lists was 9 among the 62 others. In addition to the traditional informed consent trough terms of service agreement, The Obvious Data Usage Principle [11] was applied in the application design to make it clear to users what information was being collected and how it was used. All data collected is anonymized through hashing.

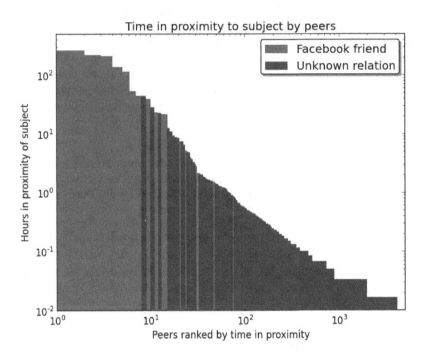

Fig. 3. Time in proximity of a single subject, and Facebook relationship

Figure 3 is a log-log plot of the time spent in proximity to one specific user versus the peers ranked by the same measure. In the plot we have colored each peer according to its relationship to the user. Red indicates a Facebook friendship relation, while blue means that the relationship is unknown, since that peer is not registered in the whoowns registry. A peer colored in blue could still be a Facebook friend of the user, but we have no information about this. This means that the time this user spent with Facebook friends was significantly larger than with friends with unknown relationships. An interpretation of this is that Facebook friendship is not only used to keep in touch with distant friends, but also a relationship users have with the people they actually spend time with. More work is needed to determine the generality of this result to other users.

4 Conclusion and Future Work

We have presented an architecture for proximity based services on smartphones, that is power efficient, easy to deploy, delegates social network management and scales well due to using direct proximity sensing rather than location and distance calculations. It also has other privacy properties than location sensing that needs further investigation.

We have shown that Proximates can be used in real world applications by means of the SmartTodos application.

Furthermore, we have shown that Proximates can be used for research applications by showing that we can measure the time users spend in proximity of Facebook friends. We also reported on how many users actually use Facebook friends lists. Further work is needed to investigate if Facebook friends list labels has the potential to be used as ground truth for classification of social context when Facebook friends labels are not available. We will also study how to improve usability by reducing the complexity of the setup of Bluetooth visibility and user ids in different social networks. We are about to launch SmartTodos on Google Play in order to scale up the amount of users and data collected.

Acknowledgements. This work was partly funded by the Industrial Excellence Center EASE – Embedded Applications Software Engineering, (http://ease.cs.lth.se) and the European 7th Framework Program, under grant VENTURI (FP7-288238).

References

1. Alani, H., Szomszor, M., Cattuto, C., Van den Broeck, W., Correndo, G., Barrat, A.: Live social semantics. In: Bernstein, A., Karger, D.R., Heath, T., Feigenbaum, L., Maynard, D., Motta, E., Thirunarayan, K. (eds.) ISWC 2009. LNCS, vol. 5823, pp. 698–714. Springer, Heidelberg (2009),
   http://link.springer.com/chapter/10.1007/978-3-642-04930-9_44
2. Barrat, A., Cattuto, C.: Temporal networks of face-to-face human interactions. Temporal Networks, pp. 50–55 (2013),
   http://link.springer.com/chapter/10.1007/978-3-642-36461-7_10
3. Beach, A., Gartrell, M., Akkala, S., Elston, J., Kelley, J., Nishimoto, K., Ray, B., Razgulin, S., Sundaresan, K., Surendar, B., Terada, M., Han, R.: WhozThat? Evolving an ecosystem for context-aware mobile social networks. Network IEEE 22(4), 50–55 (2008),
   http://dx.doi.org/10.1109/MNET.2008.4579771
4. Beach, A., Gartrell, M., Xing, X., Han, R., Lv, Q., Mishra, S., Seada, K.: Fusing mobile, sensor, and social data to fully enable context-aware computing. In: Proceedings of the Eleventh Workshop on Mobile Computing Systems Applications HotMobile 2010, p. 60 (2010), http://portal.acm.org/citation.cfm?doid=1734583.1734599
5. Blom, J., Gatica-perez, D., Kiukkonen, N.: People-Centric Mobile Sensing with a Pragmatic Twist: from Behavioral Data Points to Active User Involvement. In: Mobile Devices and Services, pp. 381–384 (2011)
6. Cattuto, C., Broeck, W.V.D., Barrat, A., Colizza, V., Pinton, J.F., Vespignani, A.: Dynamics of person-to-person interactions from distributed RFID sensor networks. PloS One 5(7), 1–9 (2010), http://dx.plos.org/10.1371/journal.pone.0011596

7. Cranshaw, J., Toch, E., Hong, J.: Bridging the gap between physical location and online social networks. In: Proceedings of the 12th ACM International Conference on Ubiquitous Computing (2010), http://dl.acm.org/citation.cfm?id=1864380

8. Eagle, N.: Can Serendipity Be Planned? MIT Sloan Management Review 46(1), 10–14 (2004), http://www.angelfire.com/ab8/iissungminshane/smr.pdf

9. Eagle, N., Sandy Pentland, A.: Reality mining: sensing complex social systems. Personal and Ubiquitous Computing 10(4), 255–268 (2005), http://www.springerlink.com/index/10.1007/s00779-005-0046-3

10. Frank, J., Mannor, S., Precup, D.: Generating storylines from sensor data. In: Mobile Data Challenge Workshop (2012)

11. Jonsson, H.: The Data Chicken and Egg Problem. In: Proceedings of the 3rd International Workshop on Research in the Large, pp. 9–12 (2012)

12. Karam, A., Mohamed, N.: Middleware for mobile social networks: A survey. In: 45th Hawaii International Conference on System Sciences Middleware, pp. 1482–1490. IEEE (2012), http://ieeexplore.ieee.org/lpdocs/epic03/wrapper.htm?arnumber+6149064, http://ieeexplore.ieee.org/xpls/abs_all.jsp?arnumber=6149064

13. Kiukkonen, N., Blom, J., Dousse, O., Gatica-perez, D., Laurila, J.: Towards rich mobile phone datasets: Lausanne data collection campaign. In: Proceeding of International Conference on Pervasive Services ICPS (2002)

14. Liu, S., Striegel, A.: Accurate Extraction of Face-to-Face Proximity Using Smartphones and Bluetooth. In: 2011 Proceedings of 20th International Conference on Computer Communications and Networks, ICCCN, pp. 1–5. IEEE (2011), http://ieeexplore.ieee.org/xpls/abs_all.jsp?arnumber=6006081

15. Mokhtar, S.B., Mcnamara, L., Capra, L.: A Middleware Service for Pervasive Social Networking. In: Proceedings of the International Workshop on Middleware for Pervasive Mobile and Embedded Computing, pp. 1–6 (2009)

16. Scholz, C., Atzmueller, M., Stumme, G.: New Insights and Methods for Predicting Face-to-Face Contacts. In: 7th Intl. AAAI Conference on Weblogs and Social Media (2013), http://www.aaai.org/ocs/index.php/ICWSM/ICWSM13/paper/viewPDFInterstitial/6097/6396

17. Schuster, D., Rosi, A., Mamei, M., Springer, T., Endler, M., Zambonelli, F.: Pervasive Social Context - Taxonomy and Survey. ACM Transactions on Intelligent Systems and Technology 9(4) (2012)

18. Tran, M.H., Han, J., Colman, A.: Social context: Supporting interaction awareness in ubiquitous environments. In: MobiQuitous, vol. 9, pp. 1–10. IEEE (2009), http://researchbank.swinburne.edu.au/vital/access/services/Download/swin:15475/SOURCE1

Context-Aware Systems and Adaptive User Authentication

Kimmo Halunen and Antti Evesti

VTT Technical Research Centre of Finland, Oulu, Finland
{kimmo.halunen,antti.evesti}@vtt.fi

Abstract. In this paper we discuss the possibilities of context-aware systems in providing more secure user authentication. We describe some approaches in using context information in adaptive security systems, especially in adaptive user authentication. In addition, we discuss some recent results in applying the context itself as an authentication factor. Recent advances in cryptographic protocol design and adaptive, context-aware systems enable the linking of the context information to the cryptographic keys and authentication. Furthermore, new protocols make adaptive user authentication easier as it is possible to combine several different factors in a single protocol. We give some examples of this and discuss the further potential of these methods.

1 Introduction

Reliable user authentication is crucial for many services that are provided over networks. In many cases, the devices that the users apply to gain access to the services provide a context that the context-aware services utilise. Furthermore, the service providers and devices have profile information on the users. The combination of these two information sources can be used in many different ways. One application area is the user authentication mentioned earlier.

Context-aware systems have become more prominent in recent years and there are many different ways that these systems can be designed and utilised [1]. From security perspective these systems offer both increased risks as well as benefits. Risks come from the fact that more and more different types of devices and sensors are networked and thus are subject to possible abuse by remote attackers. One benefit of these systems is the possibility to adapt the security of the system based on the context information.

Adaptive security systems utilise some form of security monitoring and modify the system behaviour according to the monitored security state of the system. Thus, adaptive security systems use various forms of contextual information. With the help of this information, the system provides self-protection, which defends the system against incidents and also anticipates problems [27].

Many of the adaptive security approaches use authentication as an example of a security process that can benefit from the adaptive system. However, the two domains remain separated in the sense, that although there is an adaptive process controlling the authentication, it is not utilised in or tied into the actual

M.J. O'Grady et al. (Eds.): AmI 2013 Workshops, CCIS 413, pp. 240–251, 2013.
© Springer International Publishing Switzerland 2013

authentication protocol. The adaptive process is used in setting the limits on what factors are used and how often the authentication is initiated. The authentication protocol that is used is then a separate process. In some cases this is acceptable, but it may enable the clever attacker with a way to compromise the security of the underlying authentication protocol(s) and thus undermine the security of the system as a whole.

In cryptography, authenticated key exchange (AKE) protocols are used to establish a common, secret key that is used to encrypt the communications and to authenticate the messages and their origin between two (or more) parties. Furthermore, these protocols can be usually utilised to authenticate the users or devices, even if the secret key material is not needed in the communications.

There are different ways for users and devices to authenticate themselves. These are usually called *factors* of authentication. These factors are traditionally divided into three categories. The first is *something you know* such as a password or a secret handshake. The second is *something you have* such as a key, a token or a device. The third is *something you are* or *a biometric* such as a fingerprint, DNA or some behavioral trait. Also other categories have been discussed in recent years. One is *someone you know* or someone who knows you as in e.g. [6]. Others include such ideas as proximity to friends [13] and *something you process* [32].

Several protocols have been designed to provide AKE between two parties based on one or several of the above mentioned factors. As passwords have been the dominant method of authentication there are several protocols that provide password authenticated key exchange (PAKE) such as [14] and many others. There are also authenticated key exchange protocols based on biometrics such as [5] and based on secret keys (usually stored on smart cards or other devices) and an associated PKI scheme [15,2].

The various transactions and processes that take place in the networked environment require different levels of security and different levels of authentication. As it is possible to use several different factors of authentication to gain more trust on the authenticity of the transaction, user or device, it is also important to have adaptive systems that utilise these possibilities.

1.1 Contributions and Organisation of This Paper

In this paper we discuss some possibilities of context-aware user authentication in adaptive security systems. We show that with current cryptographic protocols it is possible to link the context to the cryptographic authentication process and also to use the context in making the adaptive security decisions. We also describe and discuss the potential of some recent proposals that consider the context (or some part of it) as a separate authentication factor.

The paper is organised in the following way. In the next section we present some previous results on context-aware adaptive systems and cryptographic authentication protocols. In the third section we present different ways in which the context can be utilised in the adaptive user authentication. We illustrate some of these concepts with small examples. The fourth section briefly discusses the privacy implications of context-aware adaptive user authentication. The fifth section contains discussion and future research topics and the sixth section gives our conclusions.

2   Previous Work

In this section we present some of the most relevant previous results in context-aware systems, adaptive security and authentication.

2.1   Context-Aware and Pervasive Systems

Pervasive computing is applied in various domains to improve the life experience of people, e.g. smart spaces, healthcare and transportation. Due to these varying domains, the security requirements for different applications vary greatly together with other quality and functional requirements. Context information can be applied to deduce these requirements for the pervasive applications [25]. Moreover, context information supports the adaptive behaviour in pervasive computing. It has been stated in [8] that the adaptive behaviour is one major challenge related to pervasive environments.

It is possible to utilise the context-awareness of applications in several ways and, depending on the application, the required context information also changes. Taxonomy of security related context information for smart space purposes is presented in [10]. This taxonomy divides security related context information to three levels as follows: The bottom level consists of the physical context that describes an execution platform, e.g. operating system, utilised network connection etc. The second level constitutes of the digital context, which is intended to describe the role of the environment. For instance, the smart space can be either private or public. The highest context level is the situational context, which describes the role of the exchanged data and the user's role in the environment. For example, the user could be a healthcare professional, who is trying to retrieve work related documents from her home environment.

2.2   Adaptive Security

In an adaptive security system, the system selects the course of action among the existing security mechanisms and/or tuning parameters of these mechanisms. These modifications to the system behaviour are based on the monitored security level and the perceived context of the system. Thus, adaptive security can be seen as the capability of the system to offer self-protection. Self-protection defends the system against malicious attacks and anticipates problems [27].

Achieving adaptive security requires that the system is able to monitor its own behaviour and environment. This monitoring can be realised, for instance, by security measuring, an Intrusion Detection System (IDS) or by some other means. The monitored data is analysed further in order to recognise security breaches or other incidents, which in turn cause an adaptation need. Examples of these analyses are the calculation of security indicators [28], the calculation of authentication confidence [17] and the calculation of user's suspiciousness level [26]. Lastly, when the adaptation need is recognised, the system has to decide what parts of the system will be adapted and how. The survey in [35] reveals that this decision making part is the most uncovered area in the current security adaptation approaches.

In [9], the authors compare four security adaptation approaches from the application layer viewpoint. The compared adaptation approaches act as described above, i.e. existing security mechanisms and their parameters are adapted. Consequently, security mechanisms themselves are not made adaptive but their utilisation is adapted based on the monitored security level and context. In [35] the authors list and compare over 30 self-protection approaches in a tabular form. However, these approaches also concentrate on adapting existing security mechanisms and security policies.

2.3   Authenticated Key Exchange

In [2], Bellare and Rogaway present a framework in which they can achieve provable security for several AKE protocols that they describe and it is one of the first designs for authenticated key exchange with a proof of security. This has provided the basis on which many of the subsequent AKE protocols rely.

There has been a great amount of work done on provably secure authentication protocols with one or many factors. Single factor schemes have traditionally been password-based, as in [14], biometrics based, as in [5] or based on some public key setting as in [15]. Two-factor authenticated key exchange has been proposed for example in [22,20]. In [23] a multi-factor authenticated key exchange protocol has been introduced. Thus it can be seen that there exist many protocols, that can be used with different factors of authentication either separately or in a single protocol.

In [12] the authors describe MFAKE, a new multi-factor authentication protocol, that can be used with any number of passwords, client secret keys and biometrics. The security of MFAKE is based on sub-protocols that utilise tag-based authentication [18] for each authentication factor. This modular approach enables a security proof for the MFAKE protocol. MFAKE facilitates also mutual authentication between the client and the server.

Some form of contextual information has been proposed as a factor of authentication in several publications [29,6,13]. In [13] the authors propose using mobile devices users' proximity to their friends mobile devices as a suitable factor for authentication. In [6], the authors describe a system for vouching for legitimate users if they forget their security tokens. Also the authors of [29] propose a social approach to authentication. One could also argue that the proposal of [32] is a case of contextual information being applied to authentication.

It is worth noting that the above protocols provide examples of two different ways of using contextual information in authentication. The first, demonstrated in [13], means that the context itself becomes one factor in the authentication.

On the other hand, as in for example [6], the context can dictate how and when the user should authenticate herself to the system. This is also the case in some adaptive security systems such as in [17].

3 Combining Authentication and Context-Awareness

As user authentication is currently an important topic in information security and on the other hand different context-aware systems and middleware are emerging, it is important to examine the possible benefits and threats that this combination offers. In this section, we will discuss different ways to combine context-awareness provided by pervasive systems with adaptive security and entity authentication. In the next section we will discuss some of the privacy implications of these technologies.

First of all, we will give some definitions of concepts that are used later in this paper. *Context* is a set of environmental states and settings that either determines an application behaviour or in which the application even occurs and is interesting to the user [7]. From security perspective, this set can be assumed to be public.

3.1 Context as a Separate Authentication Factor

As mentioned in the previous section, there have been some recent proposals that use some contextual information as an authentication factor. For example, in [13] the authors propose to use the proximity of users friends as a possible factor for authentication. The proximity could be measured with many different methods such as GPS or some wireless connectivity. In [13] Bluetooth is proposed as the measure of users proximity with friends. However, this method does not generate enough entropy to be utilised in authenticated key generation.

In [32] the authors propose to add into the security of passwords by requiring the password to be a mathematical formula that is applied and the result used as the secret. There is very little indication that this would gain popular acceptance or that this approach would be immune to the same weaknesses that the normal passwords face.

There are some proposals ([29,6]), where the social context of the user is used in some authentication scenario. These proposals offer a very limited use of the context and do not rely on any autonomously working context-aware application.

The above examples are very interesting first steps in providing new authentication factors. It is also worth noting, that utilising contextual authentication factors could require very little user interaction and would thus be fairly easy to use from user's perspective. However, there is a need for further research on the most usable factors, as the recent proposals do not provide secure enough authentication or are not really related to context-aware systems.

3.2   Context-Awareness as an Adaptation Mechanism

Many attributes that the context-aware systems provide are by themselves insufficient for reliable authentication. For example GPS coordinates and IP address may be easily available, but are fairly useless as separate authentication factors. However, these can be used in adapting the authentication process.

Thus, in contextual authentication the client context defines the different factors and channels that the client must utilise to perform authentication to the server. For example, this context can be the time, the physical location (GPS), virtual location (IP address) or the different applications that the client is running.

As a small example we give the environmental variable provided by many web browsers. This variable contains a lot of information on the context, where the browser is running (e.g. operating system) as well as on the browser itself (browser name, version number etc.) and can be easily accessed by programmers. This information could be used to adapt the user authentication. For example, if the user has an outdated version of a browser, which is known to contain security vulnerabilities, the system might require two-factor authentication.

We made a small proof of concept application that recognises the name of the browser and, based on user preferences on trusted browsers, decides whether the user needs to provide just a password or a password and insert a valid USB token to the computer. The authentication was performed using the MFAKE protocol [12].

In our opinion, it would be beneficial to link the contextual information with the authentication and the possible keys generated in the process. In many adaptive authentication systems, the authentication process is completely separated from the underlying context-aware application except from some triggering functionality. This is of course sensible from development perspective as these two may then be developed independently.

However, with recent tag-based authentication methods, such as MFAKE [12], it is possible to link the contextual information either partly or completely to the authentication process. This could be included in the adaptive security process. Thus it would be harder to use successful (partial) authentications in different contexts.

In [11] the authors present an adaptive security architecture in a smart space. Their adaptive security solution is based on the Smart-M3 smart space architecture [16]. As an example of this adaptive security they give an authentication use case where user communicates via a smart phone with the established smart space and uses the smart space to open and close the lock on her apartment's front door. As the environment recognises the different actions in different contexts the user needs to authenticate and re-authenticate herself in order to be allowed to perform some tasks. The system is based on several predefined authentication levels that are enforced for certain actions of the user.

In [11] the authors do not delve deep into the authentication mechanisms that are invoked by the smart space. They only mention the usage of passwords, but do not specify a protocol for this password authentication. This is reasonable as the adaptive security system should work with any such protocol. However, with existing protocols, the contextual information that guides the adaptive security process is left out of the final authentication. With the help of MFAKE the information could be included in the user authentication. The context could be used at least in the computation of the tag and thus be linked to the end result of the authentication.

By realising the proposed scenario with the help of the MFAKE protocol, we could improve the adaptive security system. As the smart space already provides a rich contextual environment, one could include all of that or only the security related context to the MFAKE protocol. For example, when unlocking the door, the system requires a new authentication as the previous authentication level does not allow for this action. When re-authenticating the user, the MFAKE includes the context information (time, previous authentication level, required authentication level, etc.) to the computation of the tag used in the protocol. The system also makes the decision on the necessary authentication factors and proceeds with the necessary sub-protocols. After successful authentication, the adaptive security system updates the authentication level and allows the unlocking operation. This could also improve the user experience of the system, if the contextual information would be used to require less user interaction in the authentication.

4   Privacy Issues

Pervasive computing and monitoring of user context and behaviour raises some privacy issues. Many service providers already collect a lot of information on their users and profile them accordingly. Although these profiles may help in user authentication they also pose a risk to privacy.

There are methods that allow for anonymous authentication (e.g. [3,34]) and that allow for example attribute based authentication (or signatures) [21,30]. However, these only solve the problem partially for authentication. The problem with pervasive systems and possible cross matching of different contexts and profiles over several service providers is not solved by these authentication solutions.

There have been efforts to quantify and model the privacy issues related to context-aware systems. For example [19] presents a model for controlling users privacy. In [33] the authors propose to use metadata related to the quality of the context information to control the privacy.

However, as can be seen from [1], many systems do not facilitate security and privacy controls. This is fairly troubling, as in the light of recent news, the users cannot be certain that their context information is not misused by the different service providers or some governmental agencies or even blackhat hackers.

5   Discussion and Future Work

Because there are many areas of improvement both in user authentication and in context-aware systems and middleware, we discuss some of the more interesting future directions.

As seen in previous sections there are cryptographic protocols which can utilise context information and link it into the actual authentication and the shared secret between communicating parties. There are also some proposals that use the context information itself as an authentication factor. However, there are still many open questions on which context attributes are best suited to be used as authentication factors and how we can minimise the impact on privacy.

Especially with biometric authentication factors it is important to consider both improving the accuracy of different methods and to ensure that the original biometrics are not leaked in possible database breaches as the replacement of these is usually quite impossible. Some work towards this end has been done (e.g. fuzzy extractors, fuzzy vaults and fingerprint hashes), but some of these are very specific to a certain type of biometric or otherwise impractical to combine with existing biometrics. A good survey on the topic can be found in [24].

It is widely known that the username-password based authentication mechanisms start to show many signs of weakness. With a provably secure protocol as a backbone, we may start to devise authentication systems that employ the MFAKE protocol or some other protocol that enables the use of multiple different authentication factors. Thus, we could move from the username-password based authentication to more advanced and hopefully more secure and reliable authentication.

With context-aware applications the context information could be used in real-time fashion and thus it is very well suited for continuous authentication. This means that the authentication is performed continuously relating the user's actions to the level of security of the data and actions. Usually, authentication is a one-time action that grants access to different services for some period of time. It is also very much a binary decision of accept or reject. In continuous authentication the decision can be based on the context that is monitored frequently. Even if continuous authentication cannot be realised, with the use of adaptive security systems we may at least amplify the authentication mechanisms if the context of the user changes.

Furthermore, we could employ a more risk-based and probabilistic approach to authentication by using the context information. In these types of scenarios the authentication is not a clear cut accept or reject but a level of confidence on the legitimacy of the action performed by the user. For example in [17] the adaptive authentication system gives a trust score on the level of authentication. This trust score could be reflected against the security policy of the service provider.

The above discussion links authentication to trust. For example in [31], Schneier writes extensively about the different levels of trust we as individuals place on other individuals, different institutions and even processes and systems that we interact with . One possible direction of development in authentication systems could be systems that allow for these nuances of trust to be present even in online activities. Context-aware, adaptive authentication could help in developing systems to this end. By linking contextual information and adaptive mechanisms to provably secure authentication and key exchange protocols, we can provide more tools for building secure environments and applications on modern smart spaces.

However, there are many issues that the cryptographic protocols still leave open. One major issue is the enrollment of the different factors used in the protocol. One of the reasons passwords and usernames have become so popular is that enrolling to a new service is extremely easy. With other factors such as tokens, biometrics and even the new social factor, the enrollment process is usually more complicated or very hard to do in a secure manner over untrusted systems and networks. Solutions to this problem need to be devised in order to have access to the security features of MFAKE or other multi-factor authentication protocols. In [4] the authors present a very good framework for evaluating new methods of authentication. This methodology should be used to evaluate the possible benefits of adding different factors to authentication and the feasibility of new, possibly context-based, authentication factors.

One solution could be to have different trust levels for different types of enrollment and maybe to have an algorithm learn the trustworthiness of the different factors. This would make the process of authentication closer to the interactions we have in real life with other people. We have a different amount of trust for different people and we require more rigorous proofs of identity for some people than for others and in different contexts. This kind of system could be more secure than a system based only on a binary trust/no trust decisions, but it would also be more open to different attacks and prone to human-like errors of judgment over the trustworthiness of some entities. This type of approach is discussed for example in [36].

6   Conclusion

In this paper we presented some possibilities of utilising context aware systems in adaptive user authentication. Recent advances in both adaptive security systems and in cryptography show that it is possible to combine the context information gathered from modern pervasive systems with cryptographic authentication schemes. This information can be first used to control an adaptive security system and then linked to the authentication scheme via tags.

Furthermore, we discussed some proposals for utilising the context information itself as an authentication factor. However, this direction requires more research as the proposed methods do not achieve satisfactory security for authentication.

We have made some motivational proof of concept work in combining context information with the MFAKE [12] protocol. The next step is to include this in some pervasive computing system with adaptive security mechanisms. In this way we could improve and further validate our approach.

References

1. Baldauf, M., Dustdar, S., Rosenberg, F.: A survey on context-aware systems. International Journal of Ad Hoc and Ubiquitous Computing 2(4), 263–277 (2007)
2. Bellare, M., Rogaway, P.: Entity authentication and key distribution. In: Stinson, D.R. (ed.) CRYPTO 1993. LNCS, vol. 773, pp. 232–249. Springer, Heidelberg (1994)
3. Boneh, D., Franklin, M.: Anonymous authentication with subset queries. In: Proceedings of the 6th ACM Conference on Computer and Communications Security, pp. 113–119. ACM (1999)
4. Bonneau, J., Herley, C., van Oorschot, P., Stajano, F.: The quest to replace passwords: A framework for comparative evaluation of web authentication schemes. In: 2012 IEEE Symposium on Security and Privacy (SP), pp. 553–567 (May 2012)
5. Boyen, X., Dodis, Y., Katz, J., Ostrovsky, R., Smith, A.: Secure remote authentication using biometric data. In: Cramer, R. (ed.) EUROCRYPT 2005. LNCS, vol. 3494, pp. 147–163. Springer, Heidelberg (2005)
6. Brainard, J., Juels, A., Rivest, R.L., Szydlo, M., Yung, M.: Fourth-factor authentication: somebody you know. In: Conference on Computer and Communications Security: Proceedings of the 13th ACM Conference on Computer and Communications Security, vol. 30, pp. 168–178 (2006)
7. Chen, G., Kotz, D.: et al.: A survey of context-aware mobile computing research. Tech. rep., Technical Report TR2000-381, Dept. of Computer Science, Dartmouth College (2000)
8. Conti, M., Das, S.K., Bisdikian, C., Kumar, M., Ni, L.M., Passarella, A., Roussos, G., Tröster, G., Tsudik, G., Zambonelli, F.: Looking ahead in pervasive computing: Challenges and opportunities in the era of cyber–physical convergence. Pervasive and Mobile Computing 8(1), 2–21 (2012)
9. Elkhodary, A., Whittle, J.: A survey of approaches to adaptive application security. In: International Workshop on Software Engineering for Adaptive and Self-Managing Systems, ICSE Workshops SEAMS 2007, p. 16. IEEE (2007)
10. Evesti, A., Pantsar-Syväniemi, S.: Towards micro architecture for security adaptation. In: Proceedings of the Fourth European Conference on Software Architecture: Companion, pp. 181–188. ACM (2010)
11. Evesti, A., Suomalainen, J., Ovaska, E.: Architecture and knowledge-driven self-adaptive security in smart space. Computers 2(1), 34–66 (2013)
12. Fleischhacker, N., Manulis, M., Sadr-Azodi, A.: Modular design and analysis framework for multi-factor authentication and key exchange. Cryptology ePrint Archive, Report 2012/181 (2012), http://eprint.iacr.org/
13. Frankel, A., Maheswaran, M.: Feasibility of a socially aware authentication scheme. In: 6th IEEE Consumer Communications and Networking Conference, CCNC 2009, pp. 1–6 (January 2009)
14. Gentry, C., Mackenzie, P., Ramzan, Z.: Password authenticated key exchange using hidden smooth subgroups. In: Proceedings of the 12th ACM Conference on Computer and Communications Security, pp. 299–309. ACM (2005)
15. Hao, F.: On robust key agreement based on public key authentication. Security and Communication Networks (2012)

16. Honkola, J., Laine, H., Brown, R., Tyrkko, O.: Smart-m3 information sharing platform. In: 2010 IEEE Symposium on Computers and Communications (ISCC), pp. 1041–1046. IEEE (2010)
17. Hulsebosch, R., Bargh, M., Lenzini, G., Ebben, P., Iacob, S.: Context sensitive adaptive authentication. In: Kortuem, G., Finney, J., Lea, R., Sundramoorthy, V. (eds.) EuroSSC 2007. LNCS, vol. 4793, pp. 93–109. Springer, Heidelberg (2007)
18. Jager, T., Kohlar, F., Schäge, S., Schwenk, J.: Generic compilers for authenticated key exchange. In: Abe, M. (ed.) ASIACRYPT 2010. LNCS, vol. 6477, pp. 232–249. Springer, Heidelberg (2010)
19. Jiang, X., Landay, J.: Modeling privacy control in context-aware systems. IEEE Pervasive Computing 1(3), 59–63 (2002)
20. Lee, Y., Kim, S., Won, D.: Enhancement of two-factor authenticated key exchange protocols in public wireless LANs. Computers & Electrical Engineering 36(1), 213–223 (2010)
21. Maji, H.K., Prabhakaran, M., Rosulek, M.: Attribute-based signatures. In: Kiayias, A. (ed.) CT-RSA 2011. LNCS, vol. 6558, pp. 376–392. Springer, Heidelberg (2011)
22. Park, Y.M., Park, S.K.: Two factor authenticated key exchange (take) protocol in public wireless LANs. IEICE Transactions on Communications 87(5), 1382–1385 (2004)
23. Pointcheval, D., Zimmer, S.: Multi-factor authenticated key exchange. In: Bellovin, S.M., Gennaro, R., Keromytis, A.D., Yung, M. (eds.) ACNS 2008. LNCS, vol. 5037, pp. 277–295. Springer, Heidelberg (2008)
24. Rathgeb, C., Uhl, A.: A survey on biometric cryptosystems and cancelable biometrics. EURASIP Journal on Information Security 2011(1), 1–25 (2011)
25. Raychoudhury, V., Cao, J., Kumar, M., Zhang, D.: Middleware for pervasive computing: A survey. In: Pervasive and Mobile Computing (2012)
26. Ryutov, T., Zhou, L., Neuman, C., Leithead, T., Seamons, K.E.: Adaptive trust negotiation and access control. In: Proceedings of the Tenth ACM Symposium on Access Control Models and Technologies, pp. 139–146. ACM (2005)
27. Salehie, M., Tahvildari, L.: Self-adaptive software: Landscape and research challenges. ACM Transactions on Autonomous and Adaptive Systems (TAAS) 4(2), 14 (2009)
28. Savola, R.M., Abie, H.: Development of measurable security for a distributed messaging system. International Journal on Advances in Security 2(4), 358–380 (2010)
29. Schechter, S., Egelman, S., Reeder, R.: It's not what you know, but who you know: a social approach to last-resort authentication. In: Proceedings of the 27th International Conference on Human Factors in Computing Systems, pp. 1983–1992. ACM (2009)
30. Schläger, C., Sojer, M., Muschall, B., Pernul, G.: Attribute-based authentication and authorisation infrastructures for e-commerce providers. In: Bauknecht, K., Pröll, B., Werthner, H. (eds.) EC-Web 2006. LNCS, vol. 4082, pp. 132–141. Springer, Heidelberg (2006)
31. Schneier, B.: Liars and outliers: enabling the trust that society needs to thrive. Wiley (2012)
32. Shah, S., Minhas, A., et al.: New factor of authentication: Something you process. In: International Conference on Future Computer and Communication, ICFCC 2009, pp. 102–106. IEEE (2009)

33. Sheikh, K., Wegdam, M., Sinderen, M.V.: Quality-of-context and its use for protecting privacy in context aware systems. Journal of Software 3(3), 83–93 (2008)
34. Tsang, P.P., Au, M.H., Kapadia, A., Smith, S.W.: Perea: Towards practical ttp-free revocation in anonymous authentication. In: Proceedings of the 15th ACM Conference on Computer and Communications Security, pp. 333–344. ACM (2008)
35. Yuan, E., Malek, S.: A taxonomy and survey of self-protecting software systems. In: 2012 ICSE Workshop on Software Engineering for Adaptive and Self-Managing Systems (SEAMS), pp. 109–118. IEEE (2012)
36. Yung, M.: On the evolution of user authentication: Non-bilateral factors. In: Pei, D., Yung, M., Lin, D., Wu, C. (eds.) Inscrypt 2007. LNCS, vol. 4990, pp. 5–10. Springer, Heidelberg (2008)

An Ontology-Based Context-Aware Mobile System for On-the-Move Tourists

Saleh Alhazbi, Linah Lotfi, Rahma Ali, and Reem Suwailih

Computer Science and Engineering Dept., Qatar University, Qatar
{salhazbi,LL095810,ra1001782,Rs081123}@qu.edu.qa

Abstract. Ontology-based model in context-aware systems offers more expressiveness, semantically sharing and interoperability. It supports reasoning tasks in a better way than other approaches. However, the main concern with ontology implementation is the expensive computational request for the reasoning process which makes this model unsuitable for critical time applications. This applies to tourism recommender systems when user is moving. Late response based on current tourist location might recommend him points of his interest that are already behind him. In this paper, we propose an ontology-based tourism mobile system that uses current user location and his speed to provide him with a recommendation about points of his interest before reaching them.

Keywords: Context-aware, ontology modeling, reasoning, points of interests.

1   Introduction

In context-aware systems, context modeling specifies how contexts are organized, represented, and stored. Different approaches have been proposed for context modeling such as: key-value models, graphical models, object-oriented models, markup scheme models, logic-based models, and ontology-based models. Compared to other models, ontological context models offer more expressiveness, semantically sharing and interoperability, such models also support reasoning tasks in a better way than other approaches[1,2].

In practice, tourism domain is very well suited field for utilizing context-aware applications. Such applications support tourists on the move by providing them with the best information that suites their current location, and preferences. Among many mobile tourism guides that have been proposed, recent ones [3-9] use ontology-based approach to model context in tourism domain. However, the main concern with ontology implementation is the expensive computational request for the reasoning process. This shortcoming makes ontology unsuitable choice when modeling context in time-critical applications [10]. In tourism domain, this situation applies to a tourist who needs a recommendation while he is moving like riding a car or a bus. Late response based on current tourist location might recommend him points of his interests (POIs) that are already behind him.

M.J. O'Grady et al. (Eds.): AmI 2013 Workshops, CCIS 413, pp. 252–256, 2013.
© Springer International Publishing Switzerland 2013

In this paper, we propose an ontology-based context-aware mobile tourist system that supports on-the-move user, it provides him with a recommendation that includes the most suitable POIs. These POIs should match his preferences and located on his route ahead of him. Our proposed system does not only calculate predicted user's location when he receives recommendation but it estimates a new location ahead of that, in order to allow user to see this recommendation in advance before he reaches that location. This predicted location depends on user's speed, and network speed. Thus , our system is not only aware of user's location like many other tourism context-aware systems, but additionally it is aware of user's speed, his direction, and network speed as important factor that affects response time.

2   Ontology-Based Context Modeling

Ontology can be used to describe concepts in a specific domain, define their attributes, and specify relationships between them. According to Gruninger and Lee[11], using ontology to model concepts in any domain has many advantages: it allows knowledge sharing, deduces implicit knowledge through reasoning, and supports knowledge reusing. On the other side, the disadvantage of using ontology to model any knowledge base is the complexity of reasoning which might make that process computationally very expensive.

In tourism domain, many tourist recommendation systems[3-9] use ontology to model points of interest. However, none of them address performance overhead problem when reasoning the ontology. On the other hand, Lee and Meier [12] proposed a hybrid approach that comprises both ontology and object-oriented model in order to utilize ontology and at the same time overcome ontology deficiency. Similarly, the work in [10] addresses this challenge by proposing a hybrid approach that uses database modeling with ontology, the experimental results show that hybrid model is faster than the ontology model.

On contrary to these approaches, we do not focus on improving reasoning time, our proposed system addresses the challenge by calculating a predicted user location before reasoning the ontology. Reasoning process should return POIs that are around this new location and they should be received by user before he reaches that location.

3   System Architecture

Our system is composed of two modules: mobile module and server module.

Mobile Module. This module is installed on mobile device and used by tourist. When a user installs the application for the first time, he needs to register and specify his preferences. Then he can use the system to get recommendations about nearby POIs that match his interest. The mobile system is responsible for sensing contextual data which include user location, and network speed. GPS sensor is used to get user location at regular intervals of time. This multiple locations are used to calculate user average speed by the mobile application. Considering limited computing power on mobile devices, two of these locations are sent to the server in order to calculate user direction. Additionally, mobile system sends user ID, speed, and network speed. Then, it waits for receiving POIs from the server.

Server Module. This module is responsible of keeping track of users' profiles, calculating predicted location, and reasoning tourism ontology. When the server reasons the ontology, only POIs that are inside user's area of interest (AOI) are sent back to the mobile module.

4   Calculating User's Area of Interest (AOI)

User's AOI is a circle area located on tourist route. Its radius R is specified based on network speed as follows

$$R = \begin{cases} 1Km & if\,network\,speed < 1Mbps \\ 2Km & if\;1Mbps = < Network\,speed < 10Mbps \\ 3Km & if\;10\,Mbps = < Network\,speed < 20Mbps \\ 4Km & if\;20\,Mbps = < Network\,speed < 30Mbps \\ 5Km & if\;Network\,speed > = 30Mbps \end{cases}$$

The objective of restricting AOI is to improve system response time by limiting number of POIs according to network speed. Figure 1 shows how AOI center is predicted. The center of AOI is calculated based on current user location, and user speed. Assume the user was in location L_c when he requests a recommendation. First, the system should estimate his location when he is supposed to receive the response (L_p). In order to give the user a chance to see the recommendation before reaching the POIs, L_p is displaced ahead by a distance d in the same direction of the user move, this new location L_a is the center of AOI. Clearly, L_p depends on response time T_r, this time includes communication time T_c and ontology reasoning time T_n.

$$T_r = T_c + T_n \tag{1}$$

Communication time depends directly on network speed. Also, reasoning time is affected indirectly by network speed because of the way we have used above to specify R.

Because the tourism ontology is almost static, the average of response time T_{ra} can be calculated for each category of network speed. Therefore location L_p is calculated as follows

$$L_p = L_c + (T_{ra} X S_u) \quad \text{where } S_u \text{ is the user speed} \tag{2}$$

Then center of AOI (L_a) is evaluated as follows

$$L_a = L_p + d \tag{3}$$

Where d depends on user speed S_u as follows

$$d= \begin{cases} 0 & \text{if } S_u<10\ Km/h \\ 5\ X\ S_u/100 & 10 <= \text{if } S_u<100 \\ 5 & \text{if } S_u>=100 \end{cases}$$

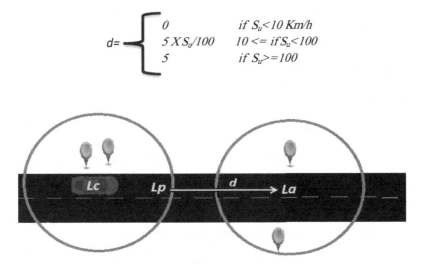

Fig. 1. Calculating user AOI

5   Conclusion

In this paper, we have proposed a context-based mobile system to notify on-the-move tourist to tourism points that match his interest. This system uses ontology modeling approach to describe tourism information. To overcome complexity of ontology reasoning, our system utilizes more contextual data such as user velocity and network speed to predict a new location ahead on user's rout so the user gets the recommendation before he reaches that location.

Acknowledgements. This publication was made possible by UREP grant # (11-111-1-022) from the Qatar national research fund (a member of Qatar foundation). The statements made herein are solely the responsibility of the author(s).

References

1. Strang, T., Linnhoff-Popien, C.: A context modeling survey. In: The Sixth International Conference on Ubiquitous Computing (UBICOMP), Nottingham (2004)
2. Bettini, C., Brdiczka, O., Henricksen, K., Indulska, J., Nicklas, D., Ranganathan, A., Riboni, D.: A survey of context modelling and reasoning techniques. Pervasive and Mobile Computing 6, 161–180 (2009)
3. Lam, T.H.W., Lee, R.S.T.: iJADE freeWalker: An ontology-based tourist guiding system. In: Gabrys, B., Howlett, R.J., Jain, L.C. (eds.) KES 2006. LNCS (LNAI), vol. 4252, pp. 644–651. Springer, Heidelberg (2006)
4. Yueh, Y., Chiu, D., Leung, H., Hung, P.: A Virtual Travel Agent System for M-Tourism with Semantic Web Service Based Design and Implementation. In: 21st International Conference on Advanced Networking and Applications (AINA 2007), Canada, pp. 142–149 (2007)

5. Song, T., Chen, S.: Establishing an Ontology-based Intelligent Agent System with Analytic Hierarchy Process to Support Tour Package Selection Service. In: International Conference on Business and Information, South Korea (2008)

6. Jakkilinki, R., Sharda, N., Ahmad, I.: Ontology-based Intelligent Tourism Information Systems: An overview of development methodology and applications. In: Proceeding of TES 2005: Tourism Enterprise Strategies: Thriving – and Surviving – in an Online Era, Melbourne, Australia (2005)

7. Kanellopoulos, D.: An ontology-based system for intelligent matching of travellers' needs for Group Package Tours. International Journal of Digital Culture and Electronic Tourism 1, 76–99 (2008)

8. Bessho, M., Kobayashi, S., Koshizuka, N., Sakamura, K.: A space-identifying ubiquitous infrastructure and its application for tour-guiding service. In: Proceeding of the 23rd ACM Symposium on Applied Computing, pp. 1616–1621 (2008)

9. Møller-Jensen, L., Egler Hansen, J.: Towards a Mobile Tourist Information System: Identifying Zones of Information Relevance. In: 10th AGILE International Conference on Geographic Information Science, Denmark, pp. 1–7 (2007)

10. Mi Park, Y., Moon, A., Il Choi, Y., Ki Kim, S., Kim, S.: An efficient context model for fast responsiveness of context-aware services in mobile networks. In: 2010 7th IEEE Consumer Communications and Networking Conference (CCNC), pp. 1–5 (2010)

11. Gruninger, M., Lee, J.: Ontology – Applications and Design. Communications of the ACM 45, 39–41 (2002)

12. Lee, D., Meier, R.: A hybrid approach to context modelling in large-scale pervasive computing environments. In: COMSWARE 2009. ACM (2009)

Modeling the Urban Context
through the Theory of Roles

Claudia Liliana Zúñiga Cañón[1,2] and Juan Carlos Burguillo Rial[1]

[1] Information Technologies Group GTI, Department of Telematics Engineering,
University of Vigo, Vigo, Spain
[2] Research Group COMBA R & D, Department of Engineering,
University of Santiago de Cali, Cali, Colombia
clzuniga@ieee.org, {clzuniga,J.C.Burguillo}@uvigo.es

Abstract. Urban environments are intelligent spaces where a wide set
of heterogeneous variables that directly influence the behavior of the individual converge. In this paper we present UrbanContext, a new model
for urban platforms that follows an individual centered approach and validates the use of the Theory of Roles to understand the behavior of the
individual within a social environment. The roles defined in UrbanContext allow the interpretation of the states of the individual, facilitating his
interaction with the environment and offering services without damaging
his privacy. We describe the UrbanContext model and the fundamental
principles that have been identified in this design; likewise we present a
first validation scenario for UrbanContext.

Keywords: Urban Computing, Urban Context, Models, Theory of Roles,
Smart Cities.

1 Introduction

Nowadays, several projects have focused their works on improving cities, with the
objective of making them more intelligent and ubiquitous. The ubiquitous city
(U-City) [1][2] is defined as a city with high technological interaction that has as
goal to offer services and information in every time and place to its inhabitants.

These urban environments become scenarios where persons, places and technologies converge. These three aspects form the so called triad [3] in urban computing. People are seen as dynamic individuals who become the main subject of
study if we want to understand these environments.

To model the context in the urban environment is complex due to the great
number of variables that converge in these spaces. This complexity demands
techniques that allow the modeling and the representation of the individuals'
behaviors in the cities.

Our contribution is UrbanContext, a new model for urban computing systems
that uses the Theory of Roles to manage the context. UrbanContext facilitates
the interpretation of the states of the individual, the development of adapted
services and the generation of positive relationships. In our work, we propose a

M.J. O'Grady et al. (Eds.): AmI 2013 Workshops, CCIS 413, pp. 257–265, 2013.
© Springer International Publishing Switzerland 2013

validation scenario in an adapted real environment, and we evaluate our roles model approach, used in UrbanContext, to understand the behavior of the individual in urban environments.

The paper is organized as follows: The first section is an introduction about the context and the theory of roles in urban computing. The second section presents the roles model used in UrbanContext and describes the dynamic of the component to model the urban context. Next, we present the validation scenario of the component and the results. Finally the conclusions and future work are presented.

2   The Context and the Theory of Roles

The *"urban atmosphere"* [4] is defined as the intersection generated between mobile and social computing, but with a specific interaction in urban spaces. In an urban atmosphere, many variables are constantly involved and mixed generating an exponential knowledge. So, to model these environments it is necessary to consider the context where they take place.

Schilit and Theimer [5] introduced the term *"context aware"*, and they consider the *"context"* as the location, identities of nearby people or objects, and the changes happening to these objects. Later, this definition was complemented in [6] where it was stated that the important aspects of context were: where are you, who are you, and what resources are near you.

Several authors refined this concept over the years. One of the broader definitions given was made by Dey [7], when he defined *"context"* as any information that can be used to characterize the situation of an entity. We must also mention that to model the context, we should include the abstraction of the situation, giving a description of the interacting states of relevant entities.

These definitions were widely discussed and subsequently improved by Dourish [8], who indicated that to really understand and model the context it was also necessary to involve social issues. Focusing on the latter idea, in Urban-Context we need a user-oriented approach that allows the identification of the individual's behavior and interaction within the urban environment.

The approach we have selected to model the context is the Theory of Roles proposed by Erving Goffman [9]. This theory considers an individual who determines his behavior according to the role he plays in a certain situation. The individual's behaviors are influenced by the interactions he experiences and he is constantly changing the roles he plays within a social environment. Besides, we considered an "own role" to model the situations when the individual is alone.

Therefore, the objectives of the UrbanContext management component, which is described in the next section, are to improve the interaction of the individual within the urban context, to identify his needs in every interaction and to provide the adequate level of privacy.

3   Roles Model for the Context in the Urban Environment

UrbanContext is a general-purpose model with a set of components, used for the design of urban computing platforms that applies the theory of roles to manage the individual's context in urban environments. UrbanContext is composed of five main components: interface, roles, semantics, services and information management (cloud).

3.1   The Management of the Context in the UrbanContext Model

In UrbanContext the management of the context and the roles assumed by the individual are modeled through the Roles Component. The Roles Component is composed of four sub-components: urban agent, urban atmosphere, context and context management. Next, we describe the main aim of all those sub-components (See Fig. 1):

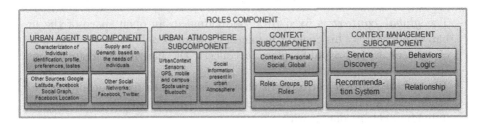

Fig. 1. Roles Component in UrbanContext

Urban Agent SubComponent. This sub-component is focused on the characterization of the user. It should collect all the information of the user directly from his interaction, as well as from different social sources he is related to.

This sub-component enables the identification of the individual through the collection of basic information that usually tends to be constant; such as name, surname, date of birth and nationality. Also, the sub-component must acquire dynamic data associated with the profile regarding preferences and tastes to generate an individual's knowledge base.

Urban Atmosphere SubComponent. This sub-component allows filtering through out all the data about the place, the environment, as well as the persons attending the space.

Context SubComponent. This sub-component is associated with the identification of the contexts in which the individual participates within the urban atmosphere. It considers that the individual can be in three different contexts: in a personal context, in a social context, and in a global context. In addition, this sub-component collects and identifies the roles of the individuals within every selected context.

Here, we must collect data from external sources such as sensors and social networks to identify the behaviors of the individual in such context.

Context Management SubComponent. This sub-component focuses on the semantic processing of all the data collected by the other components. It also achieves discovering services, establishes the logic of the individual's behaviors in the atmosphere, builds effective relationships, and eventually provides a recommendation system. Finally, this sub-component provides significant value to privacy, offering customization without forgetting about privacy threats.

3.2   Roles Component Flow

To manage the context, the first thing we do in UrbanContext is to use a multi-tier approach, which divides the context in three main parts: global, social and personal. Thus, the Roles Component provides:

- The *global context* is fixed to an individual in an open space of the urban atmosphere. This context manages all what people share through a set of services around a public place: a concert, the meeting in a square or a spontaneous congregation.
- The *social context* corresponds to what is obtained from socializing with other individuals; for example, friends, acquaintances and people the individual get in contact with.
- The *personal context* is based on the individual's own world, the one that is only available to him. In this space, the user is represented as a big bubble with some needs, fears, concerns, ideas and tastes.

At this level of abstraction, it is necessary to apply a second ranking that allows to offer customization, and most importantly user privacy. As we have said, for this approach we used the Theory of Roles described by Goffman [9], who defines that individuals are always playing roles according to the situation they are in. Applying this concept in UrbanContext (See Fig. 2), we establish that for every context in the Urban Atmosphere an individual can play different roles that we can structure hierarchically as:

Role Groups: Family, Professional or Academic, Social and Rest of the World Roles.

Role Categories: Within each Role Group we have created several categories that identify the role the individual is playing, i.e., father, uncle, teacher, friend, or just himself.

Individuals can release public information and needs according to the role and the context they are at a certain moment. This information is fed into a knowledge base that identifies the role of the individual in an urban environment to be able to provide the right services adapted to his needs.

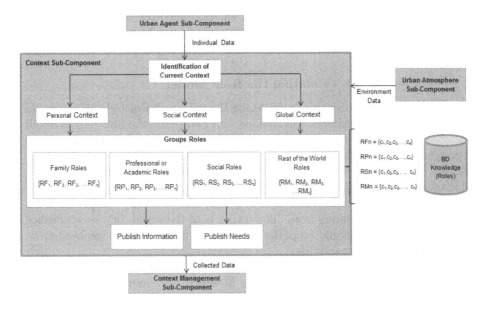

Fig. 2. Roles Description

4   Validation and Results for the Roles Model

With the aim of validating the dynamic of the roles of the individuals inside urban environments, different proposals were revised, and the developed validation plan is described in this section.

4.1   Validation of Urban Environments

The validation of urban computing models requires flexible mechanisms that adapt to every potential real environment. Different authors have stated the difficulty that emerges regarding the development of urban computing systems, when applied in real environments. Kellar [10] states that unique methodological challenges arise when the observation of context includes operations in urban environments.

On this matter, Goodman [11] shows that the experiments in the field are complex, but represent a good balance between field studies and laboratory tests. Likewise, he defines this kind of experiments as fundamental to discover behaviors that would not be recognized in a controlled environment, as these studies are highly influenced by the context in which the individual is placed.

In recent years, the scenario developed in Oulu, Finland has stand out [12][13]. The challenge in that project is to make Oulu an open ubiquitous city, in which the citizens directly participate in the development of a new city of the future.

According to all these approaches, we created a scenario through a focus group to validate the roles component within a real environment. In this way, the individuals had the freedom to interact spontaneously inside urban atmospheres; assuming roles and expressing their needs according to the situations they experienced in a normal day.

4.2 A Scenario for Validating the Role Model

We defined a validation scenario following the role model of UrbanContext. In this scenario, the experiment was divided into two parts: the first part is about the characterization of the individual and the atmosphere through the Urban Agent and Urban Atmosphere sub-components; the second part is oriented to identify the behaviors in the urban space through the Context and Context Management sub-component.

The focus group for the validation was composed of twenty people with different sex, ages and coming from different parts of the world. It was established that the experiment should be performed on very active days or weekend trips, and days with outdoor activities.

In this scenario, following tests were applied to the individuals for 24 hours aiming to identify the different contexts in which they moved, the roles they played, their needs and the information they wanted to publish.

The following items were defined for this test:

- *A basic Characterization of the individual*
- *Time Line*
- *Urban Atmosphere Characterization (Location)*
- *Contexts (Global, Social and Personal)*
- *Identification of the Group of Roles (Family Roles, Social Roles, among others)*
- *Role Category (Father, Mother, Son, Husband, Friend, among others)*
- *Information to Publish*
- *Generated Needs*

The experiment initially considered assigning to every participant a set of roles by default. The individual had the responsibility of adding new categories as needed. Likewise, another group of roles was created, it was called Rest of the World, and the individual was able to classify those category roles that did not fit in the other groups.

4.3 Validation Results

In the experiment performed, we worked with a sample group of 20 individuals, 65% men and 35% female; 90% single, 5% married and 5% separated. Among them 60% are between 18 and 27 years old, 30% between 28-40 and the rest of the participants (10%) were over 41 years old (See Fig. 3).

The experiment produced the following results:

- 15% of the participants experimented the situation of living in two contexts simultaneously; for instance, an individual felt as he was in a social and personal context at the same time.

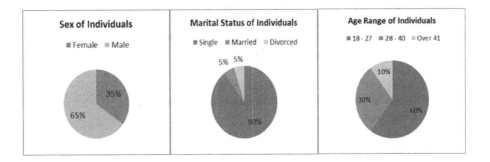

Fig. 3. Socio-demographic Data

- We identified in 90% of the provided reports, that, according to the selected context and the defined role, it was possible to determine if the person was alone or accompanied.
- The individuals could play simultaneous roles in specific moments in time. This scenario could appear inside the same role group or in different role groups. (See Fig. 4).

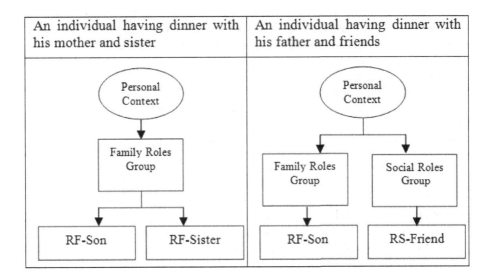

Fig. 4. Two Different Scenarios with Simultaneous Roles

- In 75% of the reports, the type of individual needs could be predicted identifying the atmosphere and the individual role he was playing at that time.
- The individuals were more willing to share information about their preferences and their likes, if they were allowed to say with whom they would

like to share them. Another positive aspect about sharing information was that they were looking for obtaining benefits, like sales or suited recommendations. For example, if a supermarket would offer sales according to his preferences, an individual would like to share it with some of the supermarkets of his choice.

- The majority of the users' necessities were related to:
  - Finding whatever they need in the least possible time.
  - Having real time assistance.
  - Finding nearby establishments.
  - Having information about the available products.
  - Having data about transportation systems.
  - Having interactive systems that allow the evaluation of services.

5   Conclusions and Future Work

In this paper we have presented UrbanContext, a new model for urban platforms that follows an individual centered approach and validates the use of the Theory of Roles to understand the individual's behavior within a social environment. We also have defined a validation scenario with individuals in a real environment for evaluating the Theory of Roles considered in UrbanContext.

We can conclude that UrbanContext and its roles model proposal, facilitates the interpretation of the states of the individual as well as his interaction with the environment. We identified that the urban atmosphere and the individual's context directly influence the needs generated by the individuals.

We have also realized, through the characterization of the individual and the urban atmosphere, that the roles model provides a knowledge base that permits the matching of states, facilitating the interaction and promoting positive relationships. Likewise, we validate that the roles model allows to classify the individual's information and can provide privacy for him.

As future work, we hope to continue the validation scenarios for UrbanContext aiming to:

- Measure the level of interaction of the individual in the urban environment.
- Identify possible services according to the atmosphere, the context and the role of the individual.
- Identify possible positive relationships in urban atmospheres.
- Use the Guacarí Living Lab [14][15] Platform as an urban collaborative environment to facilitate the application of monitoring tools that have been developed in UrbanContext.

Acknowledgements. This work was partially supported by the Xunta de Galicia under INCITE Project Number 10 PXIB 322 039 PR.

References

1. Hwang, J.: u-City: The Next Paradigm of Urban Development. In: Handbook of Research on Urban Informatics: The Practice and Promise of the Real-Time City. IGI Global (2009),
   http://www.igi-global.com/chapter/
   city-next-paradigm-urban-development/21814

2. Foth, M.: From Social Butterfly to Engaged Citizen: Urban Informatics, Social Media, Ubiquitous Computing, and Mobile Technology to Support Citizen Engagement. ch. 17. MIT Press, Cambridge (2011),
   http://mitpress.mit.edu/9780262016513

3. Foth, M., Choi, J., Satchell, C.: Urban Informatics. In: Proceedings of the ACM 2011 Conference on Computer Supported Cooperative Work (CSCW 2011). ACM, New York (2011)

4. Paulos, E., Jenkins, T.: Urban Probes: Encountering our Emerging Urban Atmospheres. In: Proceedings of the SIGCHI Conference on Human Factors in Computing Systems (CHI 2005). ACM, New York (2005)

5. Schilit, B., Theimer, M.: Disseminating Active Map Information for Mobile Host. IEEE Network 8(5) (September-October 1994)

6. Schilit, B., Adams, N., Want, R.: Context-Aware Computing Application. Mobile Computing Systems and Applications, IEEE Explore (1994)

7. Dey, A.: Understanding and Using Context. Journal Personal Ubiquitous Computing (2001)

8. Dourish, P.: What we Talk about When we Talk About Context. Journal Personal Ubiquitous Computing, V 8 (2004)

9. Goffman, E.: The Presentation of Self in Everyday Life. Doubleday & Company Inc., New York (1959)

10. Kellar, M., et al.: It's a Jungle Out There: Practical Considerations for Evaluation in the City. In: CHI 2005 Extended Abstracts on Human Factors in Computing Systems (CHI EA 2005). ACM, New York (2005)

11. Goodman, J., Brewster, S., Gray, P.: Using Field Experiments to Evaluate Mobile Guides. In: Proceedings of HCI in Mobile Guides, Workshop at Mobile HCI 2004, UK (2004)

12. Ojala, T., Kukka, H.: A Digital City Needs Open Pervasive Computing Infrastructure. In: Proc. Digital Cities 6: Concepts, Methods and Systems of Urban Informatics, State College, PA (2009)

13. Ojala, T., Kostakos, V.: UBI Challenge: Research Coopetition on Real-World Urban Computing. In: Proceedings of the 10th International Conference on Mobile and Ubiquitous Multimedia (MUM 2011). ACM, New York (2011)

14. CO-T1199: Wireless Networks and Digital Inclusion Services in the City of Guacarí. Sponsored by the IDB (Interamerican Development Bank) and the Italian Trust Fund of Information and Communication Technology for Development (2011),
    http://www.iadb.org/en/projects/
    project-description-title,1303.html?id=CO-T1199#.Ukm-S4ZWySo

15. Zuniga, C., et al.: Software Platform for Services in Colombian Cities using the Living Labs Approach. In: IEEE GLOBECOM Workshops (GC Wkshps), Houston, TX, USA (2011)

Ubiquitous Applications over Networked Femtocell

Hajer Berhouma[1], Aicha Ben Salem[2], and Kaouthar Sethom[2]

[1] ESPRIT, Institute of Engineering
[2] INNOV'COM Lab, SUPCOM, University of Carthage Tunisia

Abstract. The rapid increase in mobile data activity has raised the stakes on developing innovative new technologies and cellular topologies that can meet these demands in an efficient manner. Femtocell seems to be a good candidate that can potentially play a much broader role by enabling a new class of multimedia and family communications services. This concept may have great consumer appeal because it has the potential to transform the way people stay connected with the two things that matter most: their family (or friends) and their media. This new paradigm is called: the femto-group or Femtozone.

In this work, we present an MDA-based tool (Model driven architecture) for ubiquitous service discovery between heterogenous user's devices and services in a Femtozone.

Keywords: femtocells, MDA tool, UPnP.

1   Introduction

The femtozone or togroup is similar to peer-to-peer systems i.e. composed of devices (nodes) with different computing and communication capabilities. Each (peer) node equally acts as both, server and client. These nodes provide their services to other nodes in the Femtozone, and they are able to use remote services. The grouping may be static or dynamic. An example of an application enabled by femtocell is "friend and family", in which a parent could be notified of their child's arrival or departure from a friend's home, in addition to their own ability to share photos automatically; and ability to stream videos or TV directly to the group (football match…).

However, there is no available languages and tools, facilitating the integration and interoperability of such devices. This is strongly related to the lack of a unified service discovery mechanism that would make heterogeneous services available to the developer for composition and integration. The device and service description heterogeneity can prevent applications to use any available equivalent device on the Femto-Group to accomplish a specific task.

In fact, existing service discovery mechanisms have adopted various service-description languages, thus limiting the scope of global service discovery over neighbors -with heterogeneous equipments. Though each of them has its advantages and disadvantages in terms of expressiveness and query efficiency, they are primarily bound to the architecture of the individual discovery mechanism. A unified way for service description is needed while hiding heterogeneity.

M.J. O'Grady et al. (Eds.): AmI 2013 Workshops, CCIS 413, pp. 266–270, 2013.
© Springer International Publishing Switzerland 2013

Motivated primarily by the above considerations, this article introduces a novel methodology for application development over femtozone that is Model-driven Architecture based.

2   Problem Statement

The concepts introduced in this paper are illustrated with an example of service streaming or downloading content from a remote devices in the femto-Group:

The user A wants to watch a football match "final Monial" in life streaming from any available neighbor in the femto-Group. User B is watching the match, he can respond favorably to A. But, A Laptop used UPnP protocol to describes the TV service request while B device uses the WSDL (Web Service Description Language) to expose the service descriptions.

Other than the description format, the syntax content is not the same. The services and the actions have also different syntax, the UPnP TV offers a "Watch" service with a "read" action to read data, while the DPWS TV uses the action "steaming" to offer the similar functionality.

Devices arriving to a such environment are expected to identify other devices along with their services and integrate them regardless their protocol for service description so they can be used transparently by users, other devices or applications.

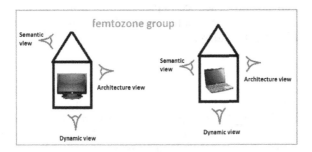

Fig. 1. Femto-group views

In order to solve this problem, we have begun by defining the different views of heterogeneity between devices in a femto group. The figure 1 presents 3 levels. The first level is the semantic view. It represents static elements like the structure of data stored in a node of the group or the way the services of a node are described (xml, wsdl...). The second level is the dynamic level. It refers to the behavior of each device protocol. The third level is the architecture view. It refers to communication between nodes. We can have a peer to peer architecture like in the protocol p2pJini. Or a centralized architecture with a control point like in UPnP. In this work we have only focus on the semantic view specifically in service description [1].

3   Service Model Discussion

To mask the devices heterogeneity in the femtozone scenario, we propose to use models. Models provide abstractions of a physical system that allow engineers to reason about that system by ignoring extraneous details while focusing on relevant ones. All forms of engineering rely on models to understand complex, real-world systems.

It is often necessary to convert to different views of the system at an equivalent level of abstraction (e.g., from a structural view to a behavioral view), and a model transformation facilitates this. In other cases, a transformation converts models offering a particular perspective from one level of abstraction to another, usually from a more abstract to less abstract view, by adding more detail supplied by the transformation rules.

Two protocols have been considered in our studies: Model Driven Architecture (MDA) [3] and Service-oriented architecture (SOA) [2].

3.1   MDA

The MDA acronym has been defined by the OMG standardization body in 2000. It means Model Driven Architecture but may represent very disparate things. In the context of service creation a model-driven approach consists primarily in the ability to generate large amounts of a service implementation from a high-level abstraction definition of the service, exploiting object-oriented modelling techniques – like MOF [4], UML [5] and QVT [6] standards.

3.2   SOA

Service-oriented architecture (SOA) is a software design and software architecture design pattern based on discrete pieces of software that provide application functionality as services, known as Service-orientation. A service is a self-contained logical representation of a repeatable function or activity. Services can be combined by other software applications that together, provide the complete functionality of a large software application. The purpose of SOA is to allow easy cooperation of a large number of computers that are connected over a network. Every computer can run an arbitrary number of services, and each service is built in a way that ensures that the service can exchange information with any other service within the reach of the network without human interaction and without the need to make changes to the underlying program itself. It defines Services as a collection of components.

3.3   SOA versus MDA

A semantic approach makes MDA simpler and more accessible than SOA. The semantic technology is again a specialist area of study and is difficult, but, now there are free software and tools available to use with the semantic technology. It enables people to experiment and learn easily and at low cost, and a growing community of people is doing just that.

MDA applications interoperate and are reusable: The MDA, designed from the start to implement in multiple middleware platforms, codes cross-platform invocations where needed, not only within a given application, but also from one to another regardless of the target platform assigned to each. This is in line with the fact the services in SOA are reusable and interoperable.

In cellular networks there is tremendous improvement expected by deployment of LTE in the near future, especially in terms of downlink/uplink rates and Quality of Service (QoS). Another key driver for offering high transfer rates and QoS is the deployment of femtocells. Using femtocells as the underlying medium layer with modeling will offer a reach solution for next generation users.

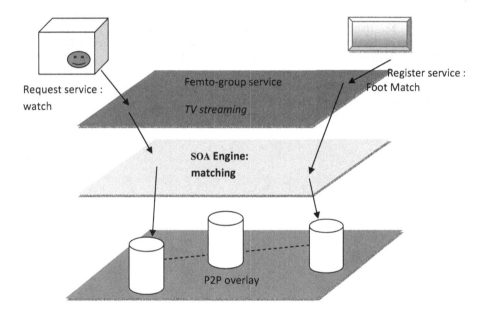

Fig. 2. Service discovery with SOA

4   Conclusion

Devices in femtozone scenario announce their hosted services each in its own description format and data content. Currently, most of the emerging semantic frameworks apply to the Web Service paradigm, without supporting directly other types of services. Our model is dedicated to femtocell environments and remains abstract enough allowing thus for extensions that are able to support new classes of services descriptions.

References

1. Tsalgatidou, A., Athanasopoulos, G., Pantazoglou, M.: Semantically enhanced discovery of heterogeneous services. In: Bramer, M., Terziyan, V. (eds.) Industrial Applications of Semantic Web. IFIP, vol. 188, pp. 275–292. Springer, Heidelberg (2005)
2. Object-Management-Group OMG. MDA Guide Version 1.0.1. (2003)
3. Hadi Valipour, M., Zafari, B.A., Niki Maleki, K., Daneshpour, N.: A Brief Survey of Software Architecture Concepts and Service Oriented Architecture. In: Proceedings of 2nd IEEE International Conference on Computer Science and Information Technology, ICCSIT 2009, China, pp. 34–38 (August 2009)
4. MOF, http://www.omg.org/mof/
5. UML, http://www.uml.org
6. Czarnecki, K., Helsen, S.: Classification of Model Transformation Approaches. In: Proceedings of the OOPSLA 2003 Workshop on the Generative Techniques in the Context Of Model-Driven Architecture, Anaheim, California, USA (2003)
7. Universal Plug and Play, http://www.upnp.org/
8. Intelligent Grouping and Resource Sharing, http://www.igrs.org/
9. Eclipse Modeling Framework Project (EMF), http://www.eclipse.org/modeling/emf/

Modeling Context-Awareness in a Pervasive Computing Middleware Using Ontologies and Data Quality Profiles

Sandra Rodríguez-Valenzuela[1,*], Juan A. Holgado-Terriza[1], Plamen Petkov[2], and Markus Helfert[2]

[1] Software Engineering Department, CITIC-UGR, University of Granada, 18071, Spain
[2] School of Computing, Dublin City University
sandra@ugr.es

Abstract. Context-awareness is one of the most relevant research areas in Pervasive Computing scope. However, in more complex environments, loosely coupled data and dynamic behavior of the environment can become a source of serious problems. These problems can spread throughout whole proactive behavior and in this way make them difficult to handle. In this paper we argue that there is a lack of research done about the data quality and quality of awareness particularly in this kind of composite systems. We investigate on how to build the semantic layer of the DOHA middleware due to reach the goal of context-awareness. To achieve that we are using a data quality approach and data profiles. In addition, we use ontologies as information representation method and to carry over the information about the profiles to the pervasive environment. By doing so, we assure proper representation of the real world and we are improving semantic data and context-awareness in such environments.

Keywords: ontology, data quality, semantic, middleware, pervasive computing, context-awareness.

1   Introduction

New software development era promotes user empowerment through accessibility of information to all, with increased security, and in the context of wider development of ambient intelligence and distributed systems. This is called pervasive (or ubiquitous) computing [3]. In a high level sense, pervasive spaces can be seen as abstract logical environments where distributed devices provide complex functionality that users claim to consume [22]. Far away from the traditional interaction between users and devices, pervasive computing reaches to deploy complex proactive behavior by means context-awareness [4].

Software Engineering and Computer Science have evolved to adapt its requirements to distributed, resource constrained devices which understand our changing needs and react to them as transparently as possible, deployed in mobile and

---

[*] Corresponding author.

M.J. O'Grady et al. (Eds.): AmI 2013 Workshops, CCIS 413, pp. 271–282, 2013.
© Springer International Publishing Switzerland 2013

pervasive environments [9]. The principles of Service Oriented Architecture paradigm (SOA) are the most widespread used to develop this kind of systems [19]. Assembling functional components into a network of loosely coupled services to create flexible, dynamic processes reinforces the use of SOA-based middleware platforms to develop pervasive applications [13].

Dynamic behavior of the environment and loosely coupled data add complexity to the composition – e.g., proactive services which act with anticipation of user desires [10]. Thus, it is important to use a high quality information model to improve the dynamic composition between context-aware services. Besides a high level information representation model it is necessary a data quality evaluation methodology to ensure the quality of the context information and the validity of the real data.

In this paper we present the analysis and design process followed to develop the semantic, context-aware layer of the middleware Dynamic Open Home-Automation (DOHA) [16]. We have designed the semantic information representation to carry out context-awareness linked with a data quality evaluation methodology. We propose an appropriate way to represent the information based on data profiles. More particularly, these profiles are carried into DOHA context by using ontology approach. The conjunction among data acquisition by DOHA services, the representation of these information using ontologies and the validation of data quality using data profiling, will help to the context-aware manager to detect problems concerned semantic data and in this way increase the context-awareness accuracy in home-automation environments. Additionally, the approach will remain loyal to Design Science methodology for conducting research.

The paper is organized as follows: we first review in Section 2 some of the most relevant works as the background to our research; then, in Section 3, we introduce some important aspects of DOHA middleware, such as its service composition model; Section 4 outlines the details of the modeling process carried out to add context-awareness to DOHA middleware; in Section 5 we present the case study and the evaluation criteria that we are using along the development of the context-aware layer of the DOHA middleware; and lastly we present our conclusions and future research in Section 6.

2   Background

Context-aware systems are able to adapt their operations to current context without explicit user intervention and thus aim at increasing usability and effectiveness by taking environmental context into account [1]. At this point, one of the first steps to build a context-aware middleware should be to define what context is. At the beginning of context-aware platforms development the context was related mainly with the location. The definition of context has evolved to our days and now the term includes not only the location or time, but also any other information that can be relevant in the interaction between users and applications. However, this information must be machine understandable and it is in this point where the information techniques appear as context representation models.

Since the Strang and Linnhoff-Popien' review paper in 2004 [20], other surveys about context modeling for context-awareness have analyzed the appropriateness of different information representation methods in pervasive computing [1] [2]. In these works a comparison between different existing models is carried out taking into account models such as key-value, markup scheme, graphical, object oriented, logic and ontology based. In all of them ontology-based models have the best positions on the evaluation due to their expressiveness.

Ontologies are a knowledge representation model being used in a wide range of research works in context-aware pervasive computing. Service Oriented Context-Aware Middleware (SOCAM) developed by Gu et al. [6] collects some representative aspects we should take into account to develop a right context-aware middleware. A context aware infrastructure requires a common context model that can be shared by all devices and services and a set of services that perform context acquisition, context discovery, context interpretation and context dissemination. Also, context modeling and reasoning using ontologies requires a formal context model, design of context ontology and context classification and dependency. In CoCA [5], a services platform is implemented as Collaboration Manager, a module that works based on peer-to-peer negotiation and communication protocols. The role of the Collaboration Manager in CoCA services platform is to share computing resources like context, rules, ontology, etc., to solve computing problems and to provide comprehensive context-aware services, which would otherwise be difficult and sometimes impossible for a single pervasive device to solve. This module uses the principle of virtual network overlay. Among the basic requirements for collaborative computing between CoCA services in the neighborhood space is the ability to self-organize into groups, discover each other and each other's services and resources, for what is used JXTA. However, the central figure of the Collaboration Manager in CoCA can be a bottleneck in the system operations. Other related work is SOAM of Vazquez et al. [21]. SOAM is an experimental model for the creation of smart objects using ontologies on the web – i.e., Semantic Web technologies to enable communication between the semantic context and reasoning processes in order to provide an adaptation of the environment to user preferences. It also uses behavioral profiles. Based on these profiles, it provides a service collaborative model between different semantic objects in the environment.

In the work of Ye et al. a deep analysis about ontology-based models in pervasive computing systems is carried out [23]. They study and analyze several ontologies developed specifically for use in pervasive computing and why none of them appears to cover adequately all the aspects in this scope. Using these arguments, they have been identified the main points to be addressed in order to apply the ontological techniques successfully in pervasive systems: context and programming support, privacy and trust, discovery, interaction design and modeling uncertainty.

Context information is gathered from a variety of sources that differ in the quality of information they produce and that are often failure prone [2]. We shall see in this paper that the development of context-aware systems must be linked with an adequate context information modeling and data quality evaluation methodology. We can summary that there are two main general questions to be answered by developers of context-aware applications: (a) what will be the acquisition method used, and (b) what will be the information representation method. We also think that is relevant to answer a third one, (c) what will be the methodology used to determine correctness of the information or data quality.

3   DOHA Middleware

With new spaces of living and interaction associated with pervasive computing new software development paradigms have appeared. There are several aspects to solve related with these new spaces of interaction. Based on an extended literature review and as software engineers and researchers, we try to solve these tasks developing a well-defined software model based on distributed services. These services are capable to deploy complex and collaborative tasks and to be executed in embedded devices with constrained resources. The main objective of our research is to design and develop a complete service-based middleware for pervasive computing. However, to develop this middleware we have to take into account several restrictions that we should to resolve step by step – i.e., dynamicity and distributed character of the services, collaboration between services and use the environment information to achieve proactive behavior without the user intervention (context-aware services).

We have developed the Dynamic Open Home-Automation middleware (DOHA) [16]. It is based on the SOA paradigm and on the peer-to-peer (P2P) middleware JXTA at communication level. We choose a P2P-based solution because we were looking for a full decentralized, distributed approach, breaking with the client/server architecture which was the most common in service-based platforms. The P2P architecture also makes easier the interoperability between different devices and is transparent with respect gateways and firewalls. DOHA has been developed taking into account the constraints imposed by the use of devices with limited resources. As Fig. 1 shows, DOHA abstracts the physical distribution of devices and its management by a set of high-level collaborative services which are physically distributed in autonomous and independent nodes.

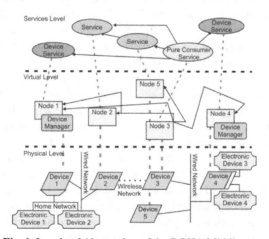

Fig. 1. Levels of Abstraction of the DOHA Middleware

3.1 DOHA Services

A DOHA Service is an autonomous self-contained component capable of performing specific activities or functions independently, that accepts one or more requests and returns one or more responses through a well-defined, standard interface.

A DOHA service has an internal structure organized in a set of software layers which form its anatomy. Fig. 2 shows the reduced class diagram of the DOHA middleware where are represented these layers. The *Interface Layer* is the public access point of the service. The *Application Layer* is the real core of the service. It is responsible to process the required operations received by the Interface Layer. Finally the *Interaction Layer* is responsible of managing the collaboration with other services, acting as a client of them.

In addition, there are three descriptive documents which form the base of the service specification: contract, composition map and configuration. S*ervice contract* describes the properties and the operations available in the service as service provider. *Service composition map* defines the composite operations that the distributed services can achieve collaboratively using a graph based representation. Finally, *service configuration* specifies the initial configuration parameters required to execute the service properly. The configuration parameters are related to the type of connectivity or physical location of the node where the service is running.

3.2 DOHA Service Composition Model

The collaboration between services in DOHA is solved by means of a service composition model. This composition model is based on orchestration principles – i.e., the control of the interaction is responsibility of each service, as well as the execution order of operations and flow of messages and transactions required in the collaboration.

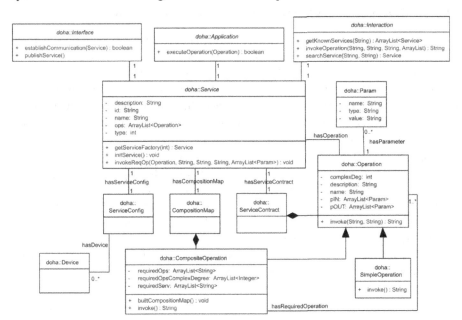

Fig. 2. Reduced Class Diagram of the DOHA Middleware

Service composition model in DOHA has two types of operations, simple and composite. A simple operation is a single transaction that the service can perform by itself. On the other hand, a composite operation involves the invocation of one or more operations in one or more services. The service that owns the composite operation is responsible of its execution and it must interact with the other services involved in the operation, the required services.

The composite operations are the base of the collaboration model of the platform and are listed by the *Service Composition Map*. We have developed a well-defined graph based model to ensure the acyclicity and correctness of the collaborative behavior of the DOHA services which was previously published in [8].

4   Modeling Context-Awareness in DOHA

DOHA services platform allows us to build pervasive applications based on a set of independent services. New services can be added without to know how are implemented or what are the operations of the rest of services in the platform. Each service in DOHA is built on the principle of decoupling the interface with respect of its implementation obtaining a component that is self-governing and self-contained. The functionality of DOHA services can be requested by any other services using its well-defined interface. The objective of this paper is to analyze how a new semantic high level layer will be added to DOHA platform and used by DOHA services to reach the goal of context-awareness.

4.1   Methodology: Software Engineering Using Design Science

Software has become a pervasive part of both our personal and professional lives [15]. Software Engineering (SE) as research discipline is a prerequisite for delivering high quality and robust software applications. The use of SE in the pervasive software development process ensures that the context-aware behavior of the end pervasive application conforms with user expectations and the design and implementation are reusable. In addition, verification and validation techniques are used to guaranty that we are building the correct application in the correct way.

Design Science (DS) approach is a methodology that proposes a set of analytical techniques and perspectives for conducting research in Information Systems (IS) [7]. DS research involves the design of novel or innovative artifacts and the analysis of the use and/or performance of such artifacts to improve and understand the behavior of aspects of IS. Such artifacts include algorithms (e.g. for information retrieval), system design methodologies, languages, etc.

We have developed the semantic, context-aware high level layer of DOHA platform following a SE design process using DS methodology.

4.2   Analysis and Design

As we introduced in Section 2, there are different architectures and frameworks trying to solve context-awareness in pervasive computing, and we included there three important questions to answer at previous stage on the development of context-aware systems.

In DOHA case, the acquisition method is directly linked with the use of DOHA services. The information of the environment, which will form the external context of the services, will be obtained by device services. These services encapsulate sensors and actuators that have a direct contact with the real world. The context information has to be represented electronically to be interpreted by services. We have studied different information representation methods, as we can see in Table 1. Using an extended literature review, included briefly in the background section of this paper, we choose ontologies and logic rules as information representation method. Finally, we have used context information processing using data profiling as methodology to determine the correctness of the information and data quality. We have extended DOHA platform using ontologies and DQ profiling. All the information related with services, operations and context data will be represented using ontologies and evaluated by means DQ profiling.

Including semantic information in DOHA platform by means ontologies brings the concept of semantic services. Using contextual information from physical world has several implications to consider related with how to obtain and process this information. Moreover, it is also necessary take into account the quality of the information involved in the context-awareness procedure. In this scope, we apply a data quality evaluation process before reasoning over data to obtain an effective proactive behavior in context-aware systems, as we can see in Fig. 3, which represents the context information processing flow. When an environment change is produced the system has to update the context information. After that, we apply a data quality evaluation process before reasoning over the data to obtain an effective proactive behavior applying an adequate action over the environment.

We propose a data quality approach for identifying semantic inaccuracies in the dynamic service composition result of the context-awareness [14]. Data profiling is a process of examining the existing data according to the environmental requirements

Table 1. Information representation methods

Artificial Intelligence	Systems modeling	Information systems
Data mining	Petri Network	Logic rules
Fuzzy logic	State machines	Ontologies

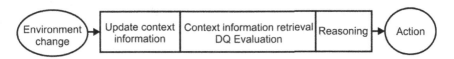

Fig. 3. Context information processing

and composing data profiles by the user of DOHA. Profiling is the stage of the DQ methodology where quality is defined [12]. Profiling helps to understand anomalies and to assess data quality, but also to discover, register, and assess contextual metadata [11]. Other benefits of the process of profiling also includes improving data quality, reducing the time for implementation of major projects, and the most important, improving the understanding of the data. Understanding of the data is vital criterion which lays the foundation of assessing DQ process. The idea of profiling in this paper is to build information profiles of the data used by services and operations. In order to do so in DOHA context, we consider the following characteristics: services involved in the composite process, data including data types/attributes and data format/structure; operations including the steps and activities in charge of data modification and transformation; and environmental/user requirement or condition needed to put the data into context. In Table 2, the contextual data (metadata) is classified of 'who', 'when', 'how' and 'what' format. This will serve as an input for the assessment stage and will enable detecting the semantically inaccurate data. This also will be foundation for the ontology that we are going to use to represent the service related information in DOHA.

In order to make good use of the context information we have analyzed the main requirements of context-aware systems, taking into account users and users preferences, embedded devices and environment data. Semantic services works with context information which has been represented considering different information models: *service model, space model* and *user model.* The *service model* describes and classifies the information elements which will be represented as services and processed by the system. The *space model* describes the physical space where the system is running and locates the *service model* in this space. Finally, the *user model* describes users' knowledge, interests and preferences. Each single information model has its own semantic representation using ontologies.

Service Functionality and Data Profiling

We have represented the data profiling schema (service, process, entity, information elements and requirements) using ontologies. Data profiling in DOHA is being implemented adding new classes to the middleware. Each element represented in the ontology of the data profiling is a new class in DOHA platform integrated with other classes which form the middleware. Data profiling in DOHA middleware will be also used to set the user preferences based on the services functionality.

Table 2. Data profiling in ubiquitous spaces

Who	How	What		When
Service	Process	Information Type/Entity	Information Elements	Requirements
Service name	Operation instance	Data Object	Data Attribute	Condition

Modeling data profiles using high level classes in DOHA helps us to keep independent the software model of the DOHA platform with respect to the data conceptualization of the specific information domain. For example, we can test different case studies applied to resolve context-awareness in smart home, industry or healthcare using DOHA middleware but with different kind of data – i.e., the data profiling representation and the data quality schema are independent of the application domain related to the final system.

Information of the Environment
The information of the environment forms the external context of the platform. This information will be captured by device services which encapsulate sensors and actuators with direct contact with the real world. This information will be represented using ontologies, too.

We are doing the design of the environment ontologies following a distributed design view. We will implement a general ontology "environment" with other specific ontologies related with each individual aspects of the environment to be used – e.g., temperature, light and humidity.

DOHA middleware has to be independent of the specific ontologies implemented to represent the information of the environment – i.e., if new elements of the real world are controlled, its ontologies will be added and recognized dynamically by DOHA.

We are using the Protégé Ontology Editor software in the design and implementation process of these ontologies [18]. Furthermore, we need to implement a parser in DOHA to pass between the format of the files built using Protégé and the DOHA classes that will use the ontologies information.

5   Case Study and Evaluation

We have used DOHA middleware in different domains of application related with pervasive computing, such as home-automation, e-health and industry. For example, in an emerging trend like the Internet of Things we have developed a case study using DOHA services to implement Data Fusion algorithms in industry domains [17]. These tests have helped us to improve the platform and to measure its applicability in distributed networks with high connectivity and a soaring number of services executing their functionality collaboratively.

We are now working building a full prototype of context-aware platform using the new version of the DOHA middleware, extended with the semantic high level layer. We have used a simple case study taking into account user preferences and simple information about the environment (light, temperature, presence and humidity), as we can see in Fig. 4. We will evaluate different scenarios in the context of an office room.

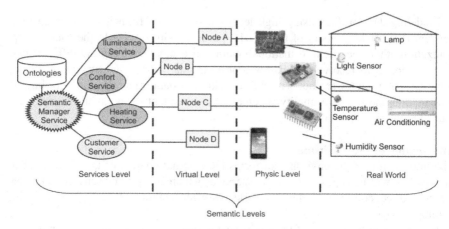

Fig. 4. Case Study

We have designed a special kind of DOHA service, the *Semantic Manager Service*. This service will be able to identify decayed data and manage the context-awareness. The *Semantic Manager Service* will share computing resources like context, rules and ontologies, to solve reasoning and to provide comprehensive context-awareness, which would otherwise be difficult and sometimes impossible for a single ubiquitous service to solve.

We are analyzing the different parts involved in the development, taking into account that the requirements will be a dynamic part related with all: data profiling, information of the environment and user preferences. Using data profiling and the information of the environment represented using ontologies, users will establish their preferences of behavior.

Also, we have defined usability, efficiency and effectiveness as operational requirements which will be used in the evaluation procedure.

To evaluate and measure *usability* we are going to use one of the fundamental metrics for that purpose called completion rates. *Completion rates metric* quantify the usability by collecting simple pass/fail metrics and reporting completion rates as a percentage. For example, related with the data profiling we would measure if the user/administrator identified the service name, process or entity involved in a given scenario. Also, related to the building of quality predicates we can measure if the user/administrator built the quality rule to constraint the office temperature or navigated through an interface to control the temperature value.

In order to measure the *efficiency* of the system developed we will use a time-based metric related with how long it takes the user/administrator and the system itself to complete a task in seconds. The Equation 1 evaluate the total task duration, where t_p is the time needed for profiling the data by the user, as well as building data quality predicates (using the ontologies in our case); and t_c is the time required to the DOHA middleware to acquire the environment information and process the context changes. This time will be influenced by the services' response and hardware speed.

$$t = t_p + t_c \tag{1}$$

6   Conclusions

DOHA is a SOA-based platform for the access, control and management of home-automation systems that facilitates the construction of dynamic, scalable and pervasive applications, based on a set of lightweight and independent services. In this paper we have expose the steps carried out in the process to model the context-aware layer in DOHA. To achieve that we are using a data quality approach and data profiles. In addition, we use ontologies as information representation method and to carry over the information about the profiles to the pervasive environment. By doing so, we assure proper representation of the real world and we are improving semantic data and context-awareness in such environments.

Semantic data quality problems are highly relevant for pervasive service environments. In these environments parties need to develop a shared understanding of the meaning of the data. The semantic layer of DOHA will use this as the context needed to achieve context-awareness. However, we argue that there is a lack of research about the data quality and quality of awareness particularly in these types of complex systems.

Currently, we are working to represent the information of the services from configuration, context and problem related data using service data profiling; establishing a semantic model of the real space which allows setting behavior patterns and which forms the base of the context-awareness; and designing the implementation of the user preferences linked with the requirements of the data profiling.

References

[1] Baldauf, M., Dustdar, S., Rosenberg, F.: A survey on context-aware systems. International Journal of Ad Hoc and Ubiquitous Computing 2(4), 263–277 (2007)

[2] Bettini, C., Brdiczka, O., Henricksen, K., Indulska, J., Nicklas, D., Ranganathan, A., Riboni, D.: A survey of context modelling and reasoning techniques. Pervasive and Mobile Computing 6(2), 161–180 (2010)

[3] Caire, P., van der Torre, L.: Convivial ambient technologies: Requirements, ontology and design. The Computer Journal 53(8), 1229–1256 (2010)

[4] Dey, A.K.: Understanding and using context. Personal and Ubiquitous Computing 5(1), 4–7 (2001)

[5] Ejigu, D., Scuturici, M., Brunie, L.: Hybrid approach to collaborative context-aware service platform for pervasive computing. Journal of Computers 3(1), 40–50 (2008)

[6] Gu, T., Pung, H.K., Zhang, D.Q.: A service-oriented middleware for building context-aware services. Journal of Network and Computer Applications 28(1), 1–18 (2005)

[7] Hevner, A.R., March, S.T., Park, J., Ram, S.: Design science in information systems research. MIS Q. 28(1), 75–105 (2004)

[8] Holgado-Terriza, J., Rodríguez-Valenzuela, S.: Services composition model for home-automation peer-to-peer pervasive computing. In: Proceedings of the Federated Conference on Computer Science and Information Systems, pp. 529–536 (2011)

[9] Kakousis, K., Paspallis, N., Papadopoulos, G.A.: A survey of software adaptation in mobile and ubiquitous computing. Enterp. Inf. Syst. 4(4), 355–389 (2010)

[10] Lassila, O.: Using the semantic web in mobile and ubiquitous computing. In: Bramer, M., Terziyan, V. (eds.) Industrial Applications of Semantic Web. IFIP, vol. 188, pp. 19–25. Springer, Heidelberg (2005)

[11] Loshin, D.: Enterprise knowledge management: the data quality approach. Morgan Kaufmann (2001)

[12] Oracle Inc.: Understanding Data Quality Management. In: Oracle® Warehouse Builder User's Guide (2008)

[13] Papazoglou, M., Traverso, P., Dustdar, S., Leymann, F.: Service-oriented computing: State of the art and research challenges. Computer 40(11), 38–45 (2007)

[14] Petkov, P., Helfert, M.: Bpel aided framework for constructing monitoring rules in service oriented architectures. In: 9th International Conference on Web Information Systems and Technologies, Aachen (2012)

[15] Preuveneers, D., Novais, P.: A survey of software engineering best practices for the development of smart applications in ambient intelligence. Journal of Ambient Intelligence and Smart Environments 4(3), 149–162 (2012)

[16] Rodríguez-Valenzuela, S., Holgado-Terriza, J.: A home-automation platform towards ubiquitous spaces based on a decentralized p2p architecture. In: International Symposium on Distributed Computing and Artificial Intelligence 2008 (DCAI 2008), vol. 50, pp. 304–308. Springer, Berlin (2009)

[17] Rodríguez-Valenzuela, S., Holgado-Terriza, J., Muros-Cobos, J.L., Gutiérrez-Guerrero, J.M.: Data fusion mechanism based on a service composition model for the internet of things. In: Actas de las III Jornadas de Computación Empotrada (JCE), Septiembre 19-21, vol. 1, pp. 64–69. Miguel Hernández University, Elche (2012)

[18] U. of Stanford: The protégé ontology editor and knowledge acquisition system, http://protege.stanford.edu

[19] Stojanovic, Z., Dahanayake, A.: Service-oriented software system engineering: challenges and practices. Idea (2005)

[20] Strang, T., Linnhoff-Popien, C.: A context modeling survey. In: Workshop Proceedings (2004)

[21] Vazquez, J., Sedano, I., López de Ipiua, D.: Soam: A web-powered architecture for designing and deploying pervasive semantic devices. International Journal of Web Information Systems 2(3), 212–224 (2007)

[22] Weiser, M.: The computer for the 21st century. Scientific American 256, 94–104 (1991)

[23] Ye, J., Coyle, L., Dobson, S., Nixon, P.: Ontology-based models in pervasive computing systems. Knowl. Eng. Rev. 22(4), 315–347 (2007)

Perspectives and Application of OUI Framework with SMaG Interaction Model

Sara Nabil and Atef Ghalwash

Computer Science Department, Faculty of Computer Science and Informatics,
Helwan University, Cairo, Egypt
sara.khnabil@gmail.com,
atef_ghalwash@yahoo.com

Abstract. OUI (Organic User Interface) together with NUI (Natural User Interface) and TUI (Tangible User Interface) falls under the field of Ubiquitous Computing, aiming to give the digital life a deeper human sense. Accordingly, we presented an OUI framework for designing OUIs to formalize the input and output interaction techniques for OUI users, and discuss it based on novel perspective of the organic interaction possible styles. We enhance the SMaG (Speech/ Manipulation/ air-Gesture) interaction model for organic interaction styles, in addition to our OUI design principles and design-specific guidelines in a perspective based on the usability aspects of the look, feel and design. Moreover, we propose a new usability model in this paper to enable measuring and testing the usability standards of organic systems, in which we called the 3Es usability model, referring to Efficiency, Enjoyment and Easiness.

Finally, we developed the 'OUI Sketcher' application as a case study for our proposed OUI framework and thus applying and testing the SMaG model. OUI Sketcher enables the user to create sketch figures and geometric drawings with all three OUI natural interactions (voice commands, touch and air-gestures) as interaction techniques, to apply the SMaG model perspectives and measure the usability standards against our OUI framework, using the 3Es usability model.

Keywords: Organic user interface, tangible interfaces, interaction techniques, ubiquitous computing, air gestures.

1 Introduction

Nowadays, technology is heading towards context-aware ubiquitous environments including novel forms of devices and interaction techniques for interfaces that are getting rather natural, tangible and even organic interfaces. NUI (Natural user interface) is known to have no traditional separate devices for data input (such as keyboard or mouse), but depend on natural actions and interaction techniques that opens the way for ubiquitous multi-touch multi-user systems. Today's tablets, smart phones and other various handheld devices are all examples of NUIs. TUI (Tangible user interface) is known for using graspable physical artefacts- called tangibles- to control digital information seamlessly in the user's physical environment, make use of

M.J. O'Grady et al. (Eds.): AmI 2013 Workshops, CCIS 413, pp. 283–295, 2013.
© Springer International Publishing Switzerland 2013

the already existing usability experience and haptic interaction skills that users have with real-world objects, as a subset from NUI. OUI (Organic User Interface) is not only a subset of NUI, but can be perceived as the NUI's legal heir. OUI is simply defined as interfaces that have non-planar displays that may actively or passively change shape via analog physical inputs [1].

In this paper we present our OUI interaction framework that is based on earlier frameworks of TUI and GUI, in addition to discussing our SMaG model for OUI input interaction techniques, and design principles and guidelines for organic interfaces. Then we propose an OUI usability standards model, we called the 3Es usability model for testing and measuring the SMaG interaction model for OUI systems. Finally, we introduce a software application in which we developed to apply and measure our OUI interaction model and framework using the 3Es usability model.

2   UI Frameworks

In this section we examine the related work of frameworks of earlier user interfaces, such as GUI and TUI, and our developed OUI framework based on the mentioned earlier frameworks.

2.1   GUI and TUI Frameworks

Ishii [1] presented the TUI framework as an evolution to its predecessor GUI framework, as shown in Figure 1. The GUI framework is constructed mainly from the MVC model (Model-View-Control) in which there is a clear distinction between the input and the output devices in the physical layer. On the other hand, the TUI framework is constructed from the MCRpd model (Model-Control-Representation, physical and digital). In the MCRpd framework, the 'model' is kept in the digital layer, however the 'view' is divided into both a physical representation and a digital

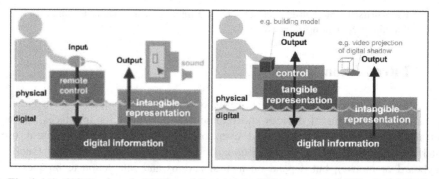

Fig. 1. left: GUI framework (MVC model) and right: TUI framework (MCRpd model) [1]

representation denoted by 'rep-p' and 'rep-d' respectively referring to tangible (such as physical objects), and intangible (such as sounds, images and video projections) representations of both physical and digital input interaction styles.

2.2   OUI Framework

Although, Ishii's TUI framework[1] shows the distinction between the two types of 'view': the tangible and intangible representation of information; that is the physical view (rep-p) and the digital view (rep-d), yet, we believe the 'control' module should be either tangible or intangible as well, as it represents all user input interaction techniques. Based on Ishii's work, we presented an OUI framework[2] that indicates the clear distinction between the 'touchable control' and 'touchless control'. The distinction between the touchable touchless control came from the fact that user interactions with organic systems does not only depend on touch, deformation and direct hand manipulation of physical objects and tangibles, but includes speech interactions and touchless air gestures as well.

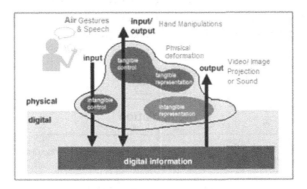

Fig. 2. OUI Framework (SMaG model)

Touchable Controls represent the physically touchable input, requiring direct interaction in which are mostly natural, anticipatory and intuitive and perceived by the user as real-world interactions,   including   hand touch, deformable and non-deformable hand manipulations of displays, physical objects and tangible devices. Touchable representation is the common area between control and representation: input and output, as shown in Figure 2. The physical input interactions of display touch, hand manipulation or deformation is responded by the system with corresponding output interactions on the same touch screen or deformable surface.

3   SMaG Interaction Model

3.1   Earlier Interaction Models

GUI frameworks depend on WIMP (window-icon-menu-pointer) interaction model for many years, providing the user with a mouse cursor pointer to select, navigate and activate required tasks, programs or processes. On the other hand, ubiquitous environments with NUI TUI and OUI interfaces evolved making the separate input devices such as keyboards and mice rather dispensable, leading to the gradual collapse of WIMP techniques. Thus, the new generation of interaction techniques appeared providing users with seamless intuitive natural experience, named by Van Dam[4] the post-WIMP interfaces, described to be rather more continuous input techniques that have natural interactions than the discrete input interactions of the earlier GUIs.

3.2   OUI Interaction Model

The OUI SMaG[2] user interaction model refers to the three main interaction categories: speech, hand manipulation and in-air gestures, as shown in Figure 3. First, speech is divided into two types: normal speech recognition and subvocal speech recognition (silent speech). Second, hand manipulations are either discrete touch, continuous touch, deformable manipulations, non-deformable manipulations, and manipulating tangibles. Third, air gestures that have different types: unimanual and bimanual hand gestures (hand wave), gaze gestures (eye tracking), face gestures (facial expressions) and other body postures and movements.

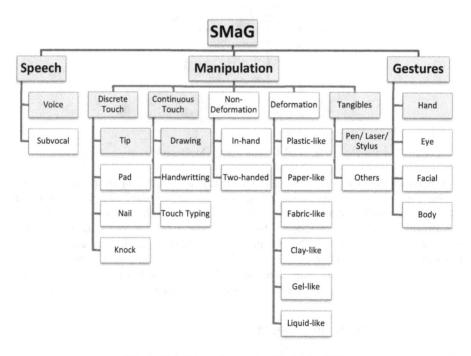

Fig. 3. SMaG input Interaction Model for OUI

Speech. Speech is one of the oldest means of interaction between human, requiring almost no effort, or even any hand, or body movement. As much as speech forms a natural way of communication between humans in their daily life, so it should be one day between human and computers, as interfaces get more natural, and computers get ubiquitous around us.

Voice Recognition. Speech recognition have been studied widely as an interaction technique for computer devices. Although it is proven hard to reach an optimum percentage of error-free speech recognition, some systems depend on speech as an essential interaction technique specially for users with speech impairments or in medical procedures where it is a must for doctors not to compromise sterility by touching buttons, keys or switches.

However, speech interaction can be very difficult or nearly impossible in crowded or noisy places. Moreover, environments that require silent interaction for either confidentiality or special-security purposes, cannot make use of normal language speech recognition technologies, but require a silent-speech recognition technology to an efficient interaction technique.

Subvocal Speech Recognition. In order to overcome the limitations of using voice recognition, some researches were made to make use of the vibrations of vocal chords of a human's silent speech. Yonck [6] described the silent speech recognition as "sub-vocal" speech recognition in which the user's silent speech forms input to the system through a small device on the user's throat reading his nerve signals directly from his throat, converting them to electric signals and sends them to a remote computer that translates them into words (commands). Subvocal interaction technique can be used with speech-impaired users, fire-fighters and special forces. Subvocal speech can be very useful in speech non-conducting medium, such as underwater for divers or in the outer space for astronauts. NASA Ames Research Center is currently developing a subvocal system for eventual use in astronauts' suits [6].

Hand Manipulations. Hand manipulations enable users to interact with the system through physical naturally affordable actions. Hand manipulations can be divided into two types: touch, and manipulations. Touch is either discrete touch or continuous touch. Manipulations are three types deformable manipulations, non-deformable manipulations, and tangibles manipulation.

Discrete and Continuous Touch. Touch interactions are two types either discrete touch or continuous touch. Discrete touch, also called 'tab', refers to single point touch in which the user touches a single point for a certain interval of time either short or long with a certain amount of pressure with the finger on the display surface. Continuous touch, such as 'drag' or 'draw', refers to finger touch moving in continuous non-stop motion on the surface of the display in an unbroken curve of motion, until the user lifts his/ her finger of the display to draw a figure or drag an icon.

Tapsense[7] enhanced the finger touch interaction by studying the different parts in a human finger, such as the tip, pad, nail and knuckle, in which presented different possible input interaction techniques for discrete touch.

In general, we highlighted in [2] the factors on which a touch input can be defined being either discrete or continuous touch, the touch type: tip, pad, nail, knuckle, the number and location of simultaneous touch points, pressure, duration, and in case of continuous touch add the shape, direction, and distance of touch path on display surface.

One kind of discrete touch is texting or touch typing. Texting does not imply keyboard typing, but indicates to the use of bare fingers to type on a graphical or projected on-screen keyboard directly on the display surface. Touch texting is often referred to as thumb typing or thumb-texting. One kind of continuous touch is free drawing. Free drawing refers to user drawing free-hand letters, numbers, figures or shapes directly on the display surface, as an input interaction style.

Deformable and Non-deformable Manipulation. Deformable manipulations are those natural actions in which the user can change the shape of the display surface with his bare hands to cope with the type of action he attempts to input to the system. For example folding a digital paper to deactivate its digital content and unfolding it to activate it.

Non-deformable manipulations are those natural actions in which the user does not change the shape of the display surface but can rather include rotation, moving or shifting its position or just change its orientation. For example stacking several digital papers or flipping one along is a non-deformable input interaction technique.

In general, these hand manipulation input interactions are based on three factors: 1) The manipulation type: deformable or non-deformable manipulations, 2) The motion axis: landscape, portrait, or diagonal, 3) The motion direction: positive, negative or dual.

In 2010, Sang-Su[8] studied the usability of four types of materials; paper, elastic cloth, and plastic by observing human manipulations when using them as deformable displays. We divided the types of deformational manipulations[2] -based on material type- as those that resemble natural manipulations: plastic-like, paper-like, fabric-like, clay-like, gel-like and liquid-like.

Tangibles Manipulations. Although, tangibles are touchable physical separate controls, tangibles are used seamlessly in the user's physical environment, with natural interactions and thus tangibles are not comparable with traditional separate input devices (keyboard and mouse). Tangible manipulations make use of the already existing usability experience and haptic interaction skills that users have with real-world physical objects. Not only does tangibles give physical representation to the digital content, but also enables this digital content -represented by the physical tangible- to be directed manipulated through the user by his bare hand.

Consequently, tangibles manipulation can be used as an interaction style in an organic system to add more intuition to the system. For example, handwriting with bare fingers can seem more awkward than handwriting with a pen. That is why using a tangible pen (stylus) in this case will be more natural to the user than his/ her own hands.

Air Gestures. Air Gestures or 'gestures' are the non-verbal form of touchless interaction that relies on visual communication of human hand, face or body. Although gestures have been used by man since the beginning of mankind as a primary means of communication that is sometimes even more efficient than speech, yet gestures has only been used in the field of human computer interaction except just recently, for the complexity of designing a system that could capture hand movements, facial expressions, eye tracking or body motion, and be always be in the ON mode for capturing such gestures. Different types of gestures can be used for different types of input interactions for performing different tasks or actions, where hand gestures can be using one or both hands. We summarized the factors[2] on which a gesture can be captured and identified by the gesture type: single hand, two hands, eye, face, feet, shoulders, body, the gesture motion axis: landscape, portrait, diagonal, the gesture direction: forward, backward, inward, or outward, and the gesture speed.

Gesture are usually captured by using infrared, colored markers and cameras for image recognition and tracking motions. Whereas, in SoundWave[9] the system uses the Doppler effect to capture gestures, by generating an inaudible tone that gets frequency-shifted when it reflects off moving objects such as the user's hand. Using the speaker and microphone already embedded inside the computer, to sense and capture different user gestures around the device, SoundWave can distinguish the basic input interactions such as: scrolling, single-tap and double-tap, activation, deactivation and rotation. For instance, SoundWave uses the walking gesture to automatically put a computer to sleep or wake it up and the Two-Handed Seesaw for rotation.

In BodyScape[11], authors presented innovative body gestural interaction techniques and classified them according to the relative location of the user's body from the input and output devices in a multi-surface environment. The body-centric free hand gestural interactions in BodyScape[11] compared between on-body touch and mid-air pointing and then combined the two together in another combined interaction technique, through defining different dominant and non-dominant body parts: torso, both arms and both legs.

In GravitySpace[12], authors presented walking recognition of users or movement of furniture using gravity pressure on pressure-sensitive interactive floor, using the capturing of unique imprints of pressure distribution caused by users walking gestures on the flat floor surface. GravitySpace also recognizes the posture gestures based on the texture and spatial arrangement of contact points on the interactive floor surface.

We conclude here that air gestures are not only about waving hands in the air at a distance from the display surface in natural gestures, but are extended to include normal body motions, leaning, walking or moving intuitively in the ubiquitous space.

Advantages of using gestures as an interaction style is that they do not need direct interaction, thus will maintain sterility in medical places such as clinics and hospitals, in contrary with direct touch or hand manipulation that can cause infections by contagious surfaces. Gestures as more suitable for distance interaction and 'large displays' than direct hand touch or manipulation. Gestures also supersede speech interactions in noisy environments. On the other hand, gestures disadvantages is basically inappropriateness in public places or multiuser systems or collaborative environments, inaccuracy –compared to speech and touch- and inefficiency of false positive and false negative gestures.

4   OUI Design Guidelines and Usability Standards

4.1   OUI Design Principles

Holman[13] introduced the three main OUI design principles that are considered the basic foundation for any guidelines or rules of OUI systems design. The OUI design principles[13] are 1) Input Equals Output: indicating that the device display is also the input device, 2) Form Equals Function: indicating that the display can take any form and be dynamic enough to change its shape to match the intended functionality as be bent inwards to zoom-in and so on, 3) Form Follows Flow: indicates that the display can change its shape and be dynamic enough so as to change according to the flow of the user interactions. Holman[14] introduced four broad rules for OUI designers, derived from the natural laws of biology, physics and human cognition. These four principles are fluidity, intuitiveness, robustness and calmness.

We discussed in [2] the drawbacks of Holman's[13] OUI design principles in which they do not comply with the input interaction techniques that does not necessarily equals the output, such as touchless gestures and speech commands, and ignored output that does not equal input, such as physical deformations of display surface as response or feedback to user input. Same applies for the second and third principles that apply only to flexible displays that can actively or passively change their shape but does not apply on all nowadays tablets and devices that enable the user to interact by touch, manipulations, speech and gestures interactions styles.

The three design principles of the organic user interface and its input interaction techniques we proposed to tackle the three points of interest: the look, feel and design successively.

P1 Natural, Intuitive Feel. OUI should feel as natural and intuitive to the user as using every-day real world objects, allowing the user to "expect output from the input".

P2 Organic, Fluid Look. OUI should look flexible and malleable (non-planer) as much as it makes it natural to see and use, being fluid enough to take any shape, change its shape (or at least contents) for visual feedback to users actions, and flow seamlessly between states.

P3 Context-aware, Calm Design. OUI should be designed -using the best suitable metaphor- to be ubiquitous, seamless and calm when not in use and aware of the context of use. Moreover, ensuring input actions must always give same responses.

4.2   OUI Design-Specific Guidelines

Based on the design guidelines for natural user interfaces[10], we proposed design-specific guidelines[2] for designing organic interfaces for each interaction style in the SMaG interaction model (Speech, Manipulation and Gesture).

The OUI design-specific guidelines are:

G1 Speech. Best fit when used with large displays, home appliances, and medical care places requiring sterility. However should be avoided in public places, multiuser systems and dangerous actions to avoid errors of high impact. Speech is captured either by voice recognition techniques or by sub-vocal speech recognition directly from the user's throat.

G2 Hand Touch and Manipulation. Best fit when used in multiuser systems, home appliances, public places, classrooms, offices, showrooms. However, should be avoided in large displays, and medical care places requiring sterility. Hand manipulations is captured either by touch-sensing, accelometers or by image or video recognition techniques.

G3 Air Gestures. Best fit when used with large displays, home appliances, medical care places requiring sterility. However, should be avoided in public places, multiuser systems and dangerous actions. Air Gestures are captured by either by image or video recognition techniques or by inaudible air frequency shift.

4.3   OUI Usability Standards

In this paper we designed a model for OUI usability standards to be able to measure the affordance and effectiveness of organic systems by users interaction through SMaG interaction model. The usability model we introduce simply contains three aspects: efficiency, enjoyment and easiness. Efficiency measures how much the system is accurate in capturing the input technique. Enjoyment measures how much the system is fun when the user interacts with. Easiness measures the simplicity of the system and the 'ease of use' from the user's point of view. We name our usability standards with the **3Es Usability Model**, referring to: Efficiency, Enjoyment, and Easiness.

Imagine the 3Es model of OUI usability standards as a triangle with its three edges representing the three usability aspects: efficiency, enjoyment and easiness, in which the triangle is meaningless without any one of its three edges.

We believe that efficiency alone creates an accurate system which is not necessarily easy to use or fun for the user. Same applies, an easy fun system loses its enjoyment when the user faces many errors or wrongfully detected input commands due to inefficient inaccurate recognition. On the other hand, the accurate easy system does not attract users nowadays if it is not quite fun and enjoying to use. Users expectations are getting higher every day with increasing requirements of fancy interfaces that are easy yet fun and for sure, quality of accuracy is a must.

5   The Application: OUI Sketcher

In this final section, we describe the software application that we developed to be a case study for our proposed OUI framework and thus applying and testing the SMaG model. We called our software application the 'OUI Sketcher', as it uses OUI interactions to help the user create sketch figures and geometric drawings.

5.1   System Description

The OUI Sketcher application is intended to help users to draw simple sketches for their and drawings using natural gestures and interaction techniques through a user-friendly interface in a context-aware medium. The user only draws simple lines, rectangles and required shapes with either their own hands or the tangible pen stylus, then the system instantly uses its pattern recognition module to render the drawn shape or irregular line into uniform perfect matching geometric shape.

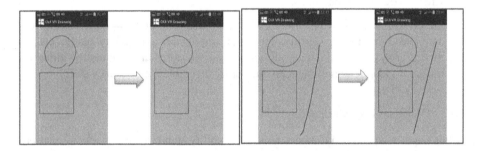

Fig. 4. a) OUI Sketcher snap shot while user drawing a free hands circle (left) and while user drawing a free hands line (left) and line automatically rendered in perfect shape (right)

5.2   System Capabilities and Constraints

The system is featured with three main capabilities: Pattern Recognition, Voice Recognition and air- Gesture recognition. The pattern recognition uses a shape matching module to be able to convert pen-based or hand-free touch drawing into perfectly rendered shapes in the same size, location and color automatically once the user lifts his/ her finger up from the surface of the display, seamlessly, as in Figure 4. The voice recognition module does not need any training or user detection, it detects only simple commands: 'DELETE', 'RED','BLUE','GREEN', as a proof-of-concept application and not a software-limitation. The gesture recognition module uses the Nanogest touchless gesture recognition SDK, with an academic research license from Nanocritical®, using the front-facing camera of device to detect hand wave to 'DELETE' as a clear, wipe or remove gesture to delete the current drawing or draft.

5.3   Applying the SMaG Model

In Figure 3, the SMaG model appears with all its categories of Speech, Manipulation and Gestures, with green highlighted types of interactions that are applied in the 'OUI Sketcher' application: voice recognition, touch (tab), handling tangible pen (stylus), and hand waves gestures. Thus we can say that the 'OUI Sketcher' makes use of all three categories of the SMaG model giving the user the variety of choice from different interaction techniques.

5.4   Usability Testing Results

To measure the users satisfactory level of the OUI Sketcher application with respect to the different SMaG interaction styles, we performed the 3Es usability testing model for OUIs. Users were chosen from different age groups and were asked to compare between different interaction styles used in the application for the same action from three aspects: efficiency, enjoyment and easiness, by simple questions rating how accurate, fun and easy was each of the three interaction techniques: voice (speech), touch (hand manipulation) and hand wave (air gesture). Table 1 shows the average results of the user survey when asked to answer on scale from 1 to 10, given 1 is the least rating and 10 is the highest rating.

Table 1. Usability testing average rating (1-10)

Interaction Style		Simplicity	Enjoyment	Efficiency	Overall Rating
Speech	Voice	9	9	8	9
Manipulation	Touch	8	8	9	8
Gesture	Wave	5	6	4	5

The average results is shown in graphical data representation in Figure 5. The results shows clearly the efficiency of touch over other interaction techniques while the simplicity of voice commands over touch and wave, and the poor overall rating of the wave gesture in the three aspects of efficiency, enjoyment and easiness. The poor overall rating of wave gesture was due to the unsure feeling of the user that he/ she is doing the right motion or expecting the right response from the system, perhaps it is the newest technology that gives the user this doubt, or may be of the inaccuracy of gesture recognition due to different lighting conditions, different motion speed of user hand, different distance of user hand from display surface, ..etc.

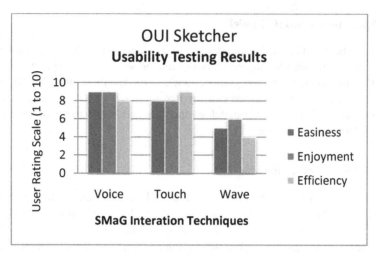

Fig. 5. Usability testing results of OUI Sketcher

6   Conclusion and Future Work

In this paper we introduced our OUI framework for organic systems design, and enhanced our SMaG interaction model for OUI input interaction techniques, to formalize input controls into their three main types: speech, hand manipulations and air gestures. In addition to the broad OUI design principles, and design-specific guidelines for each SMaG interaction type, we proposed the 3Es usability model for organic user interfaces in ubiquitous environments. We then developed a software application that implements each type of SMaG model to measure our framework against interaction techniques using the 3Es usability standards proposed in this paper. Our OUI application is a simple sketching app that automatically and instantaneously converts user's hand sketches into uniform geometrical shapes. Users were able to delete the current sketch using touch, voice command or hand wave gesture. We found that speech interaction is becoming more efficient, enjoying and easy to use often more than direct touch hand manipulation interaction. While the touchless hand wave air gesture was found to be rather less efficient or fun or easy for most of our users in the usability testing performed.

In our future work, we intend to apply our SMaG interaction model on other OUIs that are designed in the OUI framework and based on the design principles and guidelines, we will further be testing these organic systems according to the same 3Es usability standards.

References

1. Ishii, H.: Tangible Bits: Beyond Pixels. In: Proc. Of the Second International Conference on Tangible and Embedded Interaction (TEI 2008), Bonn, Germany (2008)
2. Ghalwash, A., Nabil, S.: Organic User Interfaces: Framework. Interaction model and Design Guidelines. International Journal of Ad hoc, Sensor & Ubiquitous Computing (IJASUC) 4(4) (2013)

3. Vertegaal, R., Poupyrev, I.: Organic Interaction Technologies. Communications of the ACM 51(6), 26–30 (2008)
4. Van Dam, A.: Post-WIMP User Interfaces. Communications of the ACM (1997)
5. de Vries, A.: Multi-Touch Interaction Overview., http://www.tno.nl/nui
6. Yonck, R.: The Age of the Interface. World Future Society, MD (2010)
7. Harrison, C., Schwarz, J., Hudson, S.: TapSense: Enhancing Finger Interaction on Touch Surfaces. In: ACM UIST 2011, Santa Barbara, CA, USA, October 16-19 (2011)
8. Lee, S., Kim, S., Jin, B., Choi, E., Kim, B., Jia, X., Kim, D., Lee, K.: How Users Manipulate Deformable Displays as Input Devices. In: Proc. CHI 2010. ACM, New York (2010)
9. Gupta, S., et al.: SoundWave: Using the Doppler Effect to Sense Gestures. In: CHI 2012, Austin, Texas, USA, May 5-10 (2012)
10. Wigdor, D., Wixon, D.: Brave NUI World: Designing Natural User Interfaces for Touch and Gesture (2010) ISBN 978-0-12-382231-4
11. Wagner, J., et al.: A Body-centric Design Space for Multi-surface Interaction. In: CHI 2013 - 31st International Conference on Human Factors in Computing Systems (2013)
12. Bränzel, A., et al.: GravitySpace: Tracking Users and Their Poses in a Smart Room Using a Pressure-Sensing Floor. In: CHI 2013, Paris, France (2013)
13. Holman, D., Vertegaal, R.: Organic user interfaces: designing computers in any way, shape, or form. Communications of the ACM 51 (2008)
14. Holman, D., Diehl, J., Karrer, T., Borchers, J.: Organic User Interfaces, Media Computing Group, RWTH Aachen University, Germany, http://hci.rwth-aachen.de/organic

An Open Architecture to Enhance Pervasiveness and Mobility of Health Care Services

Iván Corredor, Paula Tarrío, Ana M. Bernardos, and José R. Casar

Universidad Politécnica de Madrid, ETSI Telecomunicación,
Av. Complutense 30 28040 Madrid, Spain

Abstract. This paper describes a system for ubiquitous monitoring of health and physical parameters, suitable to run on home-based infrastructures and personal mobile settings. The system is built on a micro Web of Things Open Platform (μWoTOP), enabling easy integration of sensing and processing modules. It also facilitates building ubiquitous services by accessing biometric sensors through uniform interfaces based on REST. Additionally, the system is capable of processing user context and generate alerts based on the Common Alerting Protocol, making its output compatible with already existing medical solutions. The system has been customized to deploy a fall/faint detection solution, which enables multiple supervisors with the capability of receiving real time alerts on monitored subjects.

Keywords: Open pervasive architecture, Web of Things, user context monitoring, sensor fusion.

1 Introduction

During the last decade, research groups focused on pervasive computing have been tackling heterogeneous ecosystems of contextual sources involving sensors and actuators which are embedded in everyday and personal objects (e.g. smartphones and wearables). Currently, all those embedded devices are capable of interacting with each other in order to reason about some aspects of the user context. The *Internet of Things* paradigm has contributed with mechanisms and protocols to make possible this kind of communication. New approaches in pervasive computing are dealing with proposals to increase the ubiquity and the mobility of these IoT-based ecosystems with the aim of interconnecting isolated systems and to offer such amount of context information to external services and applications. This is considered the next step in the IoT evolution, called the *Web of Things*, which tries to integrate embedded devices into the current Internet as typical Web resources without including too much additional technology.

In this paper, we describe a system for ubiquitous monitoring of health parameters, which aims at facilitating deployments in both home and mobile personal settings. The system is capable of autonomously generating standardized alerts according to configured health parameters. The technological pillar of this system is built on the micro Web of Things Open Platform (μWoTOP), the major

M.J. O'Grady et al. (Eds.): AmI 2013 Workshops, CCIS 413, pp. 296–307, 2013.
© Springer International Publishing Switzerland 2013

research contribution of our proposal, which facilitates both connecting external sensors and developing consumer application by using REST interfaces. In order to enable interoperability, the proposed system includes an alert notification component that handles alerts in Common Alerting Protocol format. The proposal is validated through the implementation of a multi-device fall/faint detector and a remote mobile client for supervision and emergency response.

The paper is structured as follows. Section 2 contains a review of the state of the art on Web of Things platforms capable of deploying alert or event notification services. Sections 3 and 4 present the requirements and architecture of μWoTOP, respectively. Section 5 shows, through illustrative examples, how a fall/faint detector has been implemented for a specific case of use in which a supervisor service satisfactorily obtain alerts. Section 6 includes performance values for the proposed system. Conclusions and further work are in Section 7.

2   Related Work and Background

Nowadays, user devices (e.g. smartphones) equipped with sensors have become platforms enabling emergency detection tools. Among the various risky situations that may be better solved by using pervasive technologies, health ones are attracting a lot of attention in the commercial landscape [4]. For example, special attention is put on systems notifying risks in time [7]. In particular, fall detection [8] is a typical application of those systems. Many of these health systems are built on heterogeneous sensors from different manufacturers. This fact has raised the need of managing hardware and software through a unique, public and global solution. The WoT has been proposed as a feasible approach to carry out this challenge. The major characteristic of the WoT is to wrap smart things using Web interfaces so that communication barriers among *virtual* and *real* worlds can be removed. Basically, the WoT-based solutions are usually divided into two groups [11]: i) directly integrated into the Web, and ii) indirectly integrated into the Web.

On one hand, to integrate smart things directly into the Web, it is required that all of them have IP connectivity and then, to implement an embedded Web server in every smart thing. In previous research work, we have already explored such approach [2] through a Knowledge-Aware and Service-Oriented (KASO) middleware that enabled access points to expose sensors and actuators as REST resources. In the same line, Guinard et al. [5] proposed a RESTful prototype consisting of running an embedded Web server on Sun SPOT nodes. Thus, node's sensors can be accessed by invoking a GET method directly over a URI managed by a Sun SPOT. Similarly, Vazquez et al. [10] suggest deploying a tiny HTTP client on an embedded platform. In general, the major benefit of approaches integrated directly into the Web is the low latency when accessing resources provided by embedded web servers. The major weakness is the lack of scalability related to the limitations of embedded devices, in terms of energy, CPU or memory, that make difficult offering services guaranteeing a minimum Quality of Service level (e.g. latency or reliability).

On the other hand, the indirect integration of smart things into the Web consists of enabling an intermediate proxy or smart gateway to handle isolated networks of embedded devices. These smart gateways bridge the gap between embedded devices and the Web by implementing at least two protocol stacks: a full TCP/IP protocol stack to communicate with Internet-connected entities, and a proprietary protocol stack (e.g. Zigbee or Bluetooth). The latter will allow communicating with smart things. Smart gateways usually expose smart thing functionalities through uniform interfaces. An early design of a smart gateway was proposed by Trifa et al. [9] that integrated embedded devices into the Web through a system based on drivers. The *SmartThing*[1] project has recently launched a SmartThings Hub, which is a smart gateway exposing embedded and customizable devices to be mapped over RESTful interfaces.

Another common solution is to offer WoT platforms according to cloud computing premises applying the Platform as a Service (PaaS) paradigm. Xively [2], EVRYTHNG [3], Paraimpu [4] or ThingSpeak [5] are popular examples of this kind of services. These platforms provide RESTful services through which information can be managed only by accessing URIs that identify each data stream, usually called feeds or channels. The most usual set of services provided by these platforms comprise processing, sharing, mashuping and dashboards for sensors and actuators. Services provided by these platforms are specially focused on those systems needing high scalability levels. However, they strongly depend on cloud services and, thus, on the Internet infrastructure. Thus, the major weaknesses of this type of solutions are the lack of security in information transactions and unpredictable latencies when notifying events to the clients.

To overcome the above mentioned drawbacks, we propose a lightweight WoT platform, the μWoTOP, which can be deployed on everyday devices. Our proposal is explained in next Sections illustrated by means of a functional setting in which the objective is to support rapid care assessment and intervention.

3   System Requirements and Service Entities

Generally speaking, requirements of any eHealth system are very demanding since this kind of systems involves a lot of sensitive factors (e.g. general usability, wearable and low intrusive biometric sensors or management of confidential reports). Additionally, when an eHealth system is focused on stimulating independent living (as it could be a fall/faint detector application), those requirements become even more demanding. The most relevant requirements, which were considered to make proper design decisions, were classified under two groups: a) functional (focused on the system behavior) and b) non-functional (focused on

---

[1] http://www.smartthings.com/
[2] https://xively.com/
[3] http://www.evrythng.com/
[4] http://paraimpu.crs4.it/
[5] https://www.thingspeak.com/

the system constraints). The first group of requirements involves the instant detection of abnormal health-related events and its notification to applications or services interested in them. The second group includes the easy integration of non-intrusive and heterogeneous wearables (mainly biometric sensors), a high pervasiveness and integrability of the provided services into the user environment and the definition of standardized interfaces and information models in order to be accessible by as many clients as possible.

The above-mentioned requirements have driven the design decisions of the architecture for our eHealth system. Willing to provide a holistic solution both for mobile health monitoring and Ambient Home Care Systems, we hereby propose an eHealth architecture that can be customized in different application settings with minimum changes. In particular, we have worked on our existing proposals [2] to adapt them to the requirements that the health-monitoring scenario may require. The foundations of the system architecture are supported by three key elements performing different roles:

A. *Wireless wearables and their data fusion components*: A heterogeneous set of biometric sensors (e.g. heart monitor, accelerometer, body thermometer), some of which are capable of performing a previous preprocessing of sensors readings and communicate their result to other architectural elements.

B. *μWoTOP Gateways*: Their major role is to setup an event-driven message bus collecting health events detected by the wearables and transmitting urgent notifications to those entities interested in such events (e.g. medical staff at a hospital or assistants at a residence). μWoTOP Gateways can be run on two kinds of devices: infrastructure devices (i.e. fixed devices), or mobile user devices (e.g. smartphones or tablets enabled as gateways).

C. *Consumer applications*: These are pieces of software that run on user devices, both mobile and fixed (e.g. mini PCs or smart TVs). They have to implement a module to use platform services, among them the eventing service.

4 System Architecture Overview: The Micro Web of Things Open Platform

The Micro Web of Things Open Platform (μWoTOP) is based on a lightweight implementation of an open platform that was initially designed for conventional devices, i.e. PC or high capacity server. The μWoTOP Gateway has been designed according to the REST architectural paradigm [3] and Event-driven techniques. According to the "open" nature of the μWoTOP, a public REST-based API is provided allowing quick prototyping of complex applications by reusing a lot of resources, mainly sensors and actuators, in order to create mashups of real-world services.

μWoTOP follows a Platform as a Service (PaaS) approach (Fig. 1), being possible to deploy it on one or more resource-constrained computers (e.g. mini PCs or smartphones) in order to create a Peer-to-Peer (P2P) network of synchronized Gateways with standardized API. This interface provides functionalities

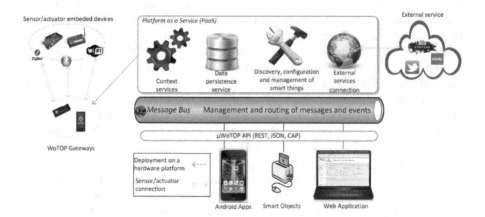

Fig. 1. μWoTOP exposed as a set of cloud services and some of the external clients that can use those services a message bus

that enable access to smart things and other contextual services (e.g. localization service) by means of a message bus. This bus enables a virtual channel offering two communication modes: *event-driven* and *on-demand*. The former dispatches events to the clients which have been previously subscribed to them. These events are usually related to an environment event detected by a smart thing through some sensor (e.g. temperature exceeding a threshold, the presence of an inhabitant, etc.). The latter works like a synchronous request-reply mechanism. The above-mentioned communication mechanisms are based on the REST architectural style and other standardized data formats as JavaScript Object Notation (JSON) or, specifically for health use cases, the Common Alert Protocol (CAP). Developers are provided with a development environment that includes a middleware defining a programming model to access the message bus that abstracts both underlying communication protocols and message formats.

Different drivers can be implemented by each Gateway in order to accept wireless connections from many different sensor/actuator devices. These devices and other contextual service being managed by a specific μWoTOP Gateway can be accessed through any other associated Gateway. This is a service offered by a discovery mechanism that notably increases the ubiquitous and scalability of the deployed services.

Finally, the μWoTOP includes a mechanism that performs data scheduling tasks in order to manage massive amounts of data generated by the smart things. The data scheduling is composed of a set of mechanisms which optimize the storage and persistence of historic data as well as the access to them. Ideally, these data will be stored in a local server or in a trusted storage cloud service.

Next Section is focused on a case study of the eHealth system that includes some details of how to use the μWoTOP.

5 Case of Use: A Fall/Faint Detector for Quick Intervention

5.1 Motivation Scenario

To demonstrate how μWoTOP can be used and to evaluate its architecture, we have built on top of it a fall/faint detection system for quick intervention. The objective of this application is to monitor outpatients, and notify possible emergency events to the adequate recipient (e.g. medical staff, family members, etc.), which will coordinate a rapid intervention when necessary.

To this end, the user will carry/wear some wearable sensors prepared to continuously measure his movements and vital signs. Some of these sensors have processing capabilities, which can be used to analyze measurements and to detect possible emergency events. The sensor measurements (related to fall detections and health status) will be sent to a μWoTOP Gateway. The Gateway will be located in the patient's home, e.g. on a mini-PC, or in the user's smartphone; it will further analyze the information, build an emergency notification according to CAP format when needed, and forward the event to the subscribed consumer applications (e.g. mobile applications managed by a family member or a medical care assistant, Fig. 2(a)). Additionally, smart objects running the μWoTOP middleware can also subscribe to those events in order to perform some action when an alert is detected (e.g. to set up a red color in a LED lamp or switch on a buzzer). These smart objects could be used, for example, to provide visual feedback on fall detection. We following describe the major parts of the developed system.

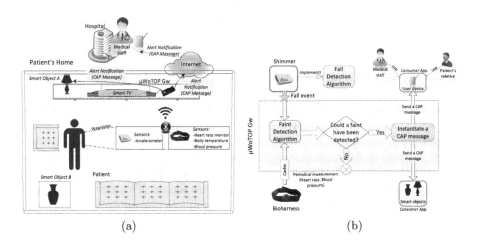

(a)   (b)

Fig. 2. a) Motivation scenario: faint/fall detection system for rapid attention; b) Faint/fall detection and notification process

5.2 Integrating Sensors into the μWoTOP: Fall / Faint Detection Algorithms

In order to detect the falls, a Shimmer device is attached to the patient's waist. This device includes an embedded 3-axis accelerometer, a programmable micro-processor and a Bluetooth radio chip, so it can be programmed to detect abnormal peaks in the acceleration measurements (falls) and transmit a Bluetooth message notifying this event. Due to the processing and memory constraints of the Shimmer device, the accelerometer signal is analyzed using a second-by-second scheme, taking the data gathered in a 1-second window. Furthermore, considering that 99% of the energy of the movements of a human body is contained below 15 Hz [1], the sampling frequency of the accelerometer is chosen to be 30 Hz (for each axis). The fall detection algorithm is based on the classifier proposed in [6] (with some differences) and consists of the following steps:

1. Low pass filtering: a third order elliptical IIR filter is used, with cut-off frequency at 0.25 Hz, 0.01 passband ripple and -100 dB stopband. The output of the filter is the component of the acceleration due to gravity (x^g, y^g, z^g), whereas the body acceleration (x^b, y^b, z^b) is obtained by subtracting this output from the original signal.

2. Calculate the Signal Magnitude Area: $SMA = \frac{1}{N} \sum_{i=1}^{N} \left(|x_i^b| + |y_i^b| + |z_i^b| \right)$, where N is the number of samples in the 1-second window, and x_i^b, y_i^b, z_i^b are the components of the i-th sample of the body acceleration.

3. If the SMA value is higher than a given threshold, the user is moving (or possibly falling). In this case, we check if the user is still in upright position by looking at the gravity component of the acceleration: if y^g is lower than 0.5 g, the user is not in upright position (in our setting, the y-axis is the one pointing to the ground when the user stands), which means that he may have fallen down. In this case, the event is notified.

This algorithm runs on the wearable device. This has the advantage that the complete raw data do not need to be transmitted continuously, which will extend the battery life of both the transmitting and the receiving device (the wearable sensor and the μWoTOP Gateway, in case it is mobile).

Faints are a special case of falls in which the vital signs of the patient are altered. In order to determine if a fall event is actually a faint, the patient has to wear a health-monitoring device. In our case, we used the Zephyr system, which includes a heart rate sensor and a blood pressure sensor. This device measures the health status of the patient and sends the complete raw information through a Bluetooth connection. In this case, as the device is not programmable, the signal needs to be analyzed externally in the μWoTOP Gateway. To this end, we have deployed an eHealth service on μWoTOP Gateways that implements a faint detection algorithm. Fig. 2(b) shows the workflow of this eHealth service.

The faint detection algorithm can be summarized as follows:

1. If a fall has been detected by the Shimmer sensor, the heart rate (HR), the systolic blood pressure (SBP) and the diastolic blood pressure (DBP) are compared with their values 60 seconds before.
2. A 'possible faint' is detected if one of the following conditions occur:
   a. SBP falls more than 20 mmHg in comparison to SBP 60 seconds before
   b. DBP falls more than 10 mmHg in comparison to DBP 60 seconds before
   c. HR falls more than 10 in comparison to HR 60 seconds before
3. If a 'possible faint' is detected an alert is sent to the consumer applications.

5.3   Alert Generation through Common Alerting Protocol (CAP)

CAP is a standardized format based on XML which was designed to communicate seamlessly different warning and emergency systems. The International Telecommunication Union, Telecommunication Standardization Sector (ITU-T) accepted CAP as Recommendation X.1303. Currently, some companies and public agencies around the world (e.g. in USA, Canada or Australia) have implemented and prototyped systems compatible with CAP.

In order to gain compatibility with such emergency systems, the μWoTOP was also designed to generate and to dispatch CAP messages to external entities when an alert is detected, as shown in Fig. 2. The CAP message structure provides substantial information about the alert. An example of a CAP message generated by the μWoTOP after processing a faint event is listed below (Fig. 3).

```
1  <?xml version = "1.0" encoding = "UTF-8"?>
2  <alert xmlns =
3  "urn:oasis:names:tc:emergency:cap:1.2">
4  <identifier>GPDS1055887203</identifier>
5  <sender>EXPLAB@GRPSS.SSR.UPM.ES</sender>
6  <sent>2013-06-15T14:57:00-07:00</sent>
7  <status>Actual</status>
8  <msgType>Alert</msgType>
9  <scope>Private</scope>
10 <info>
11 <category>Health</category>
12 <event>SEVERE </event>
13 <responseType>Execute</responseType>
14 <urgency>Immediate</urgency>
15 <severity>Severe</severity>
16 <certainty>Likely</certainty>
17 <description> A faint was detected in patient's home. Patient is currently
18 alone.Previous health measurements (60 sec): HR=75; SBP=100 ;DBP=70
19 Current health measurements: HR=60; SBP=80 ;DBP=55 </description>
20 <instruction> Patient requires attention immediately </instruction>
21 <area>
22 <areaDesc> Complutense Street #30, Madrid </areaDesc>
23 <polygon> 40.453578,-3.726057 40.453646,-3.725585 40.453301,-3.725524
24 40.453245,-3.725945 40.453578,30 -3.726057</polygon>
25 </area>
26 </info>
27 </alert>
```

Fig. 3. A CAP message describing a faint event detected at the patient's home

5.4   Middleware Mechanisms and Consumer Applications

Potential clients of our eHealth system (e.g. medical staff and smart objects) have to use specific applications to take advantage of the μWoTOP services. Every application has to implement a middleware that enables using the functionalities provided by the μWoTOP. Among these functionalities the essential one is the message bus (see Fig. 1), which supports two communication mechanisms: i) event-driven and ii) on-demand.

The event-driven mechanism supports two event notification techniques: a) condition-based: events are triggered when collected data match a specific rule or set of rules (e.g. HR<60 and fall/faint was detected); b) contract-based: events are periodically triggered to a consumer application if valid data of a specific source are available (e.g. patient blood pressure is notified every 5 minutes). For such asynchronous communication the Webhook concept is used. It consists of defining a REST-based callback to receive event notifications: clients have to specify a callback URI in the subscription that will be used by μWoTOP in order to push events by means of a POST method.

Some middleware libraries are provided in order to facilitate the programming of REST-based client applications according to the mentioned event-driven mechanism. Through this middleware, developers can manage the whole lifecycle of an application based on μWoTOP hiding the underlying complexity (e.g. protocols, message interchange, event listener instantiations, etc.). The next steps have to be follow in order to develop a simple client application that make subscriptions, consumes events and, eventually, removes the subscription:

1. Implement an event listener: The developer has to implement a component (it could be a Plain Old Java Object, POJO) which contains the logic needed for handling future events dispatched by μWoTOP Gateways. If dispatched events are related to a health emergency, they will be encapsulated in a CAP message, which has to be properly parsed.
2. Define a subscription: The subscription has to indicate, among other information, the event generator URI (Unique Resource Identifier), the event consumer URI and the rules to trigger events, i.e. a threshold, for condition-based subscriptions, or a sampling time, for contract-based subscriptions.
3. Send the subscription: The defined subscription can be sent to a specific or any μWoTOP Gateway, which will register it in a subscription table.
4. Load the event listener: Immediately after sending a subscription, an event listener associated to that subscription has to be loaded in order to start listening to every event dispatched by a μWoTOP.
5. Send an unsubscription: Finally, before application unloading, the previous subscription has to be removed by sending an unsubscription to μWoTOP Gateways indicating the code of the subscription to be ended.

This application life-cycle requires a message interchange between user devices or smart object and one or more μWoTOP Gateways. This message sequence (Fig. 4) is completely hidden to the users by the μWoTOP middleware.

On the other hand, the on-demand mechanism is much simpler than the event-driven; it is usually used to perform synchronous request for context information

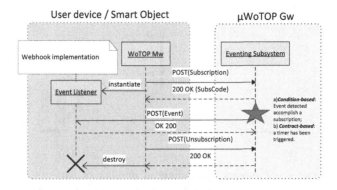

Fig. 4. Message sequence showing the event-driven mechanism offered by μWoTOP

to the μWoTOP Gateway, but also to interact with the environment by starting an action (e.g. through an actuator or modifying an execution parameter). According to the REST paradigm, GET and PUT HTTP messages will be sent during this communication mode: the former to obtain context information, and the latter to start an action over the environment.

6   Evaluation of the System Performance

In order to evaluate the performance of the proposed system we have carried out a series of experiments to obtain the latency and reliability of the event notifications.

The first experiment consisted of calculating the average latency of events dispatched by a single μWoTOP Gateway. The objective of this experiment was to test the performance of the event dispatching mechanisms implemented by μWoTOP Gateway taking into account different demanding situations. In order to facilitate these experiments, we have designed a simulation environment based on the motivation scenario shown in Fig. 2(a). This simulated scenario involves the following elements:

- *A μWoTOP Gateway*: it was deployed in a smartphone Galaxy Nexus (ARM Cortex-A9 core duo 1.2 GHz and 16 Gb) that was connected to a private Wireless Local Area Network (WLAN) at 100 Mbps.

-*Event generators*: they simulate a set of patients. We suppose that each patient generates 1 event (fall/faint) per second in order to force a much more demanding situation than usual (less than 1 fall/faint per day).

-*Event consumers*: they run on user devices connected to the same WLAN, and were simulated according to a 1:2 ratio, i.e. one consumer application per two patients (simulating e.g. a doctor supervising two patients simultaneously).

The experiment started with 2 patients and 1 consumer application, and finished with 20 patients and 10 consumer applications. Each test was running over 1 minute to compute the average event latency. Event latency was measured from

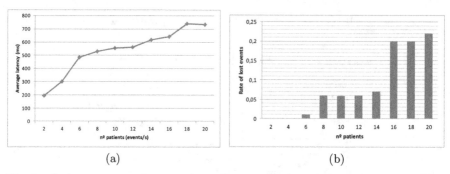

(a)   (b)

Fig. 5. a) Average event latency depending on number of patients associated to a single μWoTOP Gateway. b) Rate of lost events depending on the number of patients associated to a single μWoTOP Gateway.

the moment the event is received by the μWoTOP Gateway until the event is gathered by the consumer application. Fig. 5(a) shows the obtained results.

The minimum observed average latency during experiments was 200 ms, for 2 patients and 1 event consumer, whereas the maximum average latency (750 ms) was obtained for 20 patients and 10 consumer applications. Considering that the total time spent to carry out an emergency protocol normally ranges between 30 s and 5 minutes, the latency results are acceptable in all test cases. However, over 12 patients and 6 event consumers, the performance of μWoTOP Gateway degrades quickly.

In the described experiments, we also measured the total number of events received by consumer applications in order to measure the reliability level of the system. The reliability measurements were calculated in terms of rate of lost events (received events/generated events). Fig. 5(b) shows the rate of lost events obtained for each test case. The rate of lost events increases dramatically from 8 patients and 4 consumer applications on. Analyzing these results together with the obtained previously, we conclude that with an event throughput of more than 6 events/s, as well as more than 3 subscriptions to those events, the performance of the μWoTOP Gateway can be significantly degraded. It does not mean that the μWoTOP is a bad solution for the motivation scenario since the simulated scenario notably exceed the requirements of a real scenario where events of fall/faint will be generated once in a while.

7   Conclusions and Further Work

We have presented a ubiquitous eHealth system to assess risky situations for outpatients. The deployment of this system is only based on embedded devices and wearables to gain pervasiveness and mobility. The key element of the system is the μWoTOP, a lightweight open platform that aims at contributing to the practical combination of the Web of Things and the Internet of Things paradigms for the deployment of medium-scaled smart spaces. The latency and reliability experiments performed on a demanding simulated scenario show that μWoTOP is suitable to work in a medium-scaled real scenario, as it could be a fall/faint detection system with multiple monitored users and multiple clients.

For future work, we plan to improve the design of μWoTOP to optimize its performance in embedded and constrained devices as mini-PCs or smartphones. Moreover, we will explore deployments involving more than one μWoTOP Gateway to balance the workload and to guarantee good Quality of Service levels related to latency and reliability in order to offer this kind of services on a large scale scenario.

Acknowledgments. This work has being supported by the Government of Madrid under grant S2009/TIC-1485. The authors also acknowledge related discussions.

References

1. Antonsson, E.K., Mann, R.W.: The frequency content of gait. Journal of Biomechanics 18(1), 39–47 (1985)
2. Corredor, I., Martínez, J.F., Familiar, M.S.: Bringing pervasive embedded networks to the service cloud: A lightweight middleware approach. J. Syst. Archit. 57(10), 916–933 (2011)
3. Fielding, R.T.: Architectural styles and the design of network-based software architectures. Ph.D. thesis (2000)
4. Gómez, D., Bernardos, A.M., Portillo, J.I., Tarrío, P., Casar, J.R.: A Review on Mobile Applications for Citizen Emergency Management. In: Corchado, J.M., Bajo, J., Kozlak, J., Pawlewski, P., Molina, J.M., Julian, V., Silveira, R.A., Unland, R., Giroux, S. (eds.) PAAMS 2013. CCIS, vol. 365, pp. 190–201. Springer, Heidelberg (2013)
5. Guinard, D., Trifa, V., Pham, T., Liechti, O.: Towards physical mashups in the Web of Things. In: 6th Int. Conf. on Networked Sensing Systems, pp. 1–4 (2009)
6. Karantonis, D., Narayanan, M., Mathie, M., Lovell, N., Celler, B.: Implementation of a real-time human movement classifier using a triaxial accelerometer for ambulatory monitoring. IEEE Transactions on Information Technology in Biomedicine 10(1), 156–167 (2006)
7. Rentto, K., Korhonen, I., Väätänen, A., Pekkarinen, L., Tuomisto, T., Cluitmans, L., Lappalainen, R.: Users' preferences for ubiquitous computing applications at home. In: Aarts, E., Collier, R.W., van Loenen, E., de Ruyter, B. (eds.) EUSAI 2003. LNCS, vol. 2875, pp. 384–393. Springer, Heidelberg (2003)
8. Sposaro, F., Tyson, G.: iFall: An android application for fall monitoring and response. In: Annual Int. Conf. of the IEEE Engineering in Medicine and Biology Society, pp. 6119–6122 (2009)
9. Trifa, V., Wieland, S., Guinard, D., Bohnert, T.M.: Design and Implementation of a Gateway for Web-based Interaction and Management of Embedded Devices. In: Proc. of the 2nd Int. Workshop on Sensor Network Engineering, Marina del Rey, CA, USA (June 2009)
10. Vazquez, J., Ruiz-de Garibay, J., Eguiluz, X., Doamo, I., Renteria, S., Ayerbe, A.: Communication architectures and experiences for web-connected physical smart objects. In: 8th IEEE Int. Conf. on Pervasive Computing and Communications Workshops, pp. 684–689 (2010)
11. Zeng, D., Guo, S., Cheng, Z.: The Web of Things: A Survey. Journal of Communications 6(6) (2011) (Invited Paper)

Fiware Infrastructure for Smart Home Applications

Alia Bellabas, Fano Ramparany, and Marylin Arndt

Orange Labs, 28 chemin du vieux Chene, 38243 Meylan CEDEX, France

Abstract. This paper illustrates the interest of the technological platform developed by the European project FI-WARE for applications that are dedicated to smart home usage. Indeed, this project delivers a novel service infrastructure. This infrastructure is offering a set of Generic Enablers (GE) as generic as possible to be reused by the FI-PPP use case projects as well as by different partners of FI-WARE. In this paper, we selected two generic enablers to be tested and evaluated. This in progress study aims to better assess these generic enablers and use them to elaborate realistic innovative services.

Keywords: IoT, smart home, Generic Enabler (GE).

1 Introduction

Nowadays, most of the emerging applications are increasingly dedicated to Internet of Things (IoT) use cases. FI-WARE [4] is a European project that delivers a novel service infrastructure build upon heterogeneous architectural components called Generic Enablers (GE). The main objective of the FI-WARE project is that its generic enablers can be used within multiple applications and easily adapted to different contexts. Our objective is to test and evaluate this flexibility offered by the generic enablers. For this purpose, we have selected two generic enablers: the Complex Event Processing CEP-Proton[1] and the Publish/Subscribe Orion broker[2][3]. This selection is essentially based on the relevance they offer for home automation future services. These enablers are integrated within a proposed smart home use case that we call "Smart Home Supervision". The main idea is to supervise a home during the entire day from wake-up of a family to sleeping time and a special supervision of the children.

The paper is organized as follows. In section 2 and 3, we present the selected generic enablers within the FI-WARE project: the CEP-Proton and PubSub broker. Section 4 gives a description of the Smart Home Supervision use case. Section 5 is dedicated to the global architecture of the Smart Home Supervision and its different platforms.

2 Complex Event Processing GE

As described in Figure 1, the CEP analyses the event data in real-time, generates immediate insight and enables instant response to specific situations. A situation

M.J. O'Grady et al. (Eds.): AmI 2013 Workshops, CCIS 413, pp. 308–312, 2013.
© Springer International Publishing Switzerland 2013

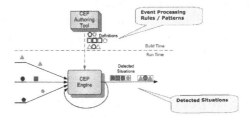

Fig. 1. Complex Event Processing architecture

is a condition that is based on a series of events that have occurred within a dynamic time window called processing context. Situations include composite events like sequences, counting operators like aggregation and absence operators.

3   Publish Subscribe Orion Broker GE

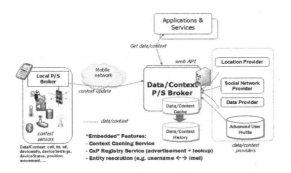

Fig. 2. Publish/Subscribe broker architecture

The pubSub broker allows the publication of the context information in push mode and to obtain the context data in pull or push mode. More precisely, Publish/Subscribe implements interface and functionality supporting context data acquisition from context sources or providers by application, services or end-users. It also allows the context providers to be registered in the systems with their specific context information and entities they are serving. Then, any external entity needing some or all available contexts of a specific entity can obtain these required information by requesting or subscribing to the instantiated Publish/Subscribe GE. Figure 2 describes the different functional blocks needed for the implementation, such as the data bases for storing the data/contexts and the related users subscriptions.

As we can see, the CEP and the PubSub GEs can collaborate closely according to their functionality. Indeed, the CEP analyses a set of events, while the PubSub broker handles subscriptions to contexts that can be detected by the CEP. This coordination is described in the next section where these two GEs are included within a use case.

4   Smart Home Supervision Use Case: Description

Among the use cases that are related to home automation, we can imagine an intelligent supervision of many events that occur when people are out of their home. Supervision activities may also be needed to take care of dependent or disabled persons and children.

Here we present a use case of smart home supervision. We use various types of sensors:

- a contact sensor: that sends an alert when a door or a window is open,
- a presence sensor: that detects persons. However, false detections may appear in case of presence of animals at home,
- a temperature sensor: that measures the temperature of home and regularly sends it to the IoT gateway,
- an on-off sensor: this sensor is particularly important to activate the managed devices like lumps or lights,
- a light sensor: that detects the luminosity degree of a given room.

The different informations are sent to the IoT gateway. Note that an IoT gateway is a device that additionally to sensing/actuating provides inter-networking and protocol conversion functionalities between devices and the Fiware platform. For our use case, we use the Happi platform, with its home gateway. The Happi platform has been developed internally to connect wireless sensors and actuators devices with to the public internet and thus makes it possible to access these devices remotely. The use case is basically related to an automated home supervision. Indeed, it describes a typical day of a family. We distinguish three main periods:

- wake up: where the home is configured to welcome the family's members by turning-on the coffee machine, the radiators in bath room, etc.
- arrival of children at home: at this time, the home is configured to be in secured mode. That means, no access to oven, to Internet and video games exceeding one hour. Also, incoming calls are redirected to the voice messaging box when the caller is not known by the children.
- sleeping time: here the home is configured to shut-down the various devices, activate the alarm, and reduce temperature for example in the living room.

5   Smart Home Supervision Use Case: Global Architecture

In order to deploy the proposed use case, we have connected two platforms: the FI-WARE platform where the CEP and PubSub GEs are deployed and the Happi platform. Within the home, a set of sensors (presence, contact, temperature, on-off and light sensors) and a Happi home box (HB) that communicates with them is required. As to manage the different subscriptions to sensors and the data transfer we use the platform of service called (PFS) and an Access Control Server (ACS).

The global implementation is divided into three main projects:

- ADAMhomeSupervision project: this project implements applications such as FireSupervision applications for managing indoor temperature, ChildSecurity for setting home on secured mode when children come home and WakeUpManagement application that puts home in alarm mode by turning off associated devices,
- HB2CEPAdapter project: this project supports interoperability between the Happi platform and the FI-WARE GEs by implementing a Rest server that receives notifications from the home box (HB) and GET requests from the CEP,
- HappiHelper project: it implements the WSDL with notifications and GetCommand sent by the home box.

More precisely, the implementation of the different communications is given as follows.

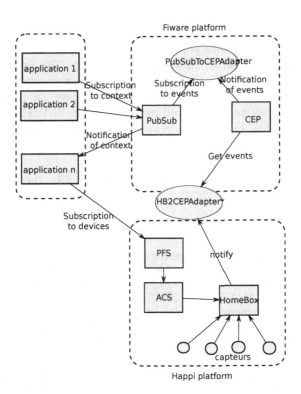

Fig. 3. Smart home supervision architecture

- the HB2CEPAdapter must be put in place to ensure the interoperability between the CEP and the Happi platform, The CEP is in this case a client that recovers the updates and recurrently analyses them according to the rules defined by the user.
- the communication between HB2CEPAdapter and the platform is established using two steps:
    - connection request to the HB via the PFS: This step is done by the different applications,
    - Each application requires a subscription to one or multiple devices stating that the notifications have to be sent to the CEP via the HB2CEPAdapter.
- once the CEP detects an abnormal context, it sends notifications to the PubSub, which notifies the applications that are subscribed for this context,
- afterwards, the applications send specific actions to actuate the devices via the home box.

6   Conclusion

In this paper, two selected generic enablers of FI-WARE have been presented: the Complex Event Processing CEP-Proton and the Publish/Subscribe broker. The CEP and the PubSub broker are frequently used to elaborate many use cases and they are directly related to home automation. They are then included within a use case dedicated to a smart home supervision. The use case is basically related to an automated home supervision. Three day periods are concerned : Wake up, children's arrival at home, and go to sleep. This implementation is presented as a beginning point and tests are in progress. Preliminary results highlight a flexibility with however some additional developing efforts. Indeed, the CEP and pubSub broker as well as most of the FI-WARE GEs are not natively interoperable. Once, all developments are done, the FI-WARE GEs offer many facilities to deploy dedicated smart applications.

Acknowledgments. This work is partially supported by the EU FI-PPP FI-WARE project [Grant no. 285248].

References

1. Etzion, O., Niblett, P.: Event Processing in Action. Manning Publications (2010)
2. Moltchanov, B., Fra', C., Valla, M., Licciardi, C.A.: Context Management Framework and Context Representation for MNO. In: Activity Context Workshop / AAAI 2012, San Francisco, USA (August 2012)
3. Moltchanov, B., Knappmeyer, M., Liaquat Kiani, S., Frá, C., Baker, N.: ContextML: A Light-Weight Context Representation and Context Management Schema. In: IEEE International Symposium on Wireless Pervasive Computing, Modena, Italy (2010)
4. Future Internet Public-Private Partnership, http://catalogue.fi-ware.eu/
5. Orange Labs group: Home Automation API's guide. Orange Labs Internal publication (2011)

Online Learning Based Contextual Model for Mobility Prediction

Munir Naveed

The University of the South Pacific Laucala Campus, Suva, Fiji

Abstract. Use of mobile devices for the personal and corporate purposes is growing rapidly. Context-awareness is an essential feature of the mobile apps. In this paper, we present an approach to predict the next place for a mobile phone by using an online learning method. We represent the model in the form of state-action representation. Each state is a distinct context and behavior of the app is represented in the form of actions applicable at that state. The results show that online learning based approach performs better than two state-of-the-art mobility prediction approaches. Performance is measured in term of accuracy to predict the next location of a mobile host.

Keywords: Context-awareness, mobility prediction, Monte-Carlo simulations.

1   Introduction

Mobile apps are widely used for the business and personal purposes these days. An app is expected to behave according to the current surroundings of the mobile device. Such a characteristic of the application makes it context-aware. The main challenging issues in building a fully context-aware app are (1) the presence of several parameters (e.g. location, user profile and device usage) that can represent a context and (2) the selection of an appropriate action that is applicable in the current context.

The paper addresses the context-awareness with the notion of identifying the location of a mobile host. The main emphasis is put on the prediction of the next place of a mobile host with respect to its current location.   The prediction the next destination of a mobile user is required for various commercial and social purposes in the mobile app development e.g. context-aware advertisements, navigation and business intelligence.

In this work, we present a Monte-Carlo based probabilistic approach, called MCPROD, to solve the prediction problem. MCPROD assumes each location of the mobile host as a state of the host. The prediction of the next place is a transition from the current state to the next state. The transition is based on a probability distribution which is built using the Monte-Carlo (MC) simulations. MCPROD applies MC simulations from an arbitrary state where each simulation traverses through all intermediate states until a terminal state is reached.   Performance of MCPROD is evaluated using CRAWDAD dataset [1].   Performance is measured using the number of observations successfully predicted.   MCPROD is compared with two rival

M.J. O'Grady et al. (Eds.): AmI 2013 Workshops, CCIS 413, pp. 313–319, 2013.
© Springer International Publishing Switzerland 2013

techniques: Naïve Bayes and logistic regression. The results show a clear advantage of using MCPROD for the prediction of next location of a mobile host.

The main contributions of this work as follow:

1. An online prediction technique for location-awareness
2. Evaluation of the technique using a well-known data set
3. Comparison with the state-of-the-art rivals technique

2   Related Work

A mobility pattern based approach is present in [2] to solve the next place prediction problem in mobile computing. Their work addresses the prediction of the next place as a learning problem where solution learns the mapping between input and output. The mobility patterns are extracted using a trajectory based approach [3] where each trajectory leads to a region of stay points. The regions are defined in a grid based representation. The transition from the current location to the next place is predicted using a probabilistic transition function. The probabilistic technique is tuned using the high level representation of the user mobility behaviour i.e. at stay regions. The results show that performance of such an algorithm largely depends on a size of the training data set.

Isaac et al. [4] presents a logistic regression and clustering based approach to identify the important places from a mobile user's mobility patterns. The main focus of their work is on identifying the key locations the user move to and then to assign semantic meanings to these places e.g. home or office etc. The clustering is applied on the user profile and Call Detail Records (CDR) to identify the important locations of a user and to classify them into home or work classes. Their work also estimates the distance between the important places which can be useful to solve the traffic related problems in large cities. The results show that their approach can identify the important location with an accuracy of 97.5%.

Xu et al. [5] present a mobile app prediction framework that mainly focuses on classification to predict the future app usage. In their work, an app usage is represented by community behavior, current sensor values (including location) and user-specific preferences. Community behavior considers a broader view of app usage where different users can share the common application e.g. a gaming user community can have the same game application to play at the same time. Community similarity learning [6] and community guided learning [7] approaches are some of the examples that this framework can use to improve the classification accuracy. The three phases of this framework capture the relationship between app usage and sensor data. The results show that framework performs better than a baseline classifier and SVM [8].

MCPROD is similar to the works of [2] in sense of calculating the probability distribution for the prediction of next place. However, MCPROD calculates such probability on the fly and does not require a processing stage like [2] and [4] does. MCPROD generates trajectory during simulation rather than in offline. There trajectories are then use to predict the next possible state for any given state.

The framework given in [5] can be a useful platform to explore MCPROD for context-awareness in a broader sense.

3   Problem Formulation

In this paper, we address the problem of predicting the next place for a mobile host if the current location is given. The problem formulation assumes that the state of a mobile host is represented by its current location. The prediction of the next place is considered as the selection of the next state s' at a given state s and action a as shown in equation (1).

$$s' = Predict(s, a) \tag{1}$$

The main challenging issues in predicting the next state are the presence of several choices for the user to move to and the random movement patterns. We present a Monte-Carlo simulation based approach to predict the next state of the user in an online style under real-time hard constraints. The problem formulation also assumes that there is a finite set of states for a mobile host to move at.

4   Notation

The finite set of states is represented by S and A is the finite set of action. T is a function $T(s, a)$ which determines if a is applicable at s where $s \in S$ and $a \in A$. $Prod(s, a, s')$ is probability distribution function that represents the probability of reaching next state s' of s when action a is applied at s.

Definition 1
$T: S \times A \rightarrow \{0, 1\}$ is defined such that it returns 0 if a is applicable at s otherwise 1 for all $s \in S$ and $a \in A$.

Definition 2
$Prod: S \times A \times S \rightarrow \,]0, 1]$ is defined using the equation (2).

$$Prod(s, a, s') = \frac{n_{s'}}{(n_s + n_a)} \qquad \forall s, s' \in S, a \in A \tag{2}$$

Where $n_{s'}$ is the number times the mobile host has been at s' when moving from s with action a. n_s is number of times the mobile host has been at state s and n_a is the number of times a has been selected at s.

Definition 3
$Next: S \times A \rightarrow 2^S$ is the deterministic state transition function.

Definition 4
$Neighbour: S \times A \rightarrow 2^S$ is a function that finds all neighbouring states of the current state s.

5   Prediction Algorithm: MCPROD

MCPROD is a real-time Monte-Carlo simulations based algorithm that predicts the next state of a mobile host. The main intuition behind using Monte-Carlo simulations for next place prediction problem is the ability of such algorithms to perform look-ahead search in a partially known environment. Such algorithms have been used successfully in partially observable environments for finding trajectories e.g. MOCART [9] and RRT [10]. Such trajectories can be used to find the important places a mobile host visits without using offline training. The many applications lack the availability of well refined training dataset to be used for tuning the predictions algorithms offline. This motivates us to use Monte-Carlo simulations for the prediction of next place in a mobile app.

The algorithm details of MCPROD are given in Figure 1. The algorithm finds the list (Π) all neighbouring states of the current state in step 1. It selects each neighbouring state s' and finds the probability of moving to s' using the statistical approach i.e. *Prod*. The long term movement probability Q is initially set to the statically calculated probability. Then MCPROD generates a trajectory of size d for each neighbouring state (step 3) and calculates a long term probability value for the given next state at step 4. When all neighbouring states are explored, then MCPROD finds the neighbouring state with the highest long term probability (step 5).

Algorithm. MCPROD *(s , A, integer d)*
1. $\Pi = Neighbour(s, A)$;
Foreach $s' \in \Pi$
2. $Q(s', d) = Prod(s, a, s')$;
3.   Real q=Simulate(s', d);
4. $Q(s', d) = q$;
End
5. $s' = \arg max_{s' \in \Pi} (Q(s', d)$;

Fig. 1. MCPROD— high level algorithm

6   Experimental Work

MCPROD is empirical evaluated using the CRAWDAD dataset available at [1]. MCPROD is implemented in C# and run on Windows 7 with Intel Core(TM) 2 processors with each 2.0GHz speed. The data is organised in such a way that MCPROD receives each entry during the runtime to training it online. MCPROD starts predicting the next places when more than one neighbouring state of the current state has $n_{s'}$ greater than 0.

There 150 observations in the refined training dataset and 75 observations are used for testing purpose. The performance is measured in terms of number of observations accurately predicted from the test data. Two rival techniques—Naive Bayes and Logistic Regression— are based on the latest works [2] and [4]. The rival algorithms are implemented and run at the same platform that is used for the evaluation of MCPROD. The same state space is used for the rival techniques and for MCPROD for a careful design of the experiments.

The initial experiments reveal that performance of MCPROD depends on the size of the look-ahead trajectory generated by MCPROD. Therefore, MCPROD is evaluated with different trajectory sizes (d) starting from $d=2, 3 \ldots 20$. The maximum trajectory size (i.e. $d=20$) is set based on the initial experiments on simulations.

7   Results

The best results from all three techniques are noted for the analysis purpose. MCPROD performs the best with $d=6$. MCPROD is trained online in such a way that it uses the training data in each simulation, to generate the trajectories. The statistical probability distribution of each state is calculated once when MCPROD see that state and is stored in a heap for future use.

Figure 2 shows a comparison of MCPROD with the rival techniques: Naïve Bayse (NB) and Logistic Regression (LR). The test results show a clear advantage of using MCPROD for the prediction of the next place at the current given position of a mobile host.

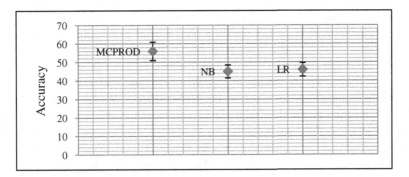

Fig. 2. Performance of MCPROD and rival techniques on test data

The main advantage that MCPROD has over the rival techniques is due to online learning of the prediction task. This feature is also benefitting in terms of the need for a large scale training dataset. However, it is not clear from the existing experiments that MCPROD can perform better than rival techniques in the presence of large scale dataset. It can be inferred from that the algorithmic detail of MCPROD that the performance of MCPROD would not be affected by the changing the size of training dataset as it depends mainly on the size of the trajectories generated during the simulations. The rival techniques can get a clear advantage in the presence of a large training dataset.

MCPROD performance highly depends on the size of trajectories generated during the simulations which requires more efforts to find an appropriate size for a dataset. To find an appropriate value for a dataset can be a time consuming task if the size of the dataset increases.

MCPROD is the best performing algorithm in the current set of experiments but it could not predict all test observations accurately. To explore it further, we identified the observations that are not accurately predicted by MCPROD. The common feature in these observations is the smaller size of the neighbouring set of the current state. In other words, MCPROD can make a wrong prediction in a case a mobile host has very limited choices. Naive Bayes (NB) has been seen successful in such instances. However, there is no orthogonal relationship between NB and MCPROD.

8   Conclusion

We present a preliminary work in the direction of the next place prediction for the mobile devices. The work presents a method that can perform well even in the presence of a small number of observations. The method is based on Monte-Carlo simulations of limited horizon. Next place prediction is commonly required in mobile computing to achieve context-awareness in the mobile apps and middleware. The existing methods heavily rely on the huge training dataset. To overcome this limitation, we prefer to design an online learning algorithm that does not require a separate offline training stage and can learn from a small set of training examples.

The results show a clear advantage of MCPROD as compared to its rival technique. However, MCPROD needs improvement in terms of its achieving better accuracy. In future, we are aiming to include a case-base reasoning approach in the Monte-Carlo simulations to improve its performance. We also aim to modify MCPROD in future to avoid its dependency on the size of the trajectories generated by the simulation model. One possible way to achieve that is to use the terminal states to determine the size of trajectories. Another objective for future work is to investigate MCPROD on large scale dataset e.g. Mobile Data Challenge 2012.

References

[1] http://crawdad.org/ctu/personal
[2] Tri Do, T.M., Gatica-Perez, D.: Contextual Conditional Models for Smartphone-based Human Mobility Prediciton. In: The Proceedings of UniComp 2012, Pittsburg, USA (2012)
[3] Zheg, V.W., Zheng, Y., Xie, X., Yang, Q.: Collaborative location and activity recommendations with gps history data. In: The Proceedings of the 19th International Conference on World Wide Web, pp. 1029–1038 (2010)
[4] Isaacman, S., Becker, R., Caceres, R., Kobourov, S., Martonosi, M., Rowland, J., Varshavsky, A.: Identifying important places in people's lives from cellular network data. In: The Proceedings of the 9th International Conference on Pervasive Computing (2011)

[5] Xu, Y., Lin, M., Lu, H., Cardone, G., Lane, N.D., Chen, Z., Campbell, A., Choudhary, T.: Preference, context and communities: A multi-facet approach to predicting smartphone app usage patterns. In: The Proceedings of ISWC 2013 (2013)

[6] Lane, N., Xu, Y., Lu, H., Hu, S., Choudhury, T., Campbell, A.T., Zhao, F.: Enabling large-scale human activity inference on smart phones using community similarity networks. In: The Proceedings of UbiComp 2011, pp. 355–364 (2011)

[7] Peebles, D., Lu, H., Lane, N.D., Choudhury, T., Campbell, A.T.: Community-guided learning: exploiting mobile sensor users to model human behavior. In: The Proceedings of 24th AAAI Conference on AI, pp. 1600–1606 (2010)

[8] Bishop, C.M.: Pattern Recognition and Machine Learning. Springer (2006)

[9] Naveed, M., Crampton, A., Kitchin, D., McCluskey, T.: Real-Time Path Planning using Simulation Based Markovian Decision Process. In: AI-2011: 31st SGAI International Conference on Artificial Intelligence (2011)

[10] LaValle, S.: Planning Algorithms. Cambridge University Press (2006)

A Mobile-Based Automation System for Maintenance Inspection and Lifesaving Support in a Smart ICT Building

Abdelkader Dekdouk

Computer Science Department, College of Arts and Applied Sciences
Dhofar University, Salalah, Oman, P.O. Box: 2509, Postal Code 211.
Laboratoire d'Informatique et de Technologie d'Information d'Oran
d_abdulkader@du.edu.om

Abstract. With the ever increasing device count and the introduction of wireless pervasive computing in building automation, in order 1) to enhance people life comfort and safety and 2) to optimize the consumption cost of public utility services like energy and water; it is becoming more than crucial to automatically manage these commonly known smart buildings. Indeed, in this research work, we propose a platform that addresses the problem of energy management of different electric devices in a smart Information and Communication Technology (ICT) building and particularly high performance computing (HPC) data centers. This platform integrates the mobile technology as a means to facilitate the maintenance operations usually executed by the mobile workforce agents on smart building electric devices. Another important issue integrated in this proposed platform deals with the monitoring of a life safety plan in case of an emergency scenario due, for instance, to fire detection. The emergency rescue monitoring is eased by the use of mobile devices such as the tablets, usually handled by people in a smart ICT building.

Keywords: Smart Building, Energy Management, Mobile Computing, Sensor Networks, Knowledge Management, Emergency Rescue and Risk management.

1 Introduction

Managing a smart building is becoming so demanding that an ordinary human is not capable of keeping track of all the offered possibilities, and hence intelligent computing support becomes a mandatory requirement for public utility efficient services (such as energy and water) and yet comfort and life safety oriented operations. The information quality available in a management system plays a crucial role for efficient sensors administration and energy consumption controlling of different electric components in a smart building. In fact, designing sufficient and concise information to the management system allows it to define better decision solutions for some given tasks like switching off the lighting when we leave a room or automatically shutting off the water valve when detecting a flood or scheduling a heat pump to start once energy from renewable sources becomes available i.e. the sun is shining on a photovoltaic installation.

M.J. O'Grady et al. (Eds.): AmI 2013 Workshops, CCIS 413, pp. 320–335, 2013.
© Springer International Publishing Switzerland 2013

In this research work, our first aim concerns the energy management in a smart building. In fact, a smart building is usually populated by multitude of sensors that cooperate in an intelligent way to particularly control the energy consumption of different devices such as lighting/shading or heating/ventilation/air-conditioning. While in functional automation, proven solution have already existed for a longer time, additional challenges arise for energy management systems that need to be tailored to some specific buildings such as academic, health-care, industrial and commercial buildings. Indeed some specific electric devices need particular energy-efficient management policies in some specific smart buildings. For instance, in health care or commercial buildings, the heating and lighting infrastructure represent the most energy-consuming systems. In industrial building, the high power machines are the main electric equipment concerned by the energy efficient management process. In academic buildings, the computing devices like the data centers, HPC machines installed in ICT spaces represent one of the most energy consuming devices and hence specific management rules are established based on the knowledge combination of ICT and HPC management experts.

The sophistication and complexity of sensor network infrastructure have made maintenance and asset management cumbersome and costly. Thus, a highly-effective mobile workforce is deemed as one of the mechanisms that can be exploited by a management system to ensure continuous and immediate services in order to meet the established requirements and standards. These operations which represent the second objective of this research work are implemented in mobile smart handhelds (such as mobile tablets) making thus this task very effective. Still based on mobile technology, the third objective of this contribution offers decision support mobile-based services that assist building occupants in monitoring their life rescue in case of situations like fire or flood detections.

In this research contribution, the proposed management platform is built on an ontology-based model unifying in a single data structure all the information related to the sensors, the devices controlled by these sensors as well as the context of an ICT building occupant defined by 1) his position in the building, 2) the events that may arise in the building and which can be life-threatening to the occupant and 3) the time of event occurrences, etc. Representing this knowledge in a machine-processable description language like OWL ensures that information can be accessed and exploited by the management system which automatically performs logical reasoning and executes control strategies based on inference rules and decision making techniques that are developed by a group of ICT and HPC management experts.

This paper is organized as follows: in Section 2, we present the architecture of our management platform. This platform is built of two main modules, namely the module of data acquisition and the module of logic reasoning and decision making. In Section 3, we present different mobile-based monitoring applications that are integrated in our management system. One of those applications is used by mobile workforce agents in order to tackle efficiently the problem of energy consumption management of the different smart building assets. Another mobile application used in this management system consists in assisting the building tenants, in case of an emergency rescue scenario. In Section 4, we investigate the HPC system monitoring (from an energy saving perspective) in an ICT building. Finally we conclude with some remarks and outline some future perspectives.

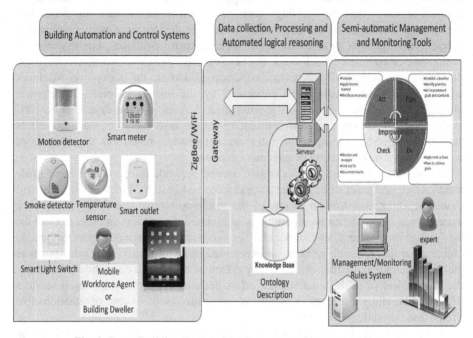

Fig. 1. Smart Building Knowledge Management System Architecture

2   Smart Building Knowledge Management System

In this section, we give an overview of the general architecture of our proposed knowledge management system of a smart building, relying on data collected by ZigBee wireless sensor network. In the literature there exist different knowledge management systems of smart buildings [1, 2, 3]; however our knowledge management system differs from the aforementioned ones, by its ability to offer mobile-based services implemented on an Android mobile tablet. The mobile-based services helps any mobile workforce agent to perform on-site management operations in an effective way. In addition to that, our platform tackles the problem of emergency response scenarios by offering mobile-based rescue solutions made on decision techniques such as logic reasoning and Bayesian networks.

2.1   Knowledge Management System Architecture

Abstract system architecture is presented here in Figure 1, based on ontology and inference engine. Sensors input data pertaining to parameters such as temperature, humidity, energy usage, carbon monoxide density, smoke density are collected and stored in sensors database. This data is filtered, summarized and converted to supply the ontology model. Based on inference rules and ontology instances we perform analysis procedures to achieve energy optimization, to avoid device degradation and to suggest solutions to some emergency rescue situations. The monitoring of HPC data centers is dealt with the help of a specific monitoring tool that is Nagios [4]. We should note by the way, that in the area of HPC data centers monitoring, there are other tools that do fairly the job (see [5, 6]). In the sequel we will discuss in more detail the HPC system monitoring.

2.2   Data Acquisition Model

This module permits to communicate with different sensors through a gateway. In building automation area, different communication protocols have been developed such as KNX, LonWorks, BACnet, Modbus, ZigBee SEP, Homeplug and 6LoWPAN [7, 8, 9]. In order to allow inter-communication between these heterogeneous technologies in a building automation system, we need to build a middleware on the top of them. However with the energy-saving purpose and for some practical reasons, regarding the installation cost of building area network (BAN), we chose to only focus on ZigBee technology for M2M communication [10] which can be easily and efficiently deployed in a BAN. In our management platform, the M2M communication network is connected to the internet through ConnectPort X2 [11] which is a small ZigBee to Ethernet/Wifi gateway providing low-cost IP networking of RF devices and sensor networks. ConnectPort X2 products feature an end-to-end development environment based on local customization via iDigi Dia framework allowing for rapid M2M-specific application development on the industry standard Python scripting engine.

Recall that the objectives of this contribution, is to manage a smart building in order 1) to optimize the energy consumption of its electric assets, and 2) to monitor the lifesaving of building occupants in the case of an emergency rescue scenario. The inherent complexity of the knowledge domain makes it hard to sufficiently cover the whole domain in detail with conventional database techniques. Thus, the semantic representation of the environment of a smart ICT building can be seen as a prerequisite of an intelligent system operating on behalf of the user.

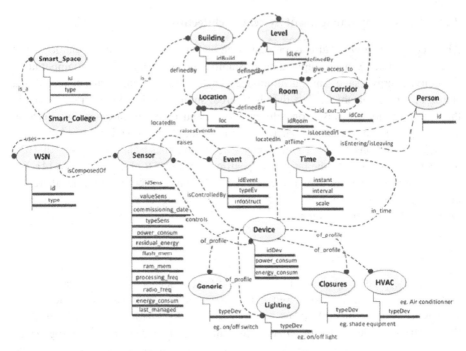

Fig. 2. Ontology Description of Smart Building Assets

2.2.1 Ontology Modeling and Logical Reasoning

To model dependencies of the different actors of a smart ICT building in an expressive way, the representation as ontology is proposed in Figure 2. Ontologies can be seen as means to describe important aspects of a knowledge domain on the basis of a formal semantic language. One possibility for an ontology representation is the Web Ontology Language OWL that can be automatically processed by a machine. Main constructs in OWL are concepts, individuals and properties. A concept denotes a construct that can have members belonging to that concept and also sub-concepts in order to form hierarchies. The concrete members of such concepts are individuals which represent entities in the modeled domain of discourse. The properties represent the attributes of these concepts. In addition to the hierarchy relationship (such as the inheritance usually defined by the "is_a" relationship), we can interconnect semantically the concepts by relations like "isLocatedIn(?x,?y)" (this relation means that a "Person" identified by the unknown parameter "?x" is located in a "Room" parameterized by "?y"). With the help of properties and relations, logical axioms can be phrased in a decidable fragment of first-order logic, that aid in describing concepts and members. By applying the defined inference rules and particularly the modus pones rule, we can deduce facts that can be added to enrich the knowledge base. Here below, we present some inference rules that are defined in our inference engine.

1. Person(?x)   and   isLeaving(?x,?y)   implies
   raiseEvent(?y,LIGHT_OFF).
2. Person(?x)   and   isEntring(?x,?y)   implies
   raiseEvent(?y, LIGHT_ON).
3. Sensor(?x) and and typeSens(?x, TEMPERATURE) and
   valueSens(?x) >THRESHOLD and isLocatedIn(?x,?y)
   implies raiseEvent(FIRE_ALARM, ?y).
4. Sensor(?x) and residualEnergy(?x) <= THREASHOLD
   implies raiseEvent(?x, ALERT_CHANGE).
5. Device(?x)   and   isControlledBy(?x,?y)   and
   powerConsum(?y)   >=   TRESHOLD   implies
   raiseEvent(ALERT_CONTROL, ?y).
6. Device(?x)   and   iscontrolledBy(?x,?y)   and
   typeDev(?x, UPS) and typeSens(?y,TEMPERATURE) and
   valueSens(?y)   >   TRESHOLD   implies
   controls(?y,?x,SHUTDOWN).
7. Device(?x)   and   isControlledBy(?x,?y)   and
   typeSens(?y, HUMIDITY) and valueSens(?y) < MIN and
   valueSens(?y)   >   MAX   implies
   raiseEvent(ALERT_HUMIDITY).
8. Person(?x)   and   isLocatedIn(?x,?y)   and
   eventCheck(FIRE_ALARM)   and
   detectSafeRoad(?y,exit,?list) implies raiseEvent(?x,
   MOVE, ?list).

Rule1 means that, when a person leaves a room, the system arises an event object with a constant value LIGHT_OFF. Rule3 means that if the temperature sensor exceeds a threshold in a given room "y", then the system arises an event object with the constant value FIRE_ALARM and the location value of this event is set to "y". Rule8 means that if a person "x" is located in a given position and a fire alarm is detected, then the systems automatically arises a MOVE event corresponding to the person "x", along with the path in the building, that "x" needs to follow in order to save his life.

2.2.2 Decision Making Using Bayesian Networks

Bayesian networks (BN), also known as belief networks belong to the family of probabilistic graphical models (GM). These graphical structures are used to represent knowledge about an uncertain domain. In particular, each node in the graph represents a random variable, while the edges between the nodes represent probabilistic dependencies among the corresponding random variables. These conditional dependencies in the graph are often estimated by using known statistical and computational methods. In Figure 3, we present the BN that illustrates a situation of a decision making in case of an alarm detection. We apply this technique to make a decision for a scenario where a building tenant is initially at position "Corridor A". For that, we evaluate the probability of safety event in corridor A, defined by the variable safety_at_A. The variable mov_safely_to_B represents the event of moving safely to corridor B. In order to decide about the safest path that leads to the exit point. We need to compute the following join probability:

```
probability(safety_at_A, mov_safely_to_E,
mov_safely_to_G, mov_safely_to_G, mov_safely_to_H,
mov_safely_to_Exit) = prob(safety_at_A)   *
prob(mov_safely_to_E | safety_at_A)   *
prob(mov_safely_to_G | mov_safely_to_E)   *
prob(mov_safely_to_H | mov_safely_to_G)   *
prob(mov_safely_to_Exit | mov_safely_to_H)
```

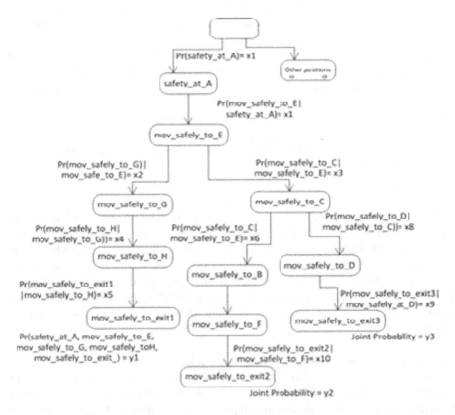

Fig. 3. Bayesian Networks Decision Making in case of an Emergency Rescue Scenario

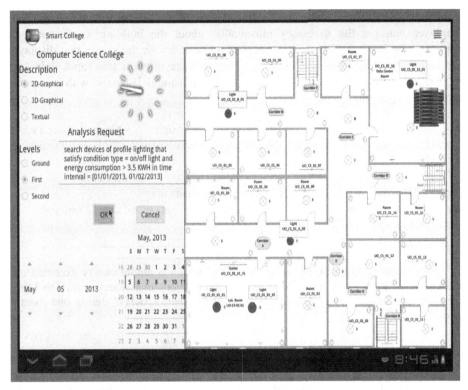

Fig. 4. Mobile Tool Interface for Energy Management in a Smart ICT Building

Based on an estimation evaluation carried out by a building safety and security expert, we can determine that the probability "y1" is greater than the probabilities "y2" and "y3" and hence we conclude that the path A-E-G-H-Exit1 is the safest one.

2.3   Mobile-Based Workforce Management Service

The sophistication and complexity of the smart buildings particularly smart ICT buildings have made maintenance and asset management cumbersome and costly. Thus, a highly-productive mobile workforce is deemed as one of the mechanisms that can be exploited by the ICT building manager to ensure that they can deliver continuous services satisfying the policies stated for the ICT building administration related to the energy consumption optimization and the comfort and safety enhancement of the ICT building occupants. Confronted by increased costs, competitive pressures, an aging workforce and today's economic challenges, many ICT buildings are looking for opportunities to reduce their costs, and improve service levels. Integrating a mobile and wireless solution that empowers employees with the information they need, to improve their job performance, is becoming inevitable [12]. Indeed a field-based employee is able to realize shorter resolution times to provide the management services. In Figure 4, we present the mobile-based tool interface that visualizes graphically the 2D-architecture design of our smart ICT building. The employee can get the necessary information about the building assets (sensor, appliance) by just touching their corresponding positions on the screen that displays the architecture design of the building. The interface offers a text input field for request acquisition. The request is expressed in a natural language with a simple grammar, as presented here:

```
1.   Request   ::=   <search>   Concept   <that   satisfy
condition> {SP} [REL Concept <that satisfy condition>
{SP}]*
2.   Concept ::= <Sensor> | <Device> | <Location> ..
3.   SP ::= simple_logic_function(params)
4.   REL   ::=   <isLocatedIn>   |   <isControlledBy>   |
<Controls> | ..
```

The request is then translated into SPARQL which is automatically executed on the Ontology knowledge base. Next we present a query that searches for ON/OFF light devices whose energy consumption is greater than 3.5KHW during one month period.

```
1. search  devices  that  satisfy  condition  {energy
   consumption > 3.5} of profile lighting that satisfy
   condition {typeDev = "on-off light"} in time that
   satisfy   condition   {interval   =   [01/01/2013,
   01/02/2013]}.
```

This query is translated into SPARQL as follows:

```
PREFIX rdf: <http://www.w3.org/1999/02/22-rdf-syntax-
ns#>

PREFIX owl: <http://www.w3.org/2002/07/owl#>

PREFIX xsd: <http://www.w3.org/2001/XMLSchema#>

PREFIX  foaf:    <http://xmlns.com/foaf/0.1/>

SELECT ?device

WHERE {

?device rdf:type foaf:Device .

?device foaf: energy_consum ?var1 .

Filter( ?var > 3.5)

lighting rdf:type foaf:Lighting .

?device foaf:of_profile ?lighting .
```

```
?lighting foaf:typeDev  "on/off light" .

?time rdf:type foaf:Time .

?device foaf:in_time ?time .

?time foaf:interval ?var2 .

FILTER (?var2 > "2013-01-01T00:00:00Z"^^xsd:dateTime)
AND (?var2 < "2012-02-01T00:00:00Z"^^xsd:dateTime> )

}
```

The following query consists in identifying the temperature sensors whose the residual energy is equal to 50% of its battery life duration.

```
2. search location of sensors that satisfy condition
   {typeSens = temperature and residual_energy = 50%}
```

Its equivalent SPARQL query is:

```
PREFIX rdf: <http://www.w3.org/1999/02/22-rdf-syntax-ns#>

PREFIX owl: <http://www.w3.org/2002/07/owl#>

PREFIX xsd: <http://www.w3.org/2001/XMLSchema#>

PREFIX foaf:   <http://xmlns.com/foaf/0.1/>

SELECT ?location

WHERE {

?location rdf:type foaf:Location .

?sensor rdf:type foaf:Sensor .

?location foaf:of ?sensor .

?sensor foaf:typeSens "temperature" .

?sensor foaf:residual_energy ?var1 .

FILTER(var1 =  50)
```

2.4   Mobile-Based Emergency Rescue Management Service

Indoor emergency response scenarios in case of an urban fire, earthquakes, gas leaks or hostage situations are in continuous enhancement particularly with the help of sensors. In fact different sensor-based intelligent emergency rescue evacuation systems have been developed [13, 14, 15, 16]. In this research work we use the mobile tablet as an asset to enhance the emergency rescue support techniques. In fact nowadays nearly most of the people have mobile smart handhelds and in the near future we predict that every student will have a mobile tablet particularly used for learning activity. Actually the mobile smart handheld includes high processing capabilities, large memory, multiple connectivity options GSM, GPRS, UMTS, LTE, WiFi. This communication stack will be enriched with low power M2M communication protocols like ZigBee Pro, BLE, in order to directly communicate with smart building sensors. In Figure 5, we present a simulation of a fire detection event in a smart ICT building. We assume an emergency scenario where the smoke has started to fill the building and spread around its rooms. In such situation, we suppose that the visibility has been reduced and hence the panic feeling has increased. The emergency rescue monitoring service offered by our management system uses the information collected from smoke sensors, movement sensors as well as mobile integrated sensors like the GPS, the accelerometer and the direction sensors. Based on this data and the Bayesian networks technique, we compute the safety probabilities of any person "P" trapped inside a building in fire at position "X" and also determine the probability to move safely from position "X" to position "Y" and hence identify the safest path to rescue that person "P" (see Figure 3).

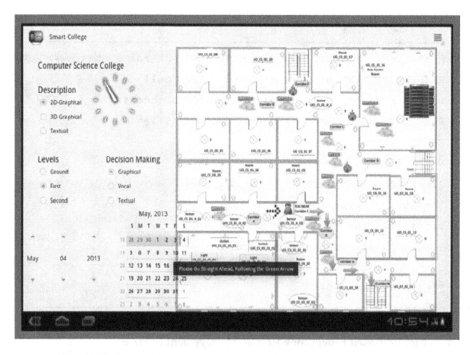

Fig. 5. Mobile Tool Interface for Monitoring Emergency Rescue Scenario

3   HPC Data Centers Energy Management in an ICT Building

HPC data centers run at their peak performance to efficiently execute scientific applications. Therefore, these HPC systems consume enormous amount of power that results in increased operational cost. The high power consumption translates into high temperature of the physical HPC systems, which in turn results in high failure rate and decreased reliability. In fact according to Arrhenius equation when applied to HPC hardware, each 10 degree increase in system's temperature doubles the system failure rate [19]. Employing an aggressive cooling system does not improve the situation, because it involves additional power consumptions and infrastructure cost.

In this section we discuss the monitoring of data centers from a green energy perspective. With the emergence of Petaflops HPC systems, we are anticipated to draw enormous amounts of electrical power. Concerns over total cost of ownership have moved the focus of the HPC system architecture from concern over peak performance towards concern over improving power efficiency [17, 18]. The increase in power consumption can be illustrated by comparing typical top 500 HPC systems. A new metric of performance in computing taking into account energy consumption has been defined representing the number of Teraflop or Petaflop execution per Watt unit. Hence based on this metric a new ranking HPC machines has been defined by the Green500 list [18]. In fact with this metric, the things changed, we notice that the IBM BlueGene which is the highest 500 top HPC machine, performs 2.1 TeraFlops/Watt, consumes 82 KWatt and hence falls to the eight rank surpassed by Appro GreenBlade taking the first rank in the Green500 list with a performance of 2.5 Teraflops/Watt.

The HPC system (named "Haytham") of our ICT Building is a BULL Cluster (Bullx R423) that is equipped with 32 nodes. Each node has 2 processor of type Intel Nehalem Ex (2.93GHz) composed of 6 cores. For every computing cycle, it can perform 4 Flops. Hence the peak performance of this supercomputer is 32*2*6*4*2.93 = 4.5 TeraFlops. This HPC machine consumes 16KW dedicated for computing and 20KW for cooling. We can hence estimate the green performance of this machine in extreme case by 4.5 TFlops/36KW = 0.125 GFlops/Watt.

In the domain of HPC system monitoring, there exists some general networking tools, such as Nagios [4], Cacti [5] and Ganglia[6] that are usually exploited to manage HPC environments. In our management framework, we particularly use Nagios to monitor Haytham HPC system. We particularly enriched Nagios tool with some monitoring shell scripts, notably the script that controls the shutting off of the nodes of the supercomputer in case of alarms detection such as the battery power is low to support the load or the maximum temperature has been violated (see appendix A).

4   Conclusion

In this paper, we propose a management system of a smart building and more specifically a smart ICT building. This system helps to manage the electric appliances of the smart building, namely the sensors and the different electric devices like the lights, HAVC equipment and particularly computing devices such as high performance computing data centers. The management process has the objectives to enhance the life comfort of the building occupants whilst also optimizing the energy consumption in the building. In order to increase the effectiveness of this management task, we developed mobile-based services that facilitate on-site interventions carried out by mobile workforce agents, in a timely and costly efficient manner. Another feature of this management system is its ability to monitor emergency response procedures based on mobile technology. In this research work, we implemented emergency rescue services based on mobile technology. In fact, these services use the mobile device features involving the

Communication, the GPS positioning sensor, the accelerometer sensor and the direction sensor along with the smoke density sensors, and the flexible visual representation of 2D and 3D architecture of the building on the mobile display. Based on these features, the emergency rescue service can draw the safest path and assists a mobile user in his rescue action. An extension of this rescue technique based on mobile technology is to consider the case of persons that might be visually impaired and deaf persons [14, 15]. Hence the offered rescue service can exploit the tactile feedback capacity that semantically enhances the mobile interface [20, 21] based on the different patterns of vibration. The management system we presented here deals with energy optimization in a smart ICT building and particularly the energy management of an HPC data center. Actually, in this area we are lacking of management experts that collectively possess sufficient knowledge on energy management and HPC administration. In [22] some challenges of HPC monitoring are presented and one of these challenges consists in analyzing the execution of different jobs on the supercomputer nodes and extracts the correlation between the jobs with respect to the energy consumption. Hence, energy consuming jobs can be launched in times where the power price is cheap or the supercomputer is not overloaded.

Appendix: Bash Script to Manage the Battery Power of a Data Center

```
#!/bin/bash

alarm1="The battery power is too low to support"
alarm2="The battery power is too low to continue to support the
load"
alarm3="On battery power in response to an input"
alarm4="In bypass in response"
alarm5="A high battery temperature exists"
alarm6="The internal battery temperature no longer exceeds the
critical threshold"
alarm7="A maximum temperature threshold violation"
clearing1="No longer on battery power"

shutcluster() {
 echo "$(date) PowerShut: (Critical) Starting a Cluster Shutdown
procedure..." >> /var/log/ups
```

```
 echo "$(date) PowerShut: (Critical) Stopping all running jobs"
>> /var/log/ups
 /usr/bin/scancel -w haytham[1-32]
 echo "$(date) PowerShut: (Critical) Shutting down Computing
Nodes" >> /var/log/ups
 /usr/sbin/nodectrl -F poweroff haytham[1-32]
 sleep 90
 for ((i=1; i <=32 ; i++))
 do
   rep=`/usr/sbin/nodectrl status haytham$i`
   if echo "$rep" | grep -q "Power is on"; then
     /usr/sbin/nodectrl -F poweroff_force haytham$i
   fi
 done
 echo "$(date) PowerShut: (Critical) Shutting down NFS Node in 3
min." >> /var/log/ups
 ssh haytham2 "shutdown -P +3" &
 echo "$(date) PowerShut (Critical) Management Node will halt
now." >> /var/log/ups
 shutdown -P now
}

echo "$(date) PowerShut: (Info) Starting PowerShut process... "
>> /var/log/ups
while true
do
 read event
 if [ -n "$event" ]; then
   echo $event >> /var/log/ups
 fi
 case $event in *"$alarm1"*|*"$alarm2"*|*"$alarm5"*|*"$alarm7"*)
shutcluster;;

     *"$alarm3"*)
        status=-1
        echo "$(date) PowerShut: (Alert) Starting a countdown
timer of 6min for a Shutdown procedure..." >> /var/log/ups
        until (( $status==1 || $status==0 )) ; do
          TMOUT=360
          read event;
          if [[ -z $event ]]; then
             status=0
          else
           if echo $event | grep -q "$clearing1"; then
             echo $event >> /var/log/ups
```

```
           echo "$(date) PowerShut: (Clearing) Shutdown is
canceled." >> /var/log/ups
           status=1
        else
          echo $event >> /var/log/ups
        fi
       fi
      done
      if (( status==0 )); then
         shutcluster
      fi
      TMOUT=0;;
 esac
done
   echo "$(date)  PowerShut:  (Alert)  Inexpected  exit  from
PowerShut process. " >> /var/log/ups
```

Special thanks go to Dr. Mejdi Kaddour for his help in the section of HPC data center monitoring.

References

1. Wei, C., Li, Y.: Design of Energy Consumption Monitoring and Energy-saving Management System of Intelligent Building based on the Internet of Things. In: IEEE Conference on Electronics, Communications and Control (ICECC) (2011)
2. Wang, L., Wang, Z., Yang, R.: Intelligent Multiagent Control System for Energy and Comfort Management in Smart and Sustainable Buildings. IEEE Transactions on Smart Grid 3(2) (2012)
3. Wicaksono, H., Rogalski, S., Kusnady, E.: Knowledge-based intelligent energy management using building automation system. In: IEEE IPEC Conference (2010)
4. Barth, W.: Nagios: System and Netwok Monitoring. No Starch Press (2008)
5. Shivakumar, P., Jouppi, N.P.: Cacti 3.0: An Integrated Cache Timing Power, and Area Model, Compaq Research Report (2001)
6. Massi, M.L., Chun, B.N., Culler, D.E.: The ganglia distributed monitoring system: design, implementation, and experience. Parallel Computing 30(7), 817–840 (2004)
7. De Craemer, K., Deconinck, G.: Analysis of State-of-the-art Smart Metering Communication Standards. In: Proceedings of the 5th Young Researchers Symposium (2010)
8. Starsinic, M.: System architecture challenges in the home M2M network. In: Applications and Technology Conference (LISAT) (2010)
9. Chen, C.-H., Gao, C.-C., Chen, J.-J.: Intelligent Home Energy Conservation System Based on WSN. In: International Conference on Electrical, Electronics and Civil Engineering (2011)
10. Fadlullah, Z.M., Fouda, M.M., Kato, N.: Toward Intelligent Machine-to-Machine Communications in Smart Grid. In: IEEE Communications Magazine (2011), http://www.digi.com/

11. Mohamed, S.F.H., Che, C.Z., Mohana, S., Mohamed, S.S.S.: Review on Mobile Workforce Management System for Electricity Supply Industries. In: IEEE Computer Science and its Applications (2009)
12. Sendra, S., Granel, E., et al.: Smart Collaborative System Using the Sensors of Mobile Devices for Montoring Disabled and Elderly People. In: 3rd IEEE International Workshop on SmArt COmmuniations in Network Technologies (2012)
13. Ito, A., Murakami, H., et al.: Universal Use of Information Delivery and Display System using Ad hoc Network for Deaf People in Times of Disaster. In: 3rd IEEE International Conference on Broadband Communications, Information Technology 1 Biomedical Applications (2008)
14. Ramlee, R., Tang, D.H.Z., Ismail, M.M.: Smart Home System for Disabled People Via Wireless Bluetooth. In: IEEE International Conference on System Engineering and Technology (2012)
15. Hayakawa, Y., Mori, K., et al.: Development of Emergency Rescue Evacuation Support System in Panic-type Disasters. In: 9th Annual IEEE Consumer Communcations and Networking Conference (2012)
16. Feng, W.C., Feng, X., Ge, R.: Green supercomputing comes of age. IT Professional 10(1), 17–23 (2008)
17. http://www.green500.org/
18. Mehrotra, R., Banicescu, I., Srivastava, S.: A Utility Based Power-Aware Autonomic Approach for Running Scientific Applications. In: IEEE 26th International Parallel and Distributed Processing Symposium Workshops & PhD Forum (2012)
19. Qian, H.: Improving access to mobile technologies using tactile feedback. ACM SIGACCESS Accessibility and Computing (102) (2012)
20. Yatani, K., Truong, K.N.: SemFeel: a user interface with semantic tactile feedback for mobile touch-screen devices. In: Proceedings of the 22nd Annual ACM Symposium on User Interface Software and Technology (2009)
21. Allcock, W., Felix, E., Lowe, M., Rheinheimer, R., Fullop, J.: Challenges of HPC Monitoring. In: ACM Super Computer Conference (2011)
22. Smith, T.F., Waterman, M.S.: Identification of Common Molecular Subsequences. J. Mol. Biol. 147, 195–197 (1981)

Author Index